D1828286

Influenza

Current Research

Edited by

Qinghua Wang

Verna and Marrs McLean Department of Biochemistry and Molecular Biology
Baylor College of Medicine
Houston, TX
USA

and

Yizhi Jane Tao

Department of BioSciences
Rice University
Houston, TX
USA

Caister Academic Press

Copyright © 2016

Caister Academic Press
Norfolk, UK

www.caister.com

British Library Cataloguing-in-Publication Data
A catalogue record for this book is available from the British Library

ISBN: 978-1-910190-43-2 (paperback)
ISBN: 978-1-910190-44-9 (ebook)

Description or mention of instrumentation, software, or other products in this book does not imply endorsement by the author or publisher. The author and publisher do not assume responsibility for the validity of any products or procedures mentioned or described in this book or for the consequences of their use.

All rights reserved. No part of this publication may be reproduced, stored in a retrieval system, or transmitted, in any form or by any means, electronic, mechanical, photocopying, recording or otherwise, without the prior permission of the publisher. No claim to original U.S. Government works.

Cover design adapted from figures courtesy of Albert Ziye Ma, 11 years old, Houston, USA.

Ebooks
Ebooks supplied to individuals are single-user only and must not be reproduced, copied, stored in a retrieval system, or distributed by any means, electronic, mechanical, photocopying, email, internet or otherwise.

Ebooks supplied to academic libraries, corporations, government organizations, public libraries, and school libraries are subject to the terms and conditions specified by the supplier.

Contents

Contributors

George F. Gao
CAS Key Laboratory of Pathogenic Microbiology and Immunology
Collaborative Innovation Center for Diagnosis and Treatment of Infectious Diseases
Institute of Microbiology
Center for Influenza Research and Early-warning
Chinese Academy of Sciences
Beijing
China

gaof@im.ac.cn

Yusong R. Guo
Department of BioSciences
Rice University
Houston, TX
USA

yrg1@rice.edu

Eike R. Hrincius
Institute of Molecular Virology (IMV)
Center for Molecular Biology of Inflammation (ZMBE)
Westfaelische Wilhelms-University Muenster
Muenster
Germany

hrincius@uni-muenster.de

Akila Jayaraman
Department of Biological Engineering
Koch Institute of Integrative Cancer Research
Massachusetts Institute of Technology
Cambridge, MA
USA

j.akila@gmail.com

James Kirui
Department of Medical Microbiology and Immunology
University of Wisconsin
Madison, WI
USA

kirui@wisc.edu

Jun Liu
National Institute for Viral Disease Control and Prevention
Chinese Center for Disease Control and Prevention
Beijing
China

liujun@ivdc.chinacdc.cn

Jonathan A. McCullers
Department of Infectious Diseases
St. Jude Children's Research Hospital; and
Department of Pediatrics
University of Tennessee Health Sciences Center
Memphis, TN
USA

jmccullers@uthsc.edu

Jaime Martin-Benito
Centro Nacional de Biotecnologia (CSIC)
Department of Macromolecular Structures
Madrid
Spain

jmartinb@cnb.csic.es

Andrew Mehle
Department of Medical Microbiology and Immunology
University of Wisconsin
Madison, WI
USA

amehle@wisc.edu

Fengyun Ni
Verna and Marrs McLean Department of Biochemistry and Molecular Biology
Baylor College of Medicine
Houston, TX
USA

fni@bcm.edu

Juan Ortin
Centro Nacional de Biotecnologia (CSIC)
Department of Macromolecular Structures
Madrid
Spain

jortin@cnb.csic.es

Rahul Raman
Department of Biological Engineering
Koch Institute of Integrative Cancer Research
Massachusetts Institute of Technology
Cambridge, MA
USA

rraman@mit.edu

Ram Sasisekharan
Department of Biological Engineering
Koch Institute of Integrative Cancer Research
Massachusetts Institute of Technology
Cambridge, MA
USA

rams@mit.edu

V. Sasisekharan
Department of Biological Engineering
Koch Institute of Integrative Cancer Research
Massachusetts Institute of Technology
Cambridge, MA
USA

sasi33@gmail.com

Yi Shi
CAS Key Laboratory of Pathogenic Microbiology and Immunology
Institute of Microbiology
Center for Influenza Research and Early-warning
Chinese Academy of Sciences
Beijing
China

shiyi@im.ac.cn

Zachary Shriver
Department of Biological Engineering
Koch Institute of Integrative Cancer Research
Massachusetts Institute of Technology
Cambridge, MA
USA

zshriver@visterrainc.com

Yizhi Jane Tao
Department of BioSciences
Rice University
Houston, TX
USA

ytao@rice.edu

Kannan Tharakaraman
Department of Biological Engineering
Koch Institute of Integrative Cancer Research
Massachusetts Institute of Technology
Cambridge, MA
USA

kannan@mit.edu

Vy Tran
Department of Medical Microbiology and Immunology
University of Wisconsin
Madison, WI
USA

vgtran@wisc.edu

Frank T. Vreede
Sir William Dunn School of Pathology
University of Oxford
Oxford
UK

frank.vreede@path.ox.ac.uk

Qinghua Wang
Verna and Marrs McLean Department of Biochemistry and Molecular Biology
Baylor College of Medicine
Houston, TX
USA

qinghuaw@bcm.edu

Yan Wu
CAS Key Laboratory of Pathogenic Microbiology and Immunology
Institute of Microbiology
Center for Influenza Research and Early-warning
Chinese Academy of Sciences
Beijing
China

wuyan@im.ac.cn

Ying Wu
CAS Key Laboratory of Pathogenic Microbiology and Immunology
Institute of Microbiology
Center for Influenza Research and Early-warning
Chinese Academy of Sciences
Beijing
China

wuying@im.ac.cn

Wenting Zhang
Department of BioSciences
Rice University
Houston, TX
USA

wentingzhang87@hotmail.com

Wenjie Zheng
Department of BioSciences
Rice University
Houston, TX
USA

pkuzwj@gmail.com

Current Books of Interest

Cyanobacteria: Omics and Manipulation	2017
Brain-eating Amoebae: Biology and Pathogenesis of *Naegleria fowleri*	2016
Foot and Mouth Disease Virus: Current Research and Emerging Trends	2017
Brain-eating Amoebae: Biology and Pathogenesis of *Naegleria fowleri*	2016
Staphylococcus: Genetics and Physiology	2016
Chloroplasts: Current Research and Future Trends	2016
Microbial Biodegradation: From Omics to Function and Application	2016
MALDI-TOF Mass Spectrometry in Microbiology	2016
Aspergillus and *Penicillium* in the Post-genomic Era	2016
Omics in Plant Disease Resistance	2016
Acidophiles: Life in Extremely Acidic Environments	2016
Climate Change and Microbial Ecology: Current Research and Future Trends	2016
Biofilms in Bioremediation: Current Research and Emerging Technologies	2016
Microalgae: Current Research and Applications	2016
Gas Plasma Sterilization in Microbiology: Theory, Applications, Pitfalls and New Perspectives	2016
Virus Evolution: Current Research and Future Directions	2016
Arboviruses: Molecular Biology, Evolution and Control	2016
Shigella: Molecular and Cellular Biology	2016
Aquatic Biofilms: Ecology, Water Quality and Wastewater Treatment	2016
Alphaviruses: Current Biology	2016
Thermophilic Microorganisms	2015
Flow Cytometry in Microbiology: Technology and Applications	2015
Probiotics and Prebiotics: Current Research and Future Trends	2015
Epigenetics: Current Research and Emerging Trends	2015
Corynebacterium glutamicum: From Systems Biology to Biotechnological Applications	2015
Advanced Vaccine Research Methods for the Decade of Vaccines	2015
Antifungals: From Genomics to Resistance and the Development of Novel Agents	2015
Bacteria-Plant Interactions: Advanced Research and Future Trends	2015
Aeromonas	2015

Full details at www.caister.com

Preface

To date there have been four types of influenza virus identified: types A, B, C and D. They are segmented, negative-strand (–) RNA viruses that constitute four out of the six genera within the *Orthomyxoviridae* family. Influenza A virus is the most troublesome one for the vast animal reservoir, the many subtypes that have been and are yet to be identified, and the tremendous ability to mutate and reassort. It is responsible for all known pandemics in human history including the three major pandemics in the last century. The most recent 'Swine flu' pandemic in 2009–2010 had an estimated global death toll of 284,000 according to US Centers for Disease Control and Prevention (CDC), demonstrating the devastating impacts of influenza A virus on our society even in modern days. Influenza A and B viruses together are responsible for seasonal epidemics each year and both have eight segments of genomic RNA. On the contrary, influenza C and D viruses only have seven segments of RNA. While influenza C virus infects human with mild symptoms, influenza D virus has only been detected in swine and cattle.

Recently, new advances in molecular biology, virology, biochemistry and structural biology have enabled the field to make many exciting discoveries that have, in some cases, conceptually revolutionized our understanding of this virus. For instance, influenza D virus, the newest member of the *Orthomyxoviridae* family, was first reported in swine in the Midwest region of the United States. The three-dimensional double-helical structure of the influenza virus RNP was finally visualized for the first time. The atomic structures of the viral polymerase complexes have now become available, thus greatly facilitating structure-based drug design targeting the viral replication. Our understanding of the host factors in influenza virus replication and antiviral responses has been significantly expanded. In addition, novel antiviral therapies have been designed against a broad array of viral proteins as well as host factors and pathways. Broadly neutralizing monoclonal antibodies against the conserved regions of haemagglutinin are currently in various stages of clinical trials. It is conceivable that these exciting new findings and development will one day translate into effective therapeutics again influenza infection.

In this book, eight chapters are showcased to illustrate some of the most important findings made in the flu field. Topics covered include stem-specific broadly neutralizing antibodies to haemagglutinin; virus replication and transcription; influenza B virus haemagglutinin; influenza A virus ribonucleoprotein complex; regulation of the virus replication machinery by host factors; evolution of receptor specificity of influenza A virus hemagglutinin; PB1-F2, a multi-functional non-structural influenza A virus protein; and avian influenza H7N9 virus. While it is mainly meant to provide a glimpse of what is currently going on in the field, this collection of work will surely show the readers how fast the field is moving forward in various directions.

We are deeply indebted to all authors for their contributions to this book. To keep up with latest discoveries, many have updated their chapters before this book went to the press. We are confident that their patience and efforts are well justified by the end results and will be appreciated by the readers! We are also grateful to Annette Griffin for her insights and patience that made this book possible.

Qinghua Wang and Yizhi Jane Tao
Houston, Texas, USA

Stem-specific Broadly Neutralizing Antibodies of Influenza Virus Haemagglutinin

1

Fengyun Ni and Qinghua Wang

Abstract

The past few years have witnessed a substantial advance in identifying novel antibodies that target conserved structural elements on influenza haemagglutinin, the receptor binding site and the stem domain, thus reviving the hope of a universal antibody. This chapter reviews the isolation of stem-specific broadly neutralizing antibodies (bnAbs), the structural basis of bnAb-mediated virus neutralization, and the novel strategies for eliciting bnAbs *in vivo*.

Introduction

Influenza virus is highly adaptive, undergoing continuous changes (antigenic drift and antigenic shift) as the result of the interplay between its error-prone RNA polymerase and antibody-mediated host selection (Noah and Noah, 2013; Webster and Govorkova, 2014). Two types of influenza virus, A and B, are the causative agents for seasonal influenza epidemics every year (Belshe, 2010; Carr, 2012). According to serological properties, influenza A viruses (IAVs) are classified into 18 antigenic subtypes of haemagglutinin (HA) and 11 antigenic subtypes of neuraminidase (NA), while influenza B virus has two co-circulating lineages that are antigenically distinct: the Yamagata and Victoria lineages (Belshe, 2010; Lin *et al.*, 2004; Wang, 2010)

HA is the most abundant glycoprotein and the major antigen on the surface of influenza virus (Julien *et al.*, 2012). The IAV HA sequence shares 40–70% sequence identity between different subtypes at amino-acid residue level. IAV HAs are further divided into two phylogenetic groups: Group 1 (H1, H2, H5, H6, H8, H9, H11, H12, H13, H16, H17, and H18) and Group 2 (H3, H4, H7, H10, H14 and H15) (Fig 1.1a). The trimeric HA is initially synthesized as a single peptide precursor (HA_0) (Chen *et al.*, 1998; Skehel and Wiley, 2000) (Fig 1.1b) that is later cleaved into disulfide-linked HA_1 and HA_2 chains (Fig 1.1c). Each HA monomer contains a globular 'head' domain that is made solely of HA_1 residues and an elongated 'stem' domain primarily consisting of an HA_2 chain that is kept in a pre-fusion conformation by the N- and C-terminal segments of HA_1 (Skehel and Wiley, 2000; Wilson *et al.*, 1981).

The HA globular 'head' domain is distal to the viral envelope and contains the receptor-binding site (RBS) that mediates the initial attachment of the virus to a host cell (de Graaf and Fouchier, 2014; Sun and Whittaker, 2013). Immunization with flu vaccines elicits antibodies that primarily target the globular head domain (Hannoun, 2013). Antibodies specific

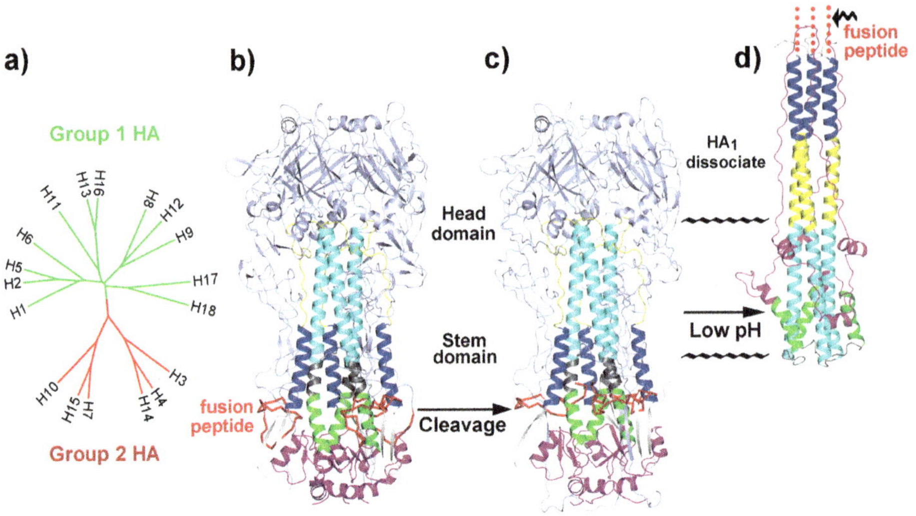

Figure 1.1 Influenza virus HA; (a) classification of IAV HAs into two phylogenetic groups; (b–d) structures of influenza A/H3 HA in different states: (b) uncleaved HA_0; (c) cleaved metastable pre-fusion HA; and (d) post-fusion HA_2.

for the globular domain usually have high neutralization efficiency; however, they tend to lose the effectiveness quickly due to the ability of influenza virus to modify the epitopes within the structurally flexible loops on the globular domain during the process of antigenic drift. Thus, the seasonal flu vaccine has to be reformulated annually (Belshe, 2010).

The HA stem domain is located proximal to the viral envelope. Low pH in endosomes induces a large-scale conformational change of HA to mediate the merger of viral envelope and host endosomal membranes and the release of viral genome into the cell (Bullough *et al.*, 1994; Chen *et al.*, 1999; Harrison, 2008; Ni *et al.*, 2014) (Fig. 1.1d). Probably owing to the scarcity of antibodies naturally elicited against this domain, the HA stem domains are better conserved across different IAV HA subtypes and between types A and B viruses. Thus, an attractive alternative to the conventional antibodies specific for the globular domain is the pursuit for stem-specific antibodies that may recognize similar epitopes among different types and subtypes of HA, which are termed as broadly neutralizing antibodies (bnAbs) (Corti and Lanzavecchia, 2013; Laursen and Wilson, 2013; Tharakaraman *et al.*, 2014). Recent advances in the field have led to the identification of a number of bnAbs that have the potential to protect human from infection by existing and newly emergent strains of influenza virus (Han and Marasco, 2011; Jegaskanda *et al.*, 2014; Laursen and Wilson, 2013; Pica and Palese, 2013; Quiñones-Parra *et al.*, 2014; Reperant *et al.*, 2014).

In this chapter, we will review the recent advances in the isolation of stem-specific bnAbs, the structural basis of bnAb-mediated virus neutralization, and the novel strategies for eliciting bnAbs *in vivo*. The reported bnAbs that neutralize IAV strains in the same subtype are not covered in this chapter (for example, Kalenik *et al.*, 2014; Whittle *et al.*, 2011). The RBS-specific heterosubtypic antibodies, such as S139/1 (Yoshida *et al.*, 2009), FE17 (Corti *et al.*, 2010), CH65 (Whittle *et al.*, 2011), C05 (Ekiert *et al.*, 2012), and H5.3 (Winarski *et al.*, 2015), are not discussed in this chapter.

Isolation of stem-specific bnAbs

The adaptive immune system produces a large and diverse population of antibodies through combinatorial rearrangement of a relatively small set of gene segments. Although the first flu vaccine was developed in early 1930s, the bnAb was not detected until 1993 (Okuno *et al.*, 1993). The limited population of bnAbs in the antibody repertoire might have hampered their identification. For instance, by analysing the serum samples from volunteers vaccinated by an H5N1 vaccine, only ~0.01% of total immunoglobulin G (IgG, the most abundant antibody isotype circulated in humans) bind to both Group 1 and 2 IAVs (Sui *et al.*, 2011).

The hybridoma technique is to obtain an immortalized hybrid cell line by fusing a B-cell with myeloma cells (cancerous B-cells) in order to produce specific monoclonal antibodies (mAbs) in a large quantity. The first stem-specific antibody C179 was isolated from an H2N2-immunized mouse in 1993 with the hybridoma technique (Okuno *et al.*, 1993). The mAbs in cultured fluids from fused cells were screened by its ability to interact with the influenza-infected cells followed by staining technique. C179 shows cross-reactivity with multiple Group 1 HA, including H1, H2, H5, H6, and H9 (Dreyfus *et al.*, 2013; Sakabe *et al.*, 2010). Recently, mouse antibody 9H10 was identified from 2,000 hybridoma cells that bound to Group 2 HAs (Tan *et al.*, 2014).

In a similar way to the hybridoma technique, antibodies PN-SIA28 and PN-SIA49 were isolated from a patient immunized with seasonal flu vaccine where the patient B-cells were immortalized by Epstein–Barr virus (EBV) transformation (Burioni *et al.*, 2010). PN-SIA28 is capable of neutralizing Group 1 HAs and some Group 2 HAs (only some old H3 viruses, but not recent H3 and H7 viruses) (Clementi *et al.*, 2011). PN-SIA49 recognizes multiple Group 1 HA, including H1, H2 and H5 (De Marco *et al.*, 2012).

Phage display is also a well-established technique that displays a protein of interest on the phage surface while containing the gene of the protein inside the phage. Two research groups independently reported the identification of bnAbs that recognize a nearly identical epitope in Group 1 HAs, CR6261 (Throsby *et al.*, 2008) and F10 (Sui *et al.*, 2009). CR6261 was obtained from the phage display library constructed from IgM memory B-cells of 10 healthy donors vaccinated with the seasonal flu vaccine (Throsby *et al.*, 2008). F10 was isolated from the library made from B-cells of 57 non-immunized donors (Sui *et al.*, 2004). In addition, the same phage display library construction method was used to identify CR9114, the most broadly neutralizing antibody known to date, which binds to a conserved epitope on the stem domain of both influenza A and B viruses (Dreyfus *et al.*, 2012).

Single-plasma B-cell culture was developed to interrogate the human plasma B-cells derived from vaccinated or infected donors in a high-throughput way (Corti *et al.*, 2011). Interleukin 6 (IL-6) was supplemented in the medium to support the survival of single plasma B-cells. The culture supernatant with secreted antibodies was analysed with parallel binding assays, and the gene of selected antibody was recovered by single-cell reverse transcription polymerase chain reaction (RT-PCR). FI6 and its designed variant FI6v3 were found to neutralize many Group 1 and 2 HA subtypes (Corti *et al.*, 2011).

Another rapid method to identify anti-HA mAbs is based on sorting the immortalized memory B-cells stained with allophycocyanin (APC)-labelled HA. Memory B-cells from donors vaccinated with seasonal flu vaccine were immortalized by retroviral transduction (Kwakkenbos *et al.*, 2010), followed by staining with APC-labelled HA. The labelled cells were sorted and measured for immune reactivity and neutralization against other HA subtypes. CR8020 (Ekiert *et al.*, 2011) and CR8043 (Friesen *et al.*, 2014) were characterized to be cross-reactive with multiple Group 2 HA subtypes.

A recent *in vivo* enrichment technique was reported to identify rare bnAbs with high frequency (Nakamura *et al.*, 2013). Human peripheral blood mononuclear cells from vaccinated donors were premixed with HA variants that are distinct from vaccine strains, followed by intrasplenic injection of the double mutant SCID/beige mouse strains that are defect in lysosomal trafficking, DNA repair and VDJ recombination. The advantage of this technique is to ensure the rapid expansion and B-cell activation, which results in intense differentiation into human plasmablasts. The spleen cells were sorted and selected for producing antibodies targeting conserved HA epitopes. Two antibodies, 39.29 and 81.39, out of 840 cloned antibodies were identified to neutralize both Group 1 and 2 HA subtypes (Nakamura *et al.*, 2013).

Structural basis of stem-specific bnAbs

The fusion mechanism is structurally and functionally conserved in influenza virus HAs. HA_2 has a much higher amino-acid sequence conservation than HA_1. This is probably because the stem domain has not yet undergone extensive antigenic drift owing to its proximal location on the virion surface that is relatively harder to access in the presence of densely packed HA molecules. The more conserved structure in the stem domain makes the identification of bnAbs possible. The binding with bnAbs inhibits the fusion process either by preventing the cleavage of the precursor HA_0 or by stabilizing the pre-fusion conformation.

Group 1 HA-specific bnAbs

Classically, characterizing escape mutants that are generated in the presence of a neutralizing antibody is used to map the epitopes on HAs that are recognized by that antibody. With the aid of crystal structures of bnAbs in complex with HAs, the structural basis of bnAb recognition can now be unequivocally defined. The structures of four Group 1 HA-specific bnAbs and HAs are available: CR6261 with H1 and H5 HAs (PDB codes: 3GBN and 3GBM), F10 with H5 HA (PDB code: 3FKU), C179 with H2 HA (PDB code: 4HLZ), and MAb 3.1 with H1 HA (PDB code: 4PY8) (Fig. 1.2). Both CR6261 and F10 utilize V_H1–69 germline gene, where only the heavy chain is involved in binding to antigens. Notably, V_H1–69 gene is used by many CD4-induced antibodies targeting HIV-1 gp120 (Huang *et al.*, 2004). In contrast, both heavy and light chains of C179 participate in the interaction with HA. The angle of MAb 3.1 (a V_H3–30 encoded antibody) in approaching the HA stem region is similar to that of C179, despite the different binding mechanisms. The epitope for these four bnAbs includes the HA_2 N-terminal residues (18–21, 38, 41–42, 45–46, 49, 52–53, 56) and HA_1 fusion subdomain residues (18, 38, 40, 42, 291–293, 318) that form a hydrophobic groove with which all these Group 1 HA-specific bnAbs bind (Fig. 1.2). The epitope partially overlaps with the fusion peptide.

All these four Group 1 HA-specific bnAbs make extensive hydrophobic interactions with HA through their heavy-chain complementarity-determining region (HCDR) 1 and HCDR3 loops: $F29^{CR6261}$, $V27^{F10}$, $F27^{C179}$, $L29^{C179}$, and $F27^{MAb\ 3.1}$, in HCDR1 loop; and $Y98^{CR6261}$, $Y102^{F10}$, $Y98^{C179}$, $F99^{C179}$, $Y100A^{C179}$, $Y99^{MAb\ 3.1}$ and $F100^{MAb\ 3.1}$ in HCDR3 loop. Further, key epitope–antibody hydrophobic interactions are contributed by F74 in frame region 3 (FR3), I53 and F54 in HCDR2 of CR6261 (Fig. 1.2a) and M54 and F55

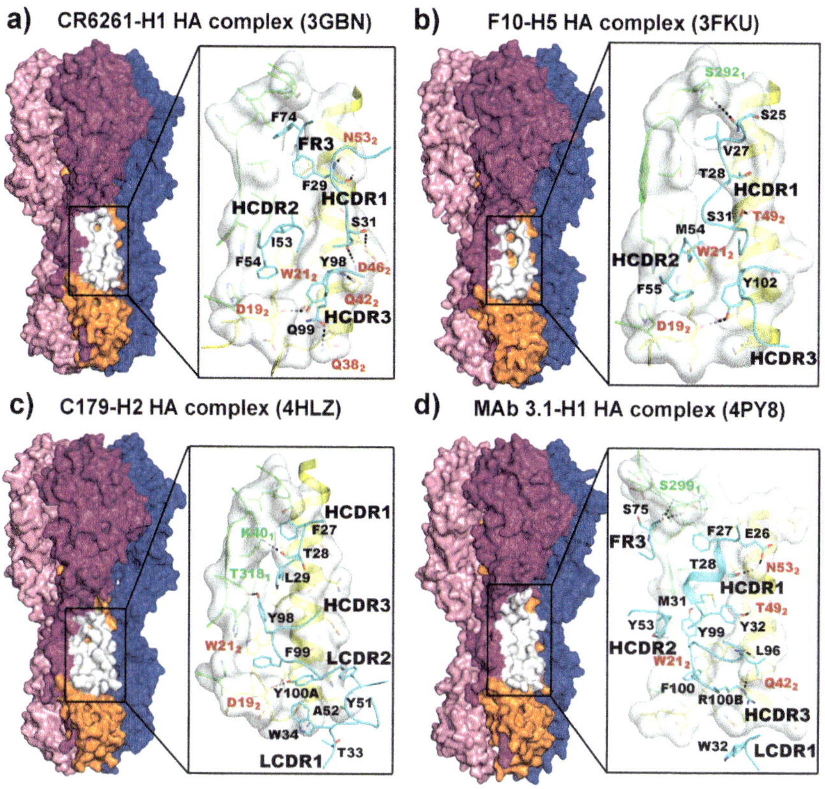

Figure 1.2 Structures of Group 1 HA-specific bnAbs. (a) CR6261–H1 HA complex; (b) F10–H5 HA complex; (c) C179–H2 HA complex; (d) MAb 3.1–H1 HA complex. For each complex, surface presentation of HA is shown on the left, with the epitope shown as white surface. The zoomed-in epitope (green for HA_1 and yellow for HA_2) and its interacting antibody fragments (cyan) are shown on the right. Representative residues from HA_1, HA_2 and the antibody are labelled in green, red and black, respectively.

in HCDR2 of F10 (Fig. 1.2b). W34 in light chain complementarity-determining region 1 (LCDR1) of C179 also interacts with HA, thus extending the buried surface area upon complex formation by ~150 Å^2 (~1460 Å^2 for C179 and ~1304 Å^2 for CR6261) (Dreyfus *et al.*, 2013; Ekiert *et al.*, 2009) (Fig. 1.2c). MAb 3.1 also employs residues 74–76 in FR3 and W32 in LCDR1 to contact with HA (Fig. 1.2d).

Group 1 HA-specific bnAbs are not reactive with Group 2 HAs. This is probably due to the presence of a conserved glycan at residue 38_1 in Group 2 HAs that may preclude the binding of antibodies. The introduction of this glycosylation site into Group 1 HAs reduced the binding with CR6261 (Throsby *et al.*, 2008). Furthermore, the side-chain orientation of $W21_2$ in the fusion peptide of HA differs by ~90° between Group 1 and 2 HAs, which may affect the favourable interactions found with Group 1 HAs (Sui *et al.*, 2009). Two H5 to H2 HA mutations within the hydrophobic groove, $L320_1P$ and $I45_2F$, are found to reduce the binding with CR6261 (Throsby *et al.*, 2008). These two residues are located at the two sides of $W21_2$ and it is unclear whether the mutations directly affect the binding with CR6261 or indirectly by influencing the side-chain orientation of $W21_2$.

The H111$_2$L escape mutant of H5 HA subtype was identified in the presence of CR6261 after 10 passages. It was speculated that this mutation might disrupt the hydrogen bond with the carbonyl group of the neighbouring T318$_1$, thus changing the hydrophobic characteristics of the epitope (Throsby *et al.*, 2008). Since H111$_2$ is very close to W21$_2$, it is also possible that the H111$_2$L mutation affects the side-chain orientation of this tryptophan, thereby weakening the interaction with Group 1 HA-specific bnAbs. Under the selection pressure of C179, escape variants of H1N1 and H2N2 strains were selected: T318$_1$K (H1N1) or V52$_2$E (H2N2) (Okuno *et al.*, 1993). Both mutations significantly change the electrostatic properties in the epitope.

Group 2 HA-specific bnAbs

Though the overall architecture of HA molecules across different subtypes is similar, they differ in the detailed structural characteristics including the distinct distribution of glycosylation sites, ionizable residues, loop conformation, and orientation of the globular head domain relative to the stem domain (Ha *et al.*, 2002; Ni *et al.*, 2014). The identification of Group 2 HA-specific antibodies appears to be less common. Until now, three stem-specific bnAbs have been structurally characterized, where two are crystal structures (Ekiert *et al.*, 2011; Friesen *et al.*, 2014) and the other was studied by a negative-stain electron microscopy (EM) reconstruction (Tan *et al.*, 2014).

CR8020 and CR8043 were identified by Wilson and colleagues and both crystallized with H3 HA (PDB codes: 3SDY and 4NM8) (Ekiert *et al.*, 2011; Friesen *et al.*, 2014). These two bnAbs bind to the base of the stem domain (Fig. 1.3), which is only about 15 Å away from the viral membrane and much lower than the epitope of Group 1 HA-specific bnAbs (Fig. 1.2). The epitope of CR8020 and CR8043 is composed of two major parts: (1) the β-sheet at HA$_2$ N-terminus in the range of 24$_2$–36$_2$ and (2) the C-terminal portion (residues 15$_2$–19$_2$) of the fusion peptide (Fig. 1.3). These two antibodies interact with the epitope by both heavy and light chains, where the heavy chain contributes 81% (CR8020) or 74% (CR8043) to the total buried surface area.

CR8020 and CR8043 interact with the C-terminal portion (residues 15$_2$–19$_2$) of the fusion peptide extensively. In CR8020, this region interacts with F32 in HCDR1, W100C in HCDR3, and Y49 in LCDR2 (Fig. 1.3a). In CR8043, this region closely contacts with Y32 in HCDR1, W100C in HCDR3, Y32 and WSO in LCDR1 (Fig. 1.3b). Both antibodies can completely block the cleavage of HA$_0$ into HA$_1$ and HA$_2$, thereby inhibiting the viral entry.

Similar to the observation that the conserved glycan at residue N38$_1$ in Group 2 HAs prevents the neutralization by CR6261, the conserved glycan at 21$_2$ in Group 1 HAs (adjacent to the HCDR1) also inhibited the binding with CR8020. Two escape variants were selected by CR8020: D19$_2$N and G33$_2$E. The mutation D19$_2$N in the fusion peptide weakens the electrostatic interaction with R53 of CR8020 light chain. The G33$_2$E mutation in the β-strand introduces a large negatively charged side chain in the HA-antibody interface. CR8043 selected R25$_2$M and Q34$_2$R escape variants, both are in the β-strand region. These mutations weaken the interactions at the centre of the epitope. Interestingly, the R25$_2$M mutation that escaped CR8043 did not affect the neutralization activity of CR8020. Similarly, the D19$_2$N and G33$_2$E mutations that reduced the binding with CR8020 can still be neutralized by CR8043. For the EM-characterized antibody 9H10, it binds to a similar epitope as CR8020 and CR8043 (Tan *et al.*, 2014) and selected R25$_2$M and D19$_2$N escape variants. Therefore, this class of antibodies uses a distinct but overlapping set of residues

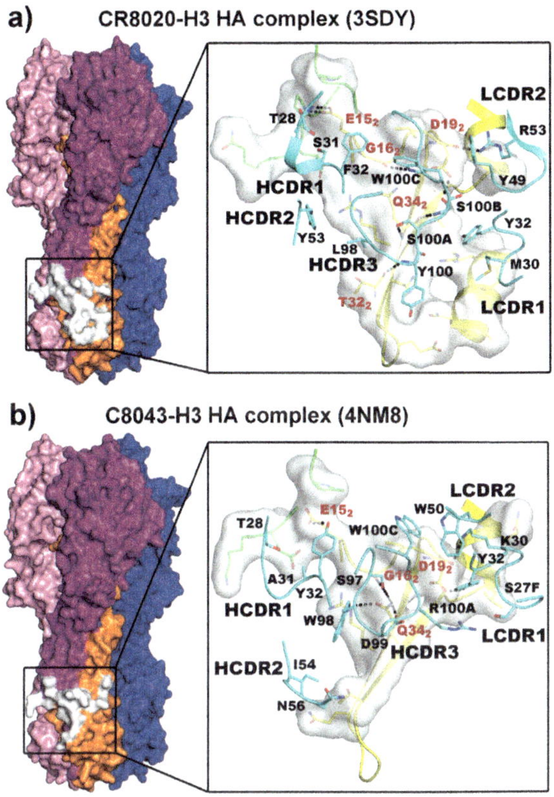

Figure 1.3 Structures of Group 2 HA-specific bnAbs. (a) CR8020–H3 HA complex; (b) CR8043–H3 HA complex. For each complex, surface presentation of HA is shown on the left, with the epitope shown as white surface. The zoomed-in epitope (green for HA_1 and yellow for HA_2) and its interacting antibody fragments (cyan) are shown on the right. Representative residues from HA_2 and the antibody are labelled in red and black, respectively.

for binding to Group 2 HA proteins. Most recently, the escape mutation $D19_2N$ has been identified in H7N9 field isolates (Tharakaraman *et al.*, 2014).

Groups 1 and 2 HA-specific bnAbs

Currently, there are two Groups 1 and 2 HA-specific bnAbs (FI6v3 and 39.29) that have been crystallized with different subtypes of HAs: FI6v3 with H1 and H3 HAs (PDB codes: 3ZTN and 3ZTJ) (Corti *et al.*, 2011) and 39.29 with H3 HA (PDB code: 4KVN) (Nakamura *et al.*, 2013). The epitopes recognized by these two bnAbs overlap with that of Group 1 HA-specific bnAbs (Fig. 1.2).

For FI6v3, both heavy and light chains interact with HA. Its long HCDR3 (22 amino acids) inserts into the shallow hydrophobic groove formed by HA_2 helix A (residues 38_2 to 57_2) and HA_1 (residues 27 to 33), and C-terminus fusion peptide (residues 17_2 to 21_2). The long HCDR3 loop of FI6v3 makes extensive contacts with HA using residues L100A, Y100C, F100D, W100F and L100G (Fig. 1.4a). On the opposite side of the hydrophobic groove, F27D, and Y29 of LCDR1 loop contacts with N-terminal of HA_2 helix A and the

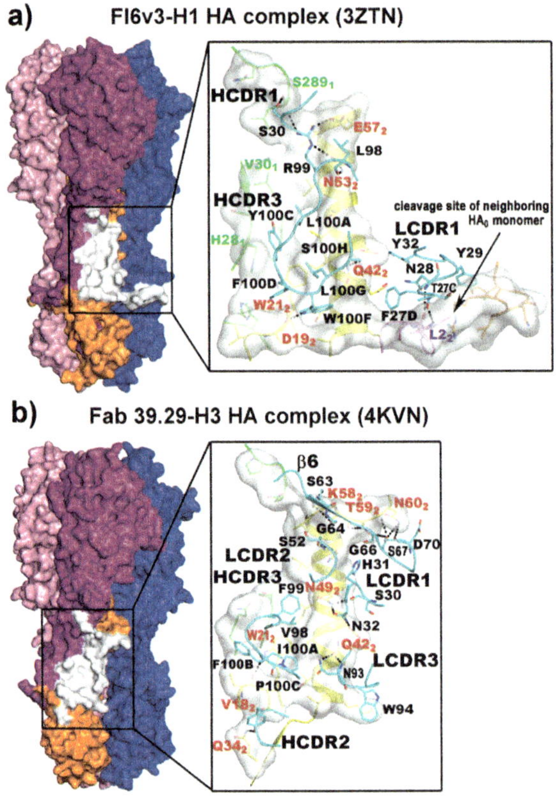

Figure 1.4 Structures of Groups 1 and 2 HA-specific bnAbs. (a) FI6v3–H1 HA complex; (b) Fab 39.29–H3 HA complex. For each complex, surface presentation of HA is shown on the left, with the epitope shown as white surface. The zoomed-in epitope (green for HA_1 and yellow for HA_2) and its interacting antibody fragments (cyan) are shown on the right. Representative residues from HA_1, HA_2 and the antibody are labelled in green, red and black, respectively.

fusion peptide of the neighbouring HA monomer when FI6v3 was co-crystallized with the uncleaved H1 HA_0 (Fig. 1.4a). The latter interaction by FI6v3 LCDR1 loop is not observed in Group 1 HA-specific bnAbs. In addition, the glycan at residue 38_1, which was speculated to prevent the binding of CR6261 with Group 2 HAs, rotates about 80° away to enable the binding of FI6v3 (Fig. 1.4a).

For antibody 39.29, despite the use of a different germline from that of FI6v3, it interacts with HA_2 helix A in a similar way as FI6v3 by both of its heavy and light chain (Fig. 1.4b). Similarly, V98, F99, I100A and P100C in HCDR3 of 39.29 makes contact with the hydrophobic groove extensively while, uniquely, all three LCDR loops of 39.29 interact with HA by predominantly polar contacts. Though the 39.29 heavy chain targets the similar position on HA as FI6v3, the 39.29 light chain positioning on HA is rotated by about 60° compared with FI6v3.

No escape mutants were yet reported under the selection pressure of FI6v3 or 39.29. However, in a study that identified another Group 1 and 2 HA-specific bnAb PN-SIA28 (Clementi *et al.*, 2011), two escape variants, $I18_2T$ and $D19_2G$, were identified. Both residues are located in the C-terminal portion of the fusion peptide and constitute the base of the hydrophobic groove formed by the helix A of HA_2. These mutations may also influence the binding with HCDR3 of FI6v3 and 39.29. Further, an alanine scanning mutagenesis study in the same report showed that the mutation in HA_1 ($H18_1A$, $H38_1A$) and the helix A of HA_2 ($T15_2A$, $M17_2A$, $I18_2A$, $D19_2A$, $G20_2A$, $W21_2A$, $T41_2A$, and $V52_2A$) affected the binding with 39.29.

Influenza A and B virus HA-specific bnAb

The identification of antibodies that broadly neutralize all influenza A and B viruses represents the ultimate goal for antibody-based influenza treatment. Like bnAbs CR6261 and F10, the influenza A and B virus-specific bnAb CR9114 also only uses its heavy chain to bind with HAs. The epitope of CR9114 is almost indistinguishable from that of CR6261 (Dreyfus *et al.*, 2012) (Fig. 1.5). The broad cross-reactivity of CR9114 is likely the consequence of the following specifics.

First, the apparent plasticity of three HCDR loops in CR9114 allows it to accommodate subtle variations in the epitope from different types of HAs. The plasticity is suggested by the different conformations of HCDRs in unbound CR9114 and CR9114-H5 HA complex structures. Especially, the more favourable orientation of F54 in HCDR2 of CR9114 may enable the high-affinity binding with HA $W21_2$ in different conformations as observed in different subtypes or types of HAs. Second, CR9114 seems to tolerate well the polymorphism at residue 49_2, $T49_2$ in Group 1 and influenza B virus HAs, and $N49_2$ in Group 2 HAs. Third, the absence of interactions between CR9114 and $T318_1$ of H5 HA may allow an alternative conformation of the conserved glycan at $N38_1$ in Group 2 HAs, and at $N332_1$ (corresponding the $T318_1$ in type A virus HAs) in influenza B virus HA to avoid steric clash with CR9114. In contrast, FI6v3 makes a hydrogen bond with $T318_1$ of both Groups 1 and 2 of influenza A virus HAs, which may prevent it from binding to influenza B virus HA (Dreyfus *et al.*, 2012).

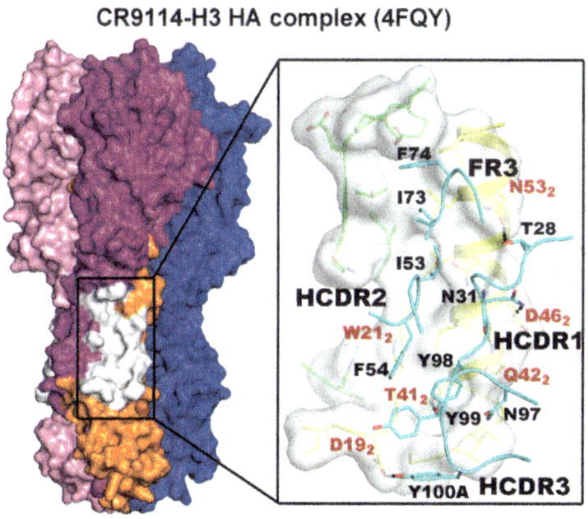

Figure 1.5 Structure of influenza A and B virus HA-specific bnAb CR9114. Surface presentation of HA is shown on the left, with the epitope shown as white surface. The zoomed-in epitope (green for HA_1 and yellow for HA_2) and its interacting antibody fragments (cyan) are shown on the right. Representative residues from HA_2 and the antibody are labelled in red and black, respectively.

No influenza B virus escape variants are generated because CR9114 could not neutralize influenza B viruses *in vitro*. However, binding experiments showed that the $D19_2N$ mutation in the fusion peptide reduces the binding of H3 and H7 HAs with CR9114. Influenza B virus HA has alanine at this position, which possibly lowers the binding affinity of CR9114 for influenza B virus. Moreover, the $I45_2F$ mutation in the helix A of HA_2 also affects the CR9114 binding.

Protection mechanism of stem-specific bnAbs

The binding of stem-specific bnAbs decreases the HA hemifusion efficiency as shown by a recent single-particle fluorescence microscopy study (Otterstrom *et al.*, 2014). About 75% of HA trimers on the viral surface bound with Group 1 HA-specific bnAb C179 (Harris *et al.*, 2013). However, *in vitro* neutralization does not correlate exactly with the *in vivo* protection. In the case of FI6, only 40% of mice are protected if FI6 lacks the complement and Fc receptor (FcR) binding region, though the *in vitro* neutralization property remains the same (Corti *et al.*, 2011). This suggests that the protection of stem-specific bnAbs may also include the Fc domain of an antibody.

FcR, a major component of the immune system, binds to the Fc domain of antibody to induce the phagocytic or cytotoxic cells for destroying the pathogens or infected cells in the processes of antibody-mediated phagocytosis or antibody-dependent cell-mediated cytotoxicity (ADCC). The protection of five stem-specific bnAbs (6F12, FI6, 2G02, 2B06, and 1F02) from lethal H1N1 challenge required FcR (DiLillo *et al.*, 2014), probably through their interactions with FcR to induce cytotoxicity of the infected cells. The efficacy of stem-specific bnAbs might be reduced if the assembly of the ternary complex, HA-bnAb-FcR, is sterically hindered by the membrane (Tharakaraman *et al.*, 2014). In addition, the complement system of the immune system complements the ability of antibodies and phagocytic cells to wipe out pathogens or infected cells. Some stem-specific bnAbs might employ complement-dependent lysis to destroy influenza-infected cells (Terajima *et al.*, 2011).

Novel strategies for eliciting bnAbs *in vivo*

The identification of stem-specific bnAbs not only renewed the hope for universal antibody therapy, but also re-ignited the pursuit for novel strategies to elicit the stem-specific bnAbs *in vivo*.

A novel immunization strategy is the prime/boost combination in which DNA vaccine encoding 2009 pandemic H1 HA was first used to prime the immune response followed by boosting with seasonal influenza vaccine. BnAbs elicited that way were able to neutralize diverse H1N1 strains of more than 70 years time span (Wei *et al.*, 2010). Similarly, it was hypothesized that sequential exposure to HAs with divergent head domains but conserved stem domains can boost the immune response towards the well-conserved stem domain (Palese and Wang, 2011). This hypothesis was subsequently confirmed in the mouse model where mice showed an increased production of stem-specific bnAbs after infection with a seasonal H1N1 virus followed by a pandemic H1N1 virus (Krammer *et al.*, 2012). Similarly, repeated immunization with chimeric HA constructs that expressed an identical stem domain but distinct head domains provided heterosubtypic protection in mice challenged with different subtypes of influenza viruses (Krammer *et al.*, 2013).

Manipulating the glycosylation state of HA is another strategy as glycans on influenza HA were reported to affect the immune response (Tate *et al.*, 2014; Wang *et al.*, 2009). One way was to reduce the fully glycosylated HA to mono-glycosylated HA to stimulate a better maturation of dendritic cells (DCs) because of the better engulfment (Chen *et al.*, 2014). The better maturation of DCs induces more CD8+ memory T cells and plasma B-cells, where antibodies with cross-strain binding ability were detected from diversely activated B-cell repertoires. Another way is to introduce more N-linked glycosylation sites in the HA head domain to create a hyper-glycosylated HA to reduce the immune response to the antigenic sites in this domain (Eggink *et al.*, 2014). The enhanced immune response directed at the more conserved stem domain was able to elicit heterosubtypic protection.

Another strategy is based on the premise that the repetitive exposure to antigens is responsible for inducing stronger immune responses (Bachmann and Zinkernagel, 1997). Ferritins are self-assembled into spherical nanoparticles consisting of 24 identical copies of ferritin (Kramer *et al.*, 2004). By inserting an HA ectodomain into the tip of each ferritin, eight HA trimers were assembled on the surface of ferritin nanoparticle (Kanekiyo *et al.*, 2013; Yassine *et al.*, 2015). Immunization with these nanoparticles improved the neutralization potency and breadth of antibody response compared to trivalent inactivated influenza vaccine.

Using the HA stem domain in the absence of head domain in the pre-fusion conformation is another novel strategy for vaccination. Such constructs generally include the ectodomain of HA_2, N- and C-terminal segments of HA_1 that interact with HA_2, and a linker to connect the N- and C-terminal segments of HA_1 (Bommakanti *et al.*, 2010). Further mutations were included to remove the exposed hydrophobic patch and destabilize the low-pH conformation. This construct was refolded from the *E. coli* inclusion body and showed the expected neutral-pH conformation. The antisera of mice immunized with this construct exhibited cross-reactivity with different subtypes (Bommakanti *et al.*, 2012). In a similar stem-only construct, the N- and C-terminal segments of HA_1 are connected by a linker with the help of a disulfide bond (Steel *et al.*, 2010). By inserting this construct to a HIV Gag-based vector, virus-like particles can be produced to elicit antisera with heterosubtypic reactivity. An adenovirus vector-based vaccine that includes codon-optimized HA_2 gene fused with CD40L ectodomain was also reported to confer complete protection against 13 subtypes of influenza A virus (Fan *et al.*, 2014). Other HA_2-based bnAbs-eliciting constructs include the central helix CD (residues 76_2–130_2) of HA_2 or a portion of HA_2 (residues 41_2–113_2), which were aimed to produce rapid scale-up of immunogens (Mallajosyula *et al.*, 2013, 2014; Wang *et al.*, 2010).

One concern related to the application of novel immunization strategies is the influenza vaccine-associated enhanced respiratory disease (VAERD) (Khurana *et al.*, 2013). When pigs were first immunized by whole inactivated H1N2 virus followed by pandemic H1N1 infection, although high titres of bnAbs were detected in the pig antisera, the pigs exhibited enhanced pneumonia and respiratory disease. This study necessitates the consideration of VAERD during the evaluation of influenza vaccines targeting HA stem domain.

Conclusions

The past few years have witnessed an exciting development in identifying novel antibodies that target conserved structural elements on influenza HA, namely the RBS and the stem domain, that are essential for effective infection of influenza virus. Owing to the conserved nature of their epitopes, these novel antibodies can broadly neutralize either a single influenza subtype over a long time period or multiple influenza subtypes. One such antibody, CR9114, neutralizes both type A and type B influenza viruses and is the most broadly neutralizing antibody identified thus far. These novel antibodies strongly renewed the long-standing hope for universal antibody therapy, and a large number of the bnAbs reviewed in this chapter are under various stages of clinical trials. Furthermore, the bnAbs specifically targeting the stem domain of HA revised the previous belief that the stem domain is essentially immune-inert. Consequently, a variety of novel strategies have been developed to elicit stem-specific bnAbs *in vivo*. Due to space limitations, in this chapter we provide only a glimpse of these exciting developments in the field. We fully expect that the excitement will last and more novel discoveries will emerge. A combined use of bnAbs and/or novel immunization strategies may soon become available to offer protection against seasonal and pandemic influenza infection. However, when that day comes, it does not mean influenza researchers can finally rest. As with any new therapeutic development against error-prone viruses such as influenza and HIV-1, resistant strains will eventually arise, and newer and smarter arms race will begin.

Acknowledgements

Q.W. thanks support from the National Institutes of Health (R01-AI067839, R01-GM116280) and the Welch Foundation (Q-1826).

References

Bachmann, M.F., and Zinkernagel, R.M. (1997). Neutralizing antiviral B-cell responses. Annu. Rev. Immunol. *15*, 235–270.

Belshe, R.B. (2010). The need for quadrivalent vaccine against seasonal influenza. Vaccine *28*, 45–53.

Bommakanti, G., Citron, M.P., Hepler, R.W., Callahan, C., Heidecker, G.J., Najar, T.A., Lu, X., Joyce, J.G., Shiver, J.W., Casimiro, D.R., *et al.* (2010). Design of an HA2-based *Escherichia coli* expressed influenza immunogen that protects mice from pathogenic challenge. Proc. Natl. Acad. Sci. U.S.A. *107*, 13701–13706.

Bommakanti, G., Lu, X., Citron, M.P., Najar, T.A., Heidecker, G.J., ter Meulen, J., Varadarajan, R., and Liang, X. (2012). design of *Escherichia coli*-expressed stalk domain immunogens of H1N1 hemagglutinin that protect mice from lethal challenge. J. Virol. *86*, 13434–13444.

Bullough, P. a, Hughson, F.M., Skehel, J.J., and Wiley, D.C. (1994). Structure of influenza haemagglutinin at the pH of membrane fusion. Nature *371*, 37–43.

Burioni, R., Canducci, F., Mancini, N., Clementi, N., Sassi, M., De Marco, D., Diotti, R.A., Saita, D., Sampaolo, M., Sautto, G., *et al.* (2010). Monoclonal antibodies isolated from human B-cells neutralize a broad range of H1 subtype influenza A viruses including swine-origin Influenza virus (S-OIV). Virology *399*, 144–152.

Carr, S. (2012). Seasonal and pandemic influenza: an overview with pediatric focus. Adv. Pediatr. *59*, 75–93.

Chen, J., Lee, K.H., Steinhauer, D.A., Stevens, D.J., Skehel, J.J., and Wiley, D.C. (1998). Structure of the hemagglutinin precursor cleavage site, a determinant of influenza pathogenicity and the origin of the labile conformation. Cell *95*, 409–417.

Chen, J., Skehel, J.J., and Wiley, D.C. (1999). N- and C-terminal residues combine in the fusion-pH influenza hemagglutinin HA(2) subunit to form an N cap that terminates the triple-stranded coiled coil. Proc. Natl. Acad. Sci. U.S.A. *96*, 8967–8972.

Chen, J.R., Yu, Y.H., Tseng, Y.C., Chiang, W.L., Chiang, M.F., Ko, Y.A., Chiu, Y.K., Ma, H.H., Wu, C.Y., Jan, J.T., *et al.* (2014). Vaccination of monoglycosylated hemagglutinin induces cross-strain protection against influenza virus infections. Proc. Natl. Acad. Sci. U.S.A. *111*, 2476–2481.

Clementi, N., De Marco, D., Mancini, N., Solforosi, L., Moreno, G.J., Gubareva, L.V., Mishin, V., Di Pietro, A., Vicenzi, E., Siccardi, A.G., *et al.* (2011). A human monoclonal antibody with neutralizing activity against highly divergent influenza subtypes. PLoS One *6*, e28001.

Corti, D., and Lanzavecchia, A. (2013). Broadly neutralizing antiviral antibodies. Annu. Rev. Immunol. *31*, 705–742.
Corti, D., Suguitan, A.L., Pinna, D., Silacci, C., Fernandez-Rodriguez, B.M., Vanzetta, F., Santos, C., Luke, C.J., Torres-Velez, F.J., Temperton, N.J., *et al.* (2010). Heterosubtypic neutralizing antibodies are produced by individuals immunized with a seasonal influenza vaccine. J. Clin. Invest. *120*, 1663–1673.
Corti, D., Voss, J., Gamblin, S.J., Codoni, G., Macagno, A., Jarrossay, D., Vachieri, S.G., Pinna, D., Minola, A., Vanzetta, F., *et al.* (2011). A neutralizing antibody selected from plasma cells that binds to group 1 and group 2 influenza A hemagglutinins. Science 333, 850–856.
DiLillo, D.J., Tan, G.S., Palese, P., and Ravetch, J.V. (2014). Broadly neutralizing hemagglutinin stalk-specific antibodies require FcγR interactions for protection against influenza virus in vivo. Nat. Med. *20*, 143–151.
Dreyfus, C., Ekiert, D.C., and Wilson, I.A. (2013). Structure of a classical broadly neutralizing stem antibody in complex with a pandemic H2 influenza virus hemagglutinin. J. Virol. *87*, 7149–7154.
Dreyfus, C., Laursen, N.S., Kwaks, T., Zuijdgeest, D., Khayat, R., Ekiert, D.C., Lee, J.H., Metlagel, Z., Bujny, M.V., Jongeneelen, M., *et al.* (2012). Highly conserved protective epitopes on influenza B viruses. Science 337, 1343–1348.
Eggink, D., Goff, P.H., and Palese, P. (2014). Guiding the immune response against influenza virus hemagglutinin towards the conserved stalk domain by hyperglycosylation of the globular head domain. J. Virol. *88*, 699–704.
Ekiert, D.C., Bhabha, G., Elsliger, M.A., Friesen, R.H.E., Jongeneelen, M., Throsby, M., Goudsmit, J., and Wilson, I.A. (2009). Antibody recognition of a highly conserved influenza virus epitope. Science *324*, 246–251.
Ekiert, D.C., Friesen, R.H.E., Bhabha, G., Kwaks, T., Jongeneelen, M., Yu, W., Ophorst, C., Cox, F., Korse, H.J.W.M., Brandenburg, B., *et al.* (2011). A highly conserved neutralizing epitope on group 2 influenza A viruses. Science *333*, 843–850.
Ekiert, D.C., Kashyap, A.K., Steel, J., Rubrum, A., Bhabha, G., Khayat, R., Lee, J.H., Dillon, M.A., O'Neil, R.E., Faynboym, A.M., *et al.* (2012). Cross-neutralization of influenza A viruses mediated by a single antibody loop. Nature *489*, 526–532.
Fan, X., Hashem, A.M., Chen, Z., Li, C., Doyle, T., Zhang, Y., Yi, Y., Farnsworth, A., Xu, K., Li, Z., *et al.* (2014). Targeting the HA2 subunit of influenza A virus hemagglutinin via CD40L provides universal protection against diverse subtypes. Mucosal Immunol. *8*, 211–220.
Friesen, R.H.E., Lee, P.S., Stoop, E.J.M., Hoffman, R.M.B., Ekiert, D.C., Bhabha, G., Yu, W., Juraszek, J., Koudstaal, W., Jongeneelen, M., *et al.* (2014). A common solution to group 2 influenza virus neutralization. Proc. Natl. Acad. Sci. U.S.A. *111*, 445–450.
De Graaf, M., and Fouchier, R.A.M. (2014). Role of receptor binding specificity in influenza A virus transmission and pathogenesis. EMBO J. 33, 823–841.
Ha, Y., Stevens, D.J., Skehel, J.J., and Wiley, D.C. (2002). H5 avian and H9 swine influenza virus haemagglutinin structures: possible origin of influenza subtypes. EMBO J. *21*, 865–875.
Han, T., and Marasco, W.A. (2011). Structural basis of influenza virus neutralization. Ann. N. Y. Acad. Sci. *1217*, 178–190.
Hannoun, C. (2013). The evolving history of influenza viruses and influenza vaccines. Expert Rev. Vaccines *12*, 1085–1094.
Harris, A.K., Meyerson, J.R., Matsuoka, Y., Kuybeda, O., Moran, A., Bliss, D., Das, S.R., Yewdell, J.W., Sapiro, G., Subbarao, K., *et al.* (2013). Structure and accessibility of HA trimers on intact 2009 H1N1 pandemic influenza virus to stem region-specific neutralizing antibodies. Proc. Natl. Acad. Sci. U.S.A. *110*, 4592–4597.
Harrison, S.C. (2008). Viral membrane fusion. Nat. Struct. Mol. Biol. *15*, 690–698.
Huang, C.C., Venturi, M., Majeed, S., Moore, M.J., Phogat, S., Zhang, M.Y., Dimitrov, D.S., Hendrickson, W.A., Robinson, J., Sodroski, J., *et al.* (2004). Structural basis of tyrosine sulfation and VH-gene usage in antibodies that recognize the HIV type 1 coreceptor-binding site on gp120. Proc. Natl. Acad. Sci. U.S.A. *101*, 2706–2711.
Jegaskanda, S., Reading, P.C., and Kent, S.J. (2014). Influenza-specific antibody-dependent cellular cytotoxicity: toward a universal influenza vaccine. J. Immunol. *193*, 469–475.
Julien, J.P., Lee, P.S., and Wilson, I.A. (2012). Structural insights into key sites of vulnerability on HIV-1 Env and influenza HA. Immunol. Rev. *250*, 180–198.
Kalenik, B., Sawicka, R., Góra-Sochacka, A., and Sirko, A. (2014). Influenza prevention and treatment by passive immunization. Acta Biochim. Pol. *61*, 573–587.

Kanekiyo, M., Wei, C.J., Yassine, H.M., McTamney, P.M., Boyington, J.C., Whittle, J.R.R., Rao, S.S., Kong, W.P., Wang, L., and Nabel, G.J. (2013). Self-assembling influenza nanoparticle vaccines elicit broadly neutralizing H1N1 antibodies. Nature *499*, 102–106.

Khurana, S., Loving, C.L., Manischewitz, J., King, L.R., Gauger, P.C., Henningson, J., Vincent, A.L., and Golding, H. (2013). Vaccine-induced anti-HA2 antibodies promote virus fusion and enhance influenza virus respiratory disease. Sci. Transl. Med. *5*, 200ra114.

Kramer, R.M., Li, C., Carter, D.C., Stone, M.O., and Naik, R.R. (2004). Engineered protein cages for nanomaterial synthesis. J. Am. Chem. Soc. *126*, 13282–13286.

Krammer, F., Pica, N., Hai, R., Tan, G.S., and Palese, P. (2012). Hemagglutinin stalk-reactive antibodies are boosted following sequential infection with seasonal and pandemic H1N1 influenza virus in mice. J. Virol. *86*, 10302–10307.

Krammer, F., Pica, N., Hai, R., Margine, I., and Palese, P. (2013). Chimeric hemagglutinin influenza virus vaccine constructs elicit broadly protective stalk-specific antibodies. J. Virol. *87*, 6542–6550.

Kwakkenbos, M.J., Diehl, S.A., Yasuda, E., Bakker, A.Q., van Geelen, C.M.M., Lukens, M.V., van Bleek, G.M., Widjojoatmodjo, M.N., Bogers, W.M.J.M., Mei, H., *et al.* (2010). Generation of stable monoclonal antibody-producing B-cell receptor-positive human memory B-cells by genetic programming. Nat. Med. *16*, 123–128.

Laursen, N.S., and Wilson, I.A. (2013). Broadly neutralizing antibodies against influenza viruses. Antiviral Res. *98*, 476–483.

Lin, Y.P., Gregory, V., Bennett, M., and Hay, A. (2004). Recent changes among human influenza viruses. Virus Res. *103*, 47–52.

Mallajosyula, V.V.A., Citron, M., Lu, X., Meulen, J.T., Varadarajan, R., and Liang, X. (2013). In vitro and in vivo characterization of designed immunogens derived from the CD-helix of the stem of influenza hemagglutinin. Proteins *81*, 1759–1775.

Mallajosyula, V.V.A., Citron, M., Ferrara, F., Lu, X., Callahan, C., Heidecker, G.J., Sarma, S.P., Flynn, J.A., Temperton, N.J., Liang, X., *et al.* (2014). Influenza hemagglutinin stem-fragment immunogen elicits broadly neutralizing antibodies and confers heterologous protection. Proc. Natl. Acad. Sci. U.S.A. *111*, E2514–E2523.

De Marco, D., Clementi, N., Mancini, N., Solforosi, L., Moreno, G.J., Sun, X., Tumpey, T.M., Gubareva, L.V., Mishin, V., Clementi, M., *et al.* (2012). A non-VH1–69 heterosubtypic neutralizing human monoclonal antibody protects mice against H1N1 and H5N1 viruses. PLoS One *7*, e34415.

Nakamura, G., Chai, N., Park, S., Chiang, N., Lin, Z., Chiu, H., Fong, R., Yan, D., Kim, J., Zhang, J., *et al.* (2013). An in vivo human-plasmablast enrichment technique allows rapid identification of therapeutic influenza A antibodies. Cell Host Microbe *14*, 93–103.

Ni, F., Chen, X., Shen, J., and Wang, Q. (2014). Structural insights into the membrane fusion mechanism mediated by influenza virus hemagglutinin. Biochemistry *53*, 846–854.

Noah, D.L., and Noah, J.W. (2013). Adapting global influenza management strategies to address emerging viruses. Am. J. Physiol. Lung Cell. Mol. Physiol. *305*, L108–L117.

Okuno, Y., Isegawa, Y., Sasao, F., and Ueda, S. (1993). A common neutralizing epitope conserved between the hemagglutinins of influenza A virus H1 and H2 strains. J. Virol. *67*, 2552–2558.

Otterstrom, J.J., Brandenburg, B., Koldijk, M.H., Juraszek, J., Tang, C., Mashaghi, S., Kwaks, T., Goudsmit, J., Vogels, R., Friesen, R.H.E., *et al.* (2014). Relating influenza virus membrane fusion kinetics to stoichiometry of neutralizing antibodies at the single-particle level. Proc. Natl. Acad. Sci. U.S.A. *111*, E5143–8.

Palese, P., and Wang, T.T. (2011). Why do influenza virus subtypes die out? A hypothesis. MBio *2*, e00150-11.

Pica, N., and Palese, P. (2013). Toward a universal influenza virus vaccine: prospects and challenges. Annu. Rev. Med. *64*, 189–202.

Quiñones-Parra, S., Loh, L., Brown, L.E., Kedzierska, K., and Valkenburg, S.A. (2014). Universal immunity to influenza must outwit immune evasion. Front. Microbiol. *5*, 285.

Reperant, L.A., Rimmelzwaan, G.F., and Osterhaus, A.D.M.E. (2014). Advances in influenza vaccination. F1000Prime Rep. *6*, 47.

Sakabe, S., Iwatsuki-Horimoto, K., Horimoto, T., Nidom, C.A., Le, M.T., Takano, R., Kubota-Koketsu, R., Okuno, Y., Ozawa, M., and Kawaoka, Y. (2010). A cross-reactive neutralizing monoclonal antibody protects mice from H5N1 and pandemic (H1N1) 2009 virus infection. Antiviral Res. *88*, 249–255.

Skehel, J.J., and Wiley, D.C. (2000). Receptor binding and membrane fusion in virus entry: the influenza hemagglutinin. Annu. Rev. Biochem. *69*, 531–569.

Steel, J., Lowen, A.C., Wang, T.T., Yondola, M., Gao, Q., Haye, K., García-Sastre, A., and Palese, P. (2010). Influenza virus vaccine based on the conserved hemagglutinin stalk domain. MBio *1*, e00018–10.

Stevens, J., Corper, A.L., Basler, C.F., Taubenberger, J.K., Palese, P., and Wilson, I.A. (2004). Structure of the uncleaved human H1 hemagglutinin from the extinct 1918 influenza virus. Science *303*, 1866–1870.

Sui, J., Li, W., Murakami, A., Tamin, A., Matthews, L.J., Wong, S.K., Moore, M.J., Tallarico, A.S.C., Olurinde, M., Choe, H., *et al.* (2004). Potent neutralization of severe acute respiratory syndrome (SARS) coronavirus by a human mAb to S1 protein that blocks receptor association. Proc. Natl. Acad. Sci. U.S.A. *101*, 2536–2541.

Sui, J., Hwang, W.C., Perez, S., Wei, G., Aird, D., Chen, L., Santelli, E., Stec, B., Cadwell, G., Ali, M., *et al.* (2009). Structural and functional bases for broad-spectrum neutralization of avian and human influenza A viruses. Nat. Struct. Mol. Biol. *16*, 265–273.

Sui, J., Sheehan, J., Hwang, W.C., Bankston, L.A., Burchett, S.K., Huang, C.Y., Liddington, R.C., Beigel, J.H., and Marasco, W.A. (2011). Wide prevalence of heterosubtypic broadly neutralizing human anti-influenza A antibodies. Clin. Infect. Dis. *52*, 1003–1009.

Sun, X., and Whittaker, G.R. (2013). Entry of influenza virus. Adv. Exp. Med. Biol. *790*, 72–82.

Tan, G.S., Lee, P.S., Hoffman, R.M.B., Mazel-Sanchez, B., Krammer, F., Leon, P.E., Ward, A.B., Wilson, I.A., and Palese, P. (2014). Characterization of a broadly neutralizing monoclonal antibody that targets the fusion domain of group 2 influenza A virus hemagglutinin. J. Virol. *88*, 13580–13592.

Tate, M.D., Job, E.R., Deng, Y.M., Gunalan, V., Maurer-Stroh, S., and Reading, P.C. (2014). Playing hide and seek: how glycosylation of the influenza virus hemagglutinin can modulate the immune response to infection. Viruses *6*, 1294–1316.

Terajima, M., Cruz, J., Co, M.D.T., Lee, J.H., Kaur, K., Wrammert, J., Wilson, P.C., and Ennis, F.A. (2011). Complement-dependent lysis of influenza a virus-infected cells by broadly cross-reactive human monoclonal antibodies. J. Virol. *85*, 13463–13467.

Tharakaraman, K., Subramanian, V., Cain, D., Sasisekharan, V., and Sasisekharan, R. (2014). Broadly neutralizing influenza hemagglutinin stem-specific antibody CR8020 targets residues that are prone to escape due to host selection pressure. Cell Host Microbe *15*, 644–651.

Throsby, M., van den Brink, E., Jongeneelen, M., Poon, L.L.M., Alard, P., Cornelissen, L., Bakker, A., Cox, F., van Deventer, E., Guan, Y., *et al.* (2008). Heterosubtypic neutralizing monoclonal antibodies cross-protective against H5N1 and H1N1 recovered from human IgM+ memory B-cells. PLoS One 3, e3942.

Wang, Q. (2010). Influenza type B virus hemagglutinin: Antigenicity, receptor binding and membrane fusion. In Influenza: Molecular Virology, Wang, Q., and Tao, Y., eds. (Caister Adademic Press: Norfolk, UK), pp. 29–52.

Wang, C.C., Chen, J.R., Tseng, Y.C., Hsu, C.H., Hung, Y.F., Chen, S.W., Chen, C.M., Khoo, K.H., Cheng, T.J., Cheng, Y.S.E., *et al.* (2009). Glycans on influenza hemagglutinin affect receptor binding and immune response. Proc. Natl. Acad. Sci. U.S.A. *106*, 18137–18142.

Wang, T.T., Tan, G.S., Hai, R., Pica, N., Ngai, L., Ekiert, D.C., Wilson, I.A., García-Sastre, A., Moran, T.M., and Palese, P. (2010). Vaccination with a synthetic peptide from the influenza virus hemagglutinin provides protection against distinct viral subtypes. Proc. Natl. Acad. Sci. U.S.A. *107*, 18979–18984.

Webster, R.G., and Govorkova, E.A. (2014). Continuing challenges in influenza. Ann. N. Y. Acad. Sci. *1323*, 115–139.

Wei, C.J., Boyington, J.C., McTamney, P.M., Kong, W.P., Pearce, M.B., Xu, L., Andersen, H., Rao, S., Tumpey, T.M., Yang, Z.Y., *et al.* (2010). Induction of broadly neutralizing H1N1 influenza antibodies by vaccination. Science *329*, 1060–1064.

Whittle, J.R., Zhang, R., Khurana, S., King, L.R., Manischewitz, J., Golding, H., Dormitzer, P.R., Haynes, B.F., Walter, E.B., Moody, M.A., *et al.* (2011). Broadly neutralizing human antibody that recognizes the receptor-binding pocket of influenza virus hemagglutinin. Proc. Natl. Acad. Sci. U.S.A. *108*, 14216–14221.

Wilson, I.A., Skehel, J.J., and Wiley, D.C. (1981). Structure of the haemagglutinin membrane glycoprotein of influenza virus at 3 Å resolution. Nature *289*, 366–373.

Winarski, K.L., Thornburg, N.J., Yu, Y., Sapparapu, G., Crowe, J.E. Jr., and Spiller, B.W. (2015). Vaccine-elicited antibody that neutralizes H5N1 influenza and variants binds the receptor site and polymorphic sites. Proc. Natl. Acad. Sci. U.S.A. *112*, 9346–9351.

Yassine, H.M., Boyington, J.C., McTamney, P.M., Wei, C.J., Kanekiyo, M., Kong, W.P., Gallagher, J.R., Wang, L., Zhang, Y., Joyce, M.G., *et al.* (2015). Hemagglutinin-stem nanoparticles generate heterosubtypic influenza protection. Nat. Med. *21*, 1065–1070.

Yoshida, R., Igarashi, M., Ozaki, H., Kishida, N., Tomabechi, D., Kida, H., Ito, K., and Takada, A. (2009). Cross-protective potential of a novel monoclonal antibody directed against antigenic site B of the hemagglutinin of influenza A viruses. PLoS Pathog. 5, e1000350.

Influenza Virus Replication and Transcription

2

Jaime Martin-Benito,* Frank T. Vreede* and Juan Ortin

Abstract

The influenza A viruses are members of the *Orthomyxoviridae* family that cause respiratory infections in humans. They appear as yearly epidemics and occasional pandemics, which constitute a serious health problem and generate an important economic burden. The virus genome consists of eight single-stranded, negative-polarity RNAs that associate to the RNA polymerase complex and the nucleoprotein to form megaDalton sized ribonucleoprotein particles (RNPs). Here we describe the structure of these RNPs, their constitutive elements and the interactions among them. In addition, we discuss the mechanisms by which the RNPs transcribe and replicate the viral genome, including the potential participation of cellular host factors.

Introduction

The influenza A viruses belong to the *Orthomyxoviridae* family and are the causative agents of yearly epidemics and more severe pandemics of respiratory disease (Shaw and Palese, 2013). They are genetically heterogeneous and can be classified in many subtypes according to their surface antigens. All influenza A viruses are endemic in wild aquatic avian species in which they replicate efficiently without causing apparent disease. From this reservoir, they can occasionally be transferred to mammalian hosts including humans, establish new viral lineages and can give rise to a new pandemic (Baigent and McCauley, 2003; Horimoto and Kawaoka, 2005). The impact of influenza pandemics depends on the virulence of the viral strain involved. Thus, the 1918 pandemic led to around 40 million deaths while the 2009 pandemic was relatively mild (Neumann and Kawaoka, 2011; Taubenberger *et al.*, 2001; Watanabe and Kawaoka, 2011). At present, viruses of the H5N1 and H7N9 subtypes, that have occasionally infected humans producing severe disease, are a continuous threat for human health (http://www.who.int/influenza/human_animal_interface/en/).

The influenza virions are enveloped particles containing in their membrane two abundant glycoproteins, haemagglutinin (HA) and neuraminidase (NA), as well as the less abundant matrix protein 2 (M2) protein. The matrix protein 1 (M1) protein, the main component of the particle, is located underneath the membrane. The viral genome consists of 8 different ribonucleoprotein complexes (RNPs), each containing a negative-polarity single-stranded RNA molecule, with a cumulative length of about 13,590 nt (Shaw and Palese, 2013). The genomic RNA in the RNPs has a circular topology, i.e. both RNA ends contact each other to

*These authors contributed equally.

form the viral promoter and are associated with the polymerase, while the rest of the RNA is bound to nucleoprotein (NP) monomers (Klumpp *et al*, 1997; Murti *et al*, 1988). The viral polymerase is a heterotrimer composed by two basic (PB1 and PB2) and one acidic (PA) protein (Detjen *et al.*, 1987; Digard *et al.*, 1989) and is responsible for virus transcription and replication (reviewed in Elton *et al.*, 2005; Fodor, 2013; Martin-Benito and Ortin, 2013; Neumann *et al.*, 2004; Resa-Infante *et al.*, 2011).

The life history of the virus ribonucleoproteins during infection

The influenza virus attaches to target cells by interaction of the surface HA with cellular sialic acid moieties linked to surface glycoproteins and glycolipids (Skehel and Wiley, 2000). Virion entry can take place either by clathrin-dependent endocytosis or macropinocytosis, depending on the shape of the particles and the type of host cell. Thus, large filamentous virions enter by macropinocytosis, while spherical particles may use either pathway (de Vries *et al.*, 2011; Rossman *et al.*, 2012). Once the virus particle is internalized, the genomic RNPs must overcome the virion and endosomal membrane barriers to reach the cytoplasm. Two viral activities are critical in this process and both depend on the acidification of the vesicle containing the virus. On the one hand, the M2 ion channel present in the virion membrane is activated by low pH and permits the transfer of proton ions into the virion, thus allowing the separation of the viral RNPs from the M1 protein layer (reviewed in Pinto and Lamb, 2006). On the other hand, the HA undergoes a strong conformational change, exposing the internal fusion peptide and inducing virion-endosomal membrane fusion (reviewed in Skehel and Wiley, 2000).

In contrast to most other RNA-containing viruses, influenza viruses transcribe and replicate their genome in the nucleus of infected cells (Herz *et al.*, 1981). This fact implies that the virus RNPs have to overcome the barrier of the nuclear envelope but allows the virus to parasitize a number of cell nuclear mechanisms to express its genome. The virus RNPs are transported to the vicinity of the nucleus as a full genome set (Chou *et al.*, 2013) and are actively transported into the nucleus by the regular cellular import pathway. Two separate nuclear localization signals have been recognized in the NP (Neumann *et al.*, 1997; Wang *et al.*, 1997) that play significant roles in the nuclear import of the RNPs (Ozawa *et al*, 2007; Wu *et al*, 2007a). Once in the nucleus, each RNP acts as an independent template for transcription and replication.

The first nuclear activity of viral RNPs is primary transcription, i.e. synthesis of viral mRNAs from the parental RNPs. This step is independent of the expression of new virus proteins, as it can take place in the presence of inhibitors of protein synthesis (Bean and Simpson, 1973; Pons, 1973), but requires active RNA polymerase II transcription, since it is inhibited by alpha-amanitin or actinomycin D (Lamb and Choppin, 1977; Rott and Scholtissek, 1970). The structure of the influenza virus mRNAs is similar to that of cellular ones, i.e. they contain a 5′-terminal cap structure and their 3′-end is polyadenylated. However, the mechanism the virus uses to generate these modifications is not post-transcriptional but rather co-transcriptional. Thus, the virus polymerase binds the cap1 structure present in nascent cellular RNA polymerase II transcripts and cleaves the pre-mRNA around 15 nt downstream. This leads to a capped-oligonucleotide that the viral polymerase uses as a primer for the initiation of virus mRNA synthesis. However, copying of the template is not complete, since the polymerase repeatedly reads a stretch of 5–7 uridines located close to the 5′-terminus of the RNP template until it eventually falls off the template. In this way, a long poly(A) tail is generated at the 3′-end of the viral mRNA.

As indicated above, the synthesis of viral proteins is a requirement for the RNPs to proceed to productive replication. At least the virus NP and the three subunits of the polymerase are necessary to generate progeny RNPs (Huang *et al.*, 1990). The first step in the replication process is the synthesis of a complementary, positive-polarity RNA copy of the parental template (cRNA) that will serve as replication intermediate. In contrast to viral mRNAs, the cRNAs do not contain a 5′-terminal cap, are not polyadenylated at their 3′-ends and are complete copies of the template. Furthermore, the cRNAs become assembled into RNP structures similar to their vRNP templates. The various cRNPs are synthesized in equimolar amounts early in the infection but do not accumulate to a large extent (Hay *et al.*, 1977). However, they are very efficient templates to generate large amounts of progeny vRNPs. The synthesis of the various viral RNPs does not take place simultaneously and is not equally efficient (Shapiro *et al.*, 1987). Some of them, such as those encoding the NP or the NS1 protein, replicate earlier than others, like those encoding the M1 protein or the HA. These RNPs all accumulate to high levels but others, like those encoding the polymerase subunits, are less abundant. In contrast to the transcription process, viral replication does not result in an RNA product but rather in a new RNP. This implies that viral replication depends on the abundant synthesis of new polymerase and NP that has to be transported to the nucleus in amounts stoichiometric with the newly synthesized progeny RNA. The progeny vRNPs can serve as templates for secondary transcription, which is first coupled to vRNP replication and later become uncoupled and ceases (Shapiro *et al.*, 1987). Hence, early replicating genes (NP or NS1) are expressed early while those replicating late (M1 or HA) are expressed later.

Progeny vRNPs will also become incorporated into nascent virions and therefore must be exported from the nucleus. This is achieved by a CRM1-dependent mechanisms relying on NESs present in NP and/or NEP proteins (Boulo *et al.*, 2007; Elton *et al.*, 2001). Each independent vRNP appears to be exported individually and then accumulates in the perinuclear region, close to the microtubule organizing centre (MTOC). Progeny vRNPs move from this location to the recycling endosomes by association to Rab11 (Amorim *et al.*, 2011; Eisfeld *et al.*, 2011). It is at this point that they interact with each other to form specific sets containing the full virus genome (Chou *et al.*, 2013) and are transported to the plasma membrane by microtubule- and actin-dependent pathways (Avilov *et al.*, 2012). These vRNP assemblies bud from the plasma membrane by association to lipid rafts containing M1 associated to the HA and NA glycoproteins and small amounts of M2 ion channel protein (reviewed in Noda and Kawaoka, 2010; Rossman and Lamb, 2011).

The architecture of the virus ribonucleoproteins

The virus RNPs are the most complex structures present in influenza virions. They contain all the elements needed to transcribe and replicate its genome: the genomic RNA, the heterotrimeric polymerase complex and multiple NP monomers, which act as a molecular scaffold of this macromolecular machine. Each of these RNPs behaves as an independent functional unit able to replicate and transcribe inside the cell (Ortega *et al.*, 2000) and can transcribe *in vitro* with the only requirement of nucleotide triphosphates and a primer donor (Bouloy *et al.*, 1978). In the RNP structure, the partially complementary ends of each single-stranded RNA segment are linked together and bound by a single copy of the viral polymerase to form a stable closed conformation decorated by NP monomers (Compans *et al*, 1972; Klumpp *et al*, 1997; Murti *et al*, 1988; Pons *et al*, 1969). The thread formed by the RNA and the NP is folded back on itself to form a double helical arrangement as outlined in Fig. 2.1A.

The genomic RNA

From the structural point of view the most variable component of the RNPs is the genomic RNA. The eight segments that constitute the viral genome have different lengths, ranging from 2341 (segment 1) to 890 nt (segment 8), which results in RNPs of distinct sizes with molecular weights varying from 2.5 to 6.4 MDa. In each RNA segment, the coding region represents the majority of its length and is associated with multiple NP molecules, in a ratio of around 24 nt per monomer (Fig. 2.1A and B) (Compans *et al.*, 1972; Ortega *et al.*, 2000). Such interaction is not sequence-specific and has been described to melt secondary structures in the RNA (Baudin *et al.*, 1994). Conversely, it has been shown that parts of the non-coding regions, located at the 5′ and 3′ ends, are highly conserved between all segments of influenza A viruses and possess partial base complementarity (Fig. 2.1B) (Desselberger *et al.*, 1980; Robertson, 1979). The interaction between the genomic RNA ends in both

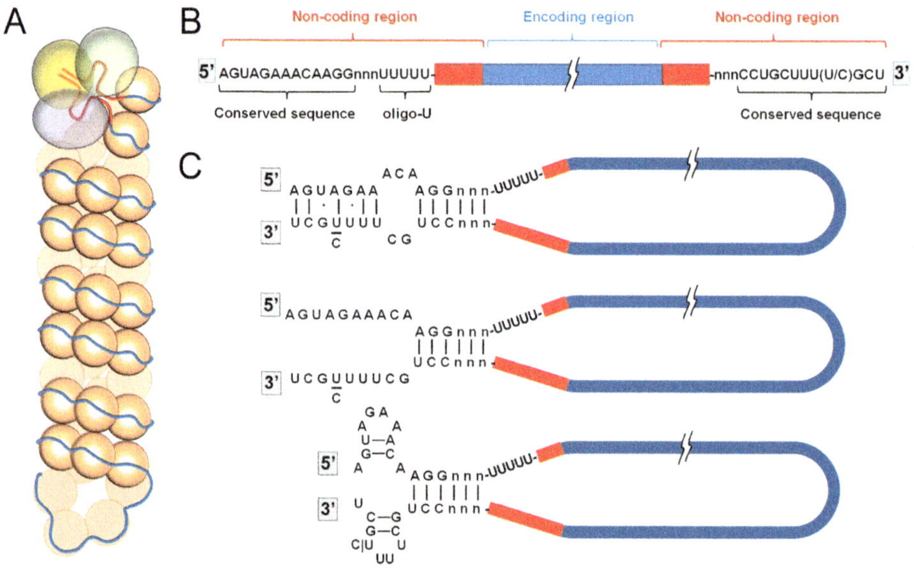

Figure 2.1 Cartoon model of the RNP structure. (A) The coding region of the single stranded RNA bound to the NP (beige circles) is depicted in blue. The non-coding regions, including the paired promoter, are depicted in red. The polymerase is shown as a group of three ellipses depicted in transparent colours. (B) Structure of the genomic vRNA. The coding and non-coding regions are depicted following the same colour code as in A. The conserved sequences, 13 and 12 nucleotides at the 5′ and 3′ ends, respectively, are shown and the only known exception, the U4C variation in the 3′ region found occasionally in segments 1, 2, 3 6 and 7, is shown in brackets. (C) Structures proposed for the vRNA promoter. From top to bottom, the panhandle, RNA-fork and corkscrew models are presented. Canonical (|) and non-canonical (·) possible base-pairings are shown.

virions and infected cells was experimentally verified by cross-linking (Hsu *et al.*, 1987), and has been shown to be stabilized by polymerase binding (Brownlee and Sharps, 2002; Klumpp *et al*, 1997) and to be required for RNA synthesis (Fodor *et al*, 1994, 1995; Hagen *et al*, 1994; Leahy *et al*, 2001a; Lee *et al*, 2003). However, the tertiary structure acquired by this promoter remains unclear and several models have been proposed, as summarized in Fig. 2.1C. The panhandle model shows the highest base-pairing and is supported by the NMR structure of a synthetic RNA obtained by joining the two conserved sequences with a tetraloop (Bae *et al.*, 2001), as well as the biophysical analysis of the isolated promoter in solution (Noble *et al.*, 2011). Nonetheless, various mutational analyses and the distinct affinity of the polymerase for the two RNA ends (González and Ortín, 1999a; Tiley *et al.*, 1994) have suggested other structural arrangements *in vivo*. Thus, the RNA-fork model proposes that the sequences close to the RNA ends remain unpaired (Fodor *et al*, 1994, 1995; Kim *et al*, 1997) and a third more elaborate structure, the corkscrew model, predicts the existence of independent hairpin loops at the 3′ and 5′ ends (Flick *et al.*, 1996). These models are not mutually exclusive, but the corkscrew arrangement is strongly favoured by several mutational analyses showing the requirement of the stem–loops at both RNA ends to maintain RNP functionality. Thus, the hairpin loop in the 3′ end is needed for the endonuclease activity (Leahy *et al.*, 2001a; Leahy *et al.*, 2001b), whereas the 5′-end loop is required for viral mRNA polyadenylation (Pritlove *et al.*, 1999). Furthermore, virus polymerase binding and stabilization depends on the presence of both loops in the promoter (Brownlee and Sharps, 2002; Flick and Hobom, 1999).

The nucleoprotein

The nucleoprotein (NP) is the major component of the RNPs. It is a 498-amino-acid-long protein that binds single stranded RNA in a co-operative, sequence-independent manner and form polymers that determine the RNP structure. The function of NP is not merely structural since it also plays several important tasks in the virus life cycle. Thus, NP mediates RNP nucleo-cytoplasmic trafficking by means of its nuclear localization signals (NLS) (Bullido *et al*, 2000; Cros *et al*, 2005; Lin and Lai, 1983; Ozawa *et al*, 2007; Wang *et al*, 1997; Wu *et al*, 2007a,b) and its nuclear export signals (NES) (Elton *et al.*, 2001; Yu *et al.*, 2012), as well as through its interaction with M1/NEP viral proteins (Boulo *et al.*, 2007). On the other hand, NP is essential to produce full-length vRNAs (Mena *et al.*, 1999; Shapiro and Krug, 1988) but it is dispensable for replication of short RNA templates *in vivo* (Resa-Infante *et al*, 2010; Turrell *et al*, 2013), suggesting that it acts as an elongation factor for the viral polymerase (Newcomb *et al.*, 2009). Finally, NP is probably involved in virus particle formation through its interaction with M1 protein (Noton *et al.*, 2007).

The atomic structures of several influenza virus NPs have been determined. They all have a crescent shape including two domains, the head and the body. A cleft enriched in basic residues is located between these domains and has been proposed as the RNA-binding site (Fig 2.2A) (Chenavas *et al*, 2013; Gerritz *et al*, 2011; Ng *et al*, 2008; Ye *et al*, 2006). The ability of NP to form oligomers is based on the presence of a tail-loop located between residues 402 and 428 that can be inserted in the body of a neighbouring NP. This interaction leads to the formation of trimers or tetramers, as described in the crystal structures (Gerritz *et al*, 2011; Ng *et al*, 2008, 2012; Ye *et al*, 2006) and ring shaped multimers or helical chains as found by electron microscopy (Ruigrok and Baudin, 1995) (Fig. 2.2B and C).

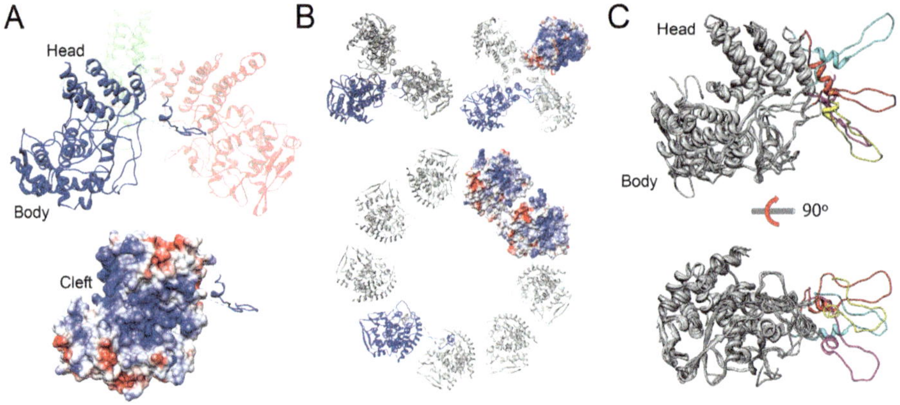

Figure 2.2 Nucleoprotein structure. (A) Atomic structure of the RNA-free NP trimer (PDB 2IQH). Only the monomer depicted in blue has been represented with solid colour to highlight the tail loop that connects two neighbouring NPs. The lower panel shows the electrostatic potential distribution of the NP surface showing the region of basic amino acids predicted as the RNA binding site in blue (Ye *et al.*, 2006). (B) Different examples of oligomers formed by the NP. At the top, raw trimeric (PDB 2IQH; influenza A virus; (Ye *et al.*, 2006) and tetrameric (PDB 3TJ0; Type B influenza virus; (Ng *et al.*, 2012)) crystallographic structures of the NP are shown. At the bottom, raw docking of the structure of the NP into the cryoelectron microscopy map determined from a mini-RNP (PDB 2WFS; (Coloma *et al.*, 2009)) is shown. The surface potential of some monomers is presented to show that the RNA binding region is located on the external part of the ring. (C) Flexibility of the tail loop connection in different crystallographic structures. The head-body domains from different NPs have been aligned to show the high flexibility of the tail-loop connection. For clarity, only the loop has been coloured according to the following code: yellow, PDB 2IQH (Ye *et al.*, 2006); pink, PDB 3RO5 (Gerritz *et al.*, 2011); cyan, PDB 2Q06 (Ng *et al*, 2008); and red, influenza B NP, PDB 3TJ0 (Ng *et al.*, 2012).

The polymerase

The influenza RNA-dependent RNA polymerase is a heterotrimer with a total molecular mass of around 250 kDa (Fig 2.3A) (Braam *et al*, 1983; Horisberger, 1980). All three subunits are essential for efficient RNA transcription and replication and multiple studies *in vivo* and *in vitro* have allowed specific functions of each subunit to be defined. The structure of the polymerase is not well known at present but it seems to be a quite flexible and dynamic complex, subject to conformational changes depending on multiple factors such as the nature of the bound promoter (vRNA or cRNA), interaction with NP or a cap donor, etc. Despite this, significant progress has been made in recent years that include the determination of the atomic structure of several subunit fragments (Fig. 2.3B) and the determination of the low/mid resolution structure of the whole polymerase complex using electron microscopy (see below).

The PB1 subunit has 757 residues and bears the polymerase activity, including the conserved SDD motif at positions 444–446 (Biswas and Nayak, 1994). It is considered the core of the complex (Digard *et al.*, 1989) and it has been shown to interact with PB2 and PA through its C- and N-terminal regions, respectively (González *et al*, 1996; He *et al*, 2008; Obayashi *et al*, 2008; Ohtsu *et al*, 2002; Sugiyama *et al*, 2009) (Fig. 2.3A). In addition, PB1 also binds the vRNA (González and Ortín, 1999a; Li *et al*, 1998) and cRNA promoter sequences (González and Ortín, 1999b). The only structural information available is limited

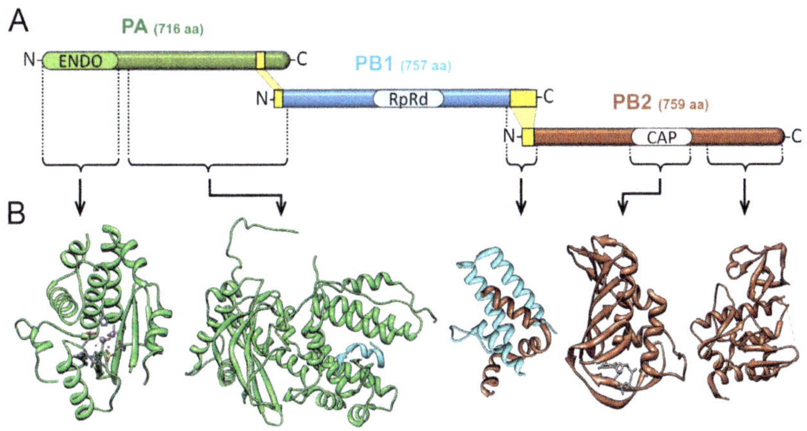

Figure 2.3 Structure of polymerase domains. (A) Classical protein interaction studies, supported by the current X ray data, have suggested an N- to C-terminal PA-PB1-PB2 consecutive arrangement of the polymerase subunits. (B) Crystallographic structure of influenza A virus polymerase domains. From left to right: PA endonuclease domain residues 1–209 (PDB 2W69; (Dias *et al*, 2009); interaction between PA C-terminus and PB1 N-terminus, residues 256–716 and 1–16, respectively (PDB 3CM8; (He *et al*., 2008); interaction between PB1 C-terminus and PB2 N-terminus, residues 679–757 and 1–37, respectively (PDB 2ZTT; (Sugiyama *et al*., 2009); PB2 CAP-binding domain residues 318–483 (PDB 2VQZ; (Guilligay *et al*., 2008), and two domains of PB2 C-terminus residues 538–667 and 686–741 (PDB 2VY6; (Tarendeau *et al*., 2008).

to the atomic structure of the first 81 N-terminal residues (He *et al*, 2008; Obayashi *et al*, 2008) and amino acids 679–757 at the C-terminus (Sugiyama *et al*., 2009) (Fig. 2.3B).

The PA subunit has 716 residues and is the best structurally characterized subunit of the complex (Fig. 2.3B). The N-terminal region harbours the endonuclease activity, which is responsible for cleaving cellular, capped pre-mRNA and is essential for viral transcription, as shown biochemically (Fodor *et al*, 2002; Hara *et al*, 2006) or by structural analyses (Dias *et al*, 2009; Yuan *et al*, 2009). The atomic structures revealed the motif PDX_nEK, between amino acids 107–134 which is characteristic of type II endonucleases. The atomic structure of the C-terminal domain of PA bound to the N-terminus of PB1 has been determined, revealing a tight interaction between the subunits (He *et al*, 2008; Obayashi *et al*, 2008). The linker region between the N- and C-terminal domains (residues 257–276) appears to be at the PA–PB1 interface, since it is stabilized by PB1 interaction (Guu *et al*., 2008). In addition to cap-snatching, PA is also involved in promoter binding (Hara *et al*, 2006; Kawaguchi *et al*, 2005) and virus particle formation (Regan *et al*., 2006) and has been associated with the proteolysis of viral and host cell proteins, although the potential active site is controversial (Hara *et al*., 2001; Perales *et al*., 2000; Rodriguez *et al*., 2007; Sanz-Ezquerro *et al*., 1996). Finally, it is worth mentioning that PA has been proposed as an antiviral target through the inhibition of its endonuclease activity (Baughman *et al*., 2012; DuBois *et al*., 2012; Kowalinski *et al*., 2012).

The PB2 subunit has 759 residues and is involved in capped RNA recognition during transcription initiation (Fechter and Brownlee, 2005). Basically, the 'cap-snatching' mechanism for transcription initiation works as follows: PB2 binds the 5′ cap-1 structures of host pre-mRNAs, PA cleaves this RNA 9–15 nucleotides downstream of the cap and the resulting fragment is used by PB1 as a primer to start the transcription process. Different regions of PB2 were proposed to be responsible for cap recognition (Fechter *et al.*, 2003; Honda *et al.*, 1999; Li *et al.*, 2001), but the determination of the atomic structure of the fragment comprising residues 318–483, bound to a m^7GTP molecule, revealed that the central portion of the protein contains the cap-binding site (Fechter *et al.*, 2003; Guilligay *et al.*, 2008). The structure of two other PB2 fragments has been solved using X-ray crystallography: the first one encompasses residues 538–676 (Tarendeau *et al.*, 2008), including the K627 residue, a key determinant of host range and pathogenicity (Subbarao *et al.*, 1993), and the second one delineates the subunit contact between PB2 and PB1 (Fig. 2.3B) (Sugiyama *et al.*, 2009). Finally, the C-terminal domain of PB2, containing the bipartite nuclear import signal (residues 738–755) has been crystallized in a complex with the importin α5 (Tarendeau *et al.*, 2007). In addition to its role in transcription, PB2 has also been associated with replication, since point mutations on its N-terminal region affect virus RNA replication but not transcription (Gastaminza *et al.*, 2003).

The complete polymerase complex has been found in infected cells in two forms, as a component of the RNP (Klumpp *et al.*, 1997) and as a free heterotrimer (Detjen *et al.*, 1987). The determination of the polymerase quaternary organization has been hampered by its high flexibility and conformational variability and the technical difficulties in obtaining the purified complex. Nevertheless, our knowledge of the polymerase arrangement has increased over the years thanks to electron microscopy studies. Thus, low-/mid-resolution structures of the isolated recombinant polymerase (Moeller *et al.*, 2012; Resa-Infante *et al.*, 2010; Torreira *et al.*, 2007), the polymerase of a mini or a full-size recombinant RNP (Area *et al.*, 2004; Coloma *et al.*, 2009; Martín-Benito *et al.*, 2001; Moeller *et al.*, 2012) and the polymerase of virion RNPs (Arranz *et al.*, 2012) (Fig. 2.4) have been obtained (see next section for details).

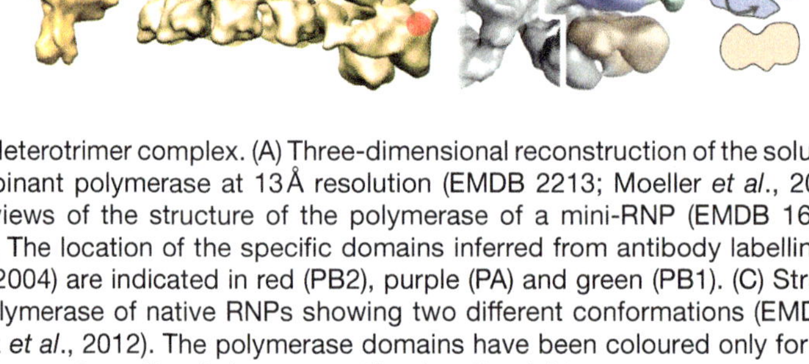

Figure 2.4 Heterotrimer complex. (A) Three-dimensional reconstruction of the soluble influenza virus recombinant polymerase at 13Å resolution (EMDB 2213; Moeller *et al.*, 2012); (B) two orthogonal views of the structure of the polymerase of a mini-RNP (EMDB 1603; (Coloma *et al.*, 2009). The location of the specific domains inferred from antibody labelling or tagging (Area *et al.*, 2004) are indicated in red (PB2), purple (PA) and green (PB1). (C) Structure of the wild type polymerase of native RNPs showing two different conformations (EMDB 2207 and 2208; Arranz *et al.*, 2012). The polymerase domains have been coloured only for the purpose of showing the conformational changes, outlined on the right.

The ribonucleoprotein complex

The genomic RNA, polymerase and NP are assembled into RNPs, which adopt a double helical conformation with one copy of the polymerase at one end and a closing loop at the other (Compans *et al*, 1972; Jennings *et al*, 1983; Klumpp *et al*, 1997; Murti *et al*, 1988; reviewed in Zheng and Tao, 2013). Native RNPs are characterized by their diversity in size, depending on the viral gene encoded, and their high flexibility, features that have hampered detailed structural analysis. In order to overcome such problems, a recombinant, biologically active mini-RNP containing a small vRNA of 248 nucleotides was generated by *in vivo* amplification (Ortega *et al.*, 2000). The single size and lower structural flexibility of this recombinant RNP allowed the generation of a three-dimensional reconstruction that revealed a nonameric ring-like structure connected to the viral polymerase (Fig. 2.4B) (Coloma *et al.*, 2009; Martín-Benito *et al.*, 2001). The resolution obtained in the cryoelectron microscopy map (12 Å) (Coloma *et al.*, 2009) did not allow the unambiguous determination of the RNA path, but docking of the NP atomic structure into the ring showed that the RNA binding cleft is located on the external side of the ring (Fig. 2.2B, lower panel), as was the case in the trimeric crystallographic structures (Ye *et al.*, 2006). Additionally, this mini-RNP was used to generate the first structural information of the polymerase complex by labelling the different subunits with monoclonal antibodies or tags (Area *et al.*, 2004) (Fig. 2.4B). However, these particles lacked the helical features typical of virion RNPs and a new approach was necessary to obtain their structure. A separate analysis of termini and central regions of the full-length RNPs was performed that allowed the three-dimensional reconstruction of the helical part and the ends containing the polymerase and the closing loop. With this experimental strategy, the structure of native RNPs isolated from virions (Arranz *et al.*, 2012) and full-size recombinant RNPs (Moeller *et al.*, 2012) were obtained (Fig. 2.5).

The structures of the central region determined in the two studies have common features: a double helical arrangement with two opposite polarity RNA-NP strands that define a minor groove, where both strands are connected, and a major groove, where the strands are not physically in contact (Fig. 2.5A). Nevertheless, the two models also present significant differences in the helical parameters and in the docking of the NP atomic structure. Thus, Arranz *et al.* (2012) proposed a left-handed helix with a rise step between NP monomers of 28.4 Å and an angle of −60°, while Moeller *et al.* (2012) suggested a right-handed helix with a rise step of 32.6 Å and an angle of +73.9°. These structural differences extend to the docking of the NP into the structures. On the one hand, Arranz *et al.* (2012) placed the head domain of the NP oriented towards the major groove, with the N-terminal regions of two NPs on opposite strands interacting at the minor groove; this layout leaves the RNA binding site of the NP mainly facing the major groove and the outer side of the RNP, where it is easily accessible during polymerization (Fig. 2.5B, left panel). On the other hand, Moeller *et al.* (2012) suggested that the interaction between opposite strands involves the NP head domains and, as a result, the RNA binding site faces the internal part of the minor groove. This arrangement does not leave the genomic RNA directly accessible for transcription or replication, and suggests that at least local disassembly of the NP–RNA complex is required for these processes to occur (Fig. 2.5B, right panel). The origin of these differences is not clear but some of the possibilities are (i) the source of the RNPs (virion-derived vs. recombinant particles), (ii) the purification protocol that could determine the compactness of the RNP or (iii) the limited resolution that could determine the alternative docking solutions. Further studies are needed to shed light on this issue.

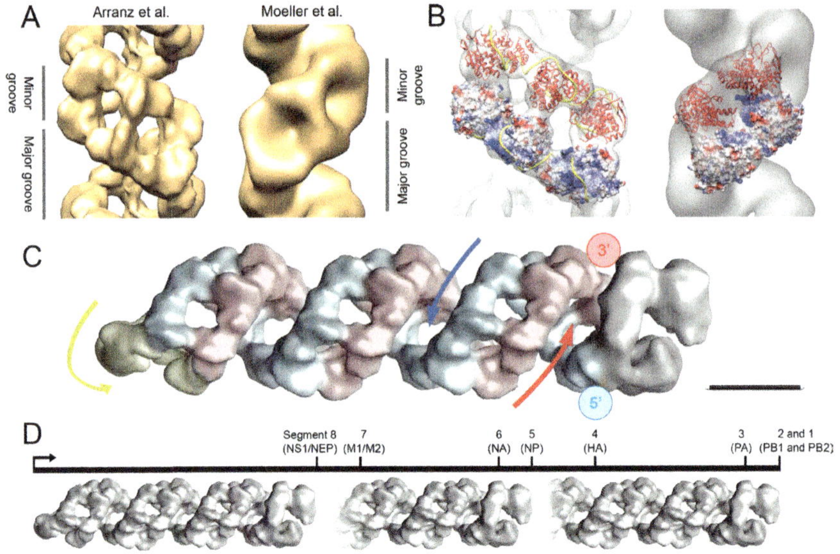

Figure 2.5 Structure of the vRNP. (A) Structure of the helical part of the RNP determined using cryoelectron microscopy by Arranz *et al*. (18 Å resolution; virion RNPs; EMDB 2205) and Moeller *et al*. (21 Å resolution; recombinant RNPs; EMDB 2209). Both maps show a double helical arrangement with a major and a minor groove, but in the first case the structure is a left-handed helix and in the second a right handed-helix (for details see Arranz *et al*., 2012; Moeller *et al*., 2012). (B) Docking of the NP monomer into the cryoelectron microscopy maps (PDBs 4BBL and 2YMN). In the upper strand of the helix a ribbon model is shown and in the lower strand the surface potential of the NP monomers is shown. The position of the predicted RNA binding region is different in the two structures. Thus, while in the model presented by Arranz *et al*. (2012) the RNA would face the major groove, with the two threads of the ascending and descending strands relatively distant (depicted in yellow), the model presented by Moeller *et al*. predicts that the RNA would be buried in the minor groove with the two threads very close to each other. (C) Structure of the complete vRNP obtained from the juxtaposition of the helical part and the two terminal regions (Arranz *et al*., 2012). The two strands of the helix have been coloured in red and blue, the polymerase in grey and the closing loop in yellow. The combination of the NP docking assays and the mutational analysis performed by Turrell *et al*. (2013) shows that the red strand corresponds to the 3′ end of the RNA and the blue strand to the 5′ end; arrows indicate the direction of the RNA from 5′ to 3′ end. The scale bar indicates 100 Å. (D) Diagram of the relative size of the RNPs present in the virion. The black line represents the length of the different segments, from 1 to 8; the main protein encoded by each one is shown in brackets. In the lower part three representative RNPs, corresponding to the small, mid and large sizes, are depicted.

The heterogeneity of the RNPs is not limited to the flexibility of the helical part but is extended to the termini. The three-dimensional reconstructions of the RNP closing loop show a rather variable structure due to the lack of inter-strand stabilization in this region (Arranz *et al*., 2012) and the possible slight variability in the number of monomers involved in this loop (Moeller *et al*., 2012). Additionally, the reconstructions of the polymerase end show two alternative conformations of the complex in the virion RNPs (Fig. 2.4C) (Arranz *et al*., 2012). The differences are depicted in Fig. 2.4C and show a rotation and displacement of the blue and green regions of the polymerase. The proportion of the two conformations is roughly 50%, but their biological relevance is unknown at present. The conformational flexibility of the polymerase is also reflected in the differences between the structure of the complex in the native RNP and in the recombinant mini-RNP. In both cases the structure shows the same general arrangement, with two masses divided by a large central groove, but part of the polymerase is twisted and tilted in the helical RNPs in comparison with the mini-RNP (compare Fig. 2.4B and C), so that is not possible to make a direct extrapolation of the subunit distribution known for the polymerase of the mini-RNP to the polymerase of the native RNP. The juxtaposition of the reconstruction of the two RNP termini and the central part yields the structure of the complete RNP (Fig. 2.5C). The final size of each segment depends on the length of the RNA and is summarized in Fig. 2.5D.

RNP formation

Information about how the nascent RNP adopts its quaternary structure is very scarce. The double helical structure of the RNP appears to be the result of a combination of three factors: (i) the inherent tendency of the NP to form helical multimers (Ruigrok and Baudin, 1995); (ii) the ability of NP to bind RNA; and (iii) the closed structure of the genomic vRNA, due to RNA–RNA and RNA–polymerase interactions (Hsu *et al*, 1987; Klumpp *et al*, 1997), which forces NP to follow an 'up and down' path 'from and to' the polymerase. The NP binds RNA without sequence specificity but it has been shown that in infected cells this binding is limited to viral RNAs. Additionally, NP interacts with the PB1 and PB2 polymerase subunits (Biswas *et al*, 1998; Coloma *et al*, 2009). For these reasons it is generally thought that the polymerase serves as a nucleation element for the assembly of nascent RNA by NP (Portela and Digard, 2002; Resa-Infante *et al*, 2011). A recent study on RNP assembly during the replication process shows that NP monomers are incorporated onto the nascent RNA chain in a 'tail loop first' orientation in a process that is independent of RNA binding (Fig. 2.5C) (Turrell *et al.*, 2013). However, it remains unknown how the NP-RNA strand folds to generate the RNP double helix arrangement, allowing interaction between NPs that are separated in the sequence.

cRNP versus vRNP

The cRNPs are the virus RNA replication intermediates and are synthesized in small amounts during the viral life cycle or during *in vivo* replication of recombinant replicons (Martin-Benito and Ortin, 2013; Ortega *et al.*, 2000). Similarly, recombinant micro-replicons devoid of NP accumulate *in vivo* as a mixture of polymerase–RNA complexes containing only a small proportion of cRNA (Resa-Infante *et al.*, 2010). Structural differences between complexes containing cRNA or vRNA are expected. Thus, biochemical studies have shown that the interaction of PB1 with cRNA or vRNA promoters is different, suggesting conformational changes in the polymerase (González and Ortín, 1999b). It has also been demonstrated that a differential role of the PA subunit exists for vRNA or cRNA binding (Maier *et al.*, 2008). Moreover, the mechanisms for initiation of replication are different for cRNP and vRNP templates (Deng *et al.*, 2006). Currently, the available information on RNP structure comes primarily from vRNPs and little is known about cRNPs. This is for two main reasons: (i) until recently, there were no efficient protocols to separate cRNPs from vRNPs and (ii) vRNPs are much more abundant than cRNPs and any structural study performed with a mixture of both species will be biased towards the predominant complex, i.e. the vRNP. However, a RNA-based affinity purification protocol has recently been reported for the isolation of cRNPs from infected cells and this strategy has allowed the first preliminary results on the cRNP structure to be obtained (York *et al.*, 2013).

The regulation of transcription and replication

During the viral life cycle, the kinetics for the accumulation of the products of viral transcription and replication in the infected cell are vastly different (Fig. 2.6). Initially upon infection, the vRNPs introduced into the cell by the infecting virions synthesize predominantly viral mRNA which accumulates rapidly to a peak at 4–6 hours post infection, whereafter mRNA levels diminish (Shapiro *et al*, 1987; Vreede *et al*, 2010). cRNA is also templated by the virion-derived vRNPs and is detectable soon after infection. The expression of viral proteins from newly synthesized mRNA enables replication of cRNA to vRNA which then forms the template for secondary transcription to mRNA and the synthesis of further cRNA (Mark *et al.*, 1979; Vreede *et al.*, 2004). However, cRNA only accumulates to a low plateau by 4–6 hours post infection, whereas vRNA continues to accumulate beyond 8 hours post infection to high levels. These observations are indicative of multiple levels of regulation of RNP activity: (i) there exists a switch from a predominantly transcription phase early in infection to a later phase of predominantly replication; (ii) vRNP activity is regulated between transcription (vRNA→mRNA) and the first step of replication (vRNA→cRNA) and (iii) vRNA-templated (vRNA→cRNA) and cRNA-templated (cRNA→vRNA) replication are differentially regulated. A large body of research has been devoted to these questions. Various models involving regulatory roles for viral and host factors have been proposed to explain the control mechanisms (reviewed in Resa-Infante *et al.*, 2011), but a unifying model which incorporates and addresses all the experimental data has proved elusive.

Elucidation of the detailed molecular mechanisms of replication and transcription suggested that the mode of initiation and termination in replication and transcription are coupled by currently unknown mechanisms. Thus, transcription requires a capped primer for initiation of viral transcription, and elongation continues until steric hindrance hypothetically caused by the continued association of the viral polymerase with the 5′ end of the vRNA template results in the addition of a poly(A) tail through reiterative stuttering on a stretch of 5–6 U residues 15–16 nucleotides from the 5′ end of the vRNA template (Fodor *et al*, 1994; Hagen *et al*, 1994; Poon *et al*, 1998). In contrast, the products of replication are full length copies of the template and possess a 5′-terminal triphosphate, indicative of de novo initiation at the 3′-terminus of the template and run-off termination

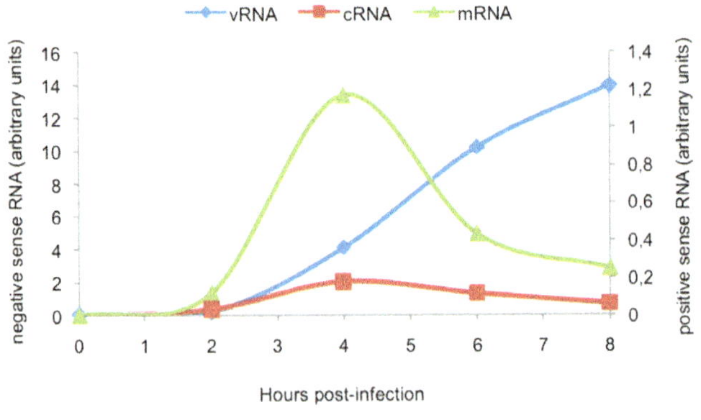

Figure 2.6 Accumulation of influenza virus RNA species in a time course of infection.

at the 5′-terminus of the template (Hay *et al.*, 1980). Such coupling of initiation and termination events in transcription and replication suggests that (i) differential regulation of vRNA-templated activity occurs primarily at the level of initiation and/or (ii) entirely distinct polymerase complexes may be responsible for replication and transcription. The former possibility had long been accepted as a likely mechanism. Thus, it has long been known that the inhibition of protein expression in an infected cell, for instance by cycloheximide treatment, allows primary viral transcription but prevents viral replication (Mark *et al.*, 1979). This suggested that viral proteins were responsible for a switch in the activity of the viral polymerase. In particular, the presence of newly expressed 'free' NP emerged from extensive biochemical and mutagenesis studies as the leading candidate responsible for directing a switch in vRNP activity from transcription to replication by interacting with the polymerase, the vRNA template or the cRNA product (reviewed in (Portela and Digard, 2002). In addition, NP was proposed to act as an anti-terminator during replication, preventing the viral polymerase from terminating prematurely at the polyadenylation signal (Beaton and Krug, 1986). However, emerging evidence suggests that NP plays no regulatory role in determining the mode of initiation or termination by the viral RNA polymerase (Resa-Infante *et al*, 2010; Turrell *et al*, 2013). In particular, short vRNA-like templates with large internal deletions but retaining the 5′ and 3′-terminal sequences were found to be efficiently transcribed and replicated in the absence of NP in cell culture-mediated RNP reconstitution experiments, yielding authentic 5′ capped and 3′ polyadenylated mRNA-like transcripts and uncapped and non-polyadenylated vRNA-like replication products. In fact, the very existence of a switch in RNP activity early during viral infection was called into question by complementation experiments in which the pre-expression of catalytically inactive polymerase and NP was shown to allow the accumulation of cRNA from infecting vRNPs in the absence of protein expression (Vreede *et al.*, 2004). However, the levels of cRNA detected were severely reduced if the RNA-binding capacity of the pre-expressed polymerase or NP was inhibited by mutagenesis (Vreede *et al*, 2004, 2011). These data were interpreted to mean that the vRNPs from an infecting virus synthesize both mRNA and cRNA, but cRNA is quickly degraded by cellular nucleases. It was proposed that viral polymerase and NP were required to stabilize cRNA in viral infections by assembly into cRNPs (Fig. 2.7). Indeed, pre-expressed polymerase and NP were shown to assemble specifically with cRNA (Vreede and Brownlee, 2007). This interpretation also correlates with the observation that purified virion-derived vRNPs can synthesize both cRNA and mRNA *in vitro* (Vreede and Brownlee, 2007). However, these studies did not address the regulatory mechanism by which either transcription or replication is initiated, hypothesizing instead that it might be stochastic, i.e. dependent on the random selection of either a capped primer or an ATP molecule for phosphodiester bond formation with GTP to initiate transcription or replication, respectively (Butcher *et al*, 2001; Olson *et al*, 2010; Vreede *et al*, 2008).

The invocation of distinct replicase and transcriptase complexes is an attractive model that has gained support in recent years (Jorba *et al.*, 2009; Moeller *et al.*, 2012). According to this model (Fig. 2.8), mRNA synthesis is performed in cis by the RNA polymerase that forms part of the vRNP. The *cis*-polymerase requires a capped primer for initiation, and creates a steric block for termination of transcription, thus favouring polyadenylation. In contrast, replication is performed in trans by an RNA polymerase that is distinct from the RNP-associated polymerase.

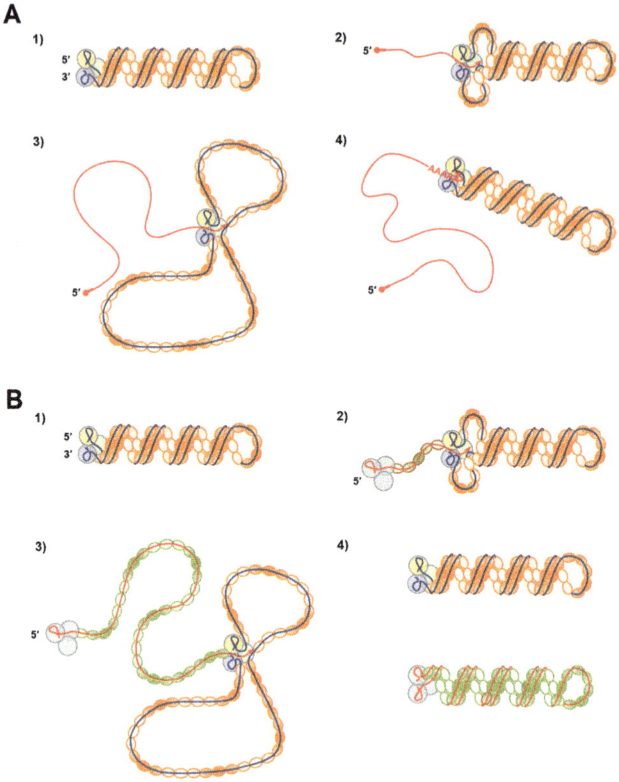

Figure 2.7 Schematic diagram of a model for RNP transcription and replication by a cis-acting polymerase. The (cis-acting) trimeric viral RNA polymerase (shaded in transparent colours) resident on the negative sense (v)RNA template (coloured dark blue) carries out both transcription to mRNA (A) and replication to cRNA (B). The resident NP is shaded orange. The RNA stem–loop structures represent the 5′ and 3′-terminal promoters. Positive sense nascent RNA transcripts are coloured red. The RNA stem–loop structures represent the 5′ and 3′ terminal promoters. The capped primer is denoted by a red keyhole. The arrow head indicates the site of polymerization. mRNA is polyadenylated by stuttering of the polymerase on the 5′ proximal poly(U) signal. cRNA is stabilized by newly expressed viral RNA polymerase (shaded grey) and NP (shaded green). The model does not attempt to address the extent or mechanism of template and product RNP unfolding or (re)folding; the intermediate conformations shown here are speculative.

The first support for such a *trans*-complementation model came from experiments carried out in cell culture using polymerase complexes that are defective in either transcription or replication to establish that a polymerase complex different from that acting during replication is incorporated into progeny RNPs (Jorba *et al.*, 2009). This allowed the rescue of recombinant RNPs that are defective in replication which were then used to examine whether the polymerase complex associated with the RNP (acting *in cis*) or a different soluble trans-acting polymerase complex is responsible for replication. The data suggested that replication occurs *in trans*, i.e. a polymerase complex distinct from that present in the template RNP can perform the replicative synthesis of viral RNA. Taken together, it was proposed that a soluble polymerase complex genetically distinguishable from that present

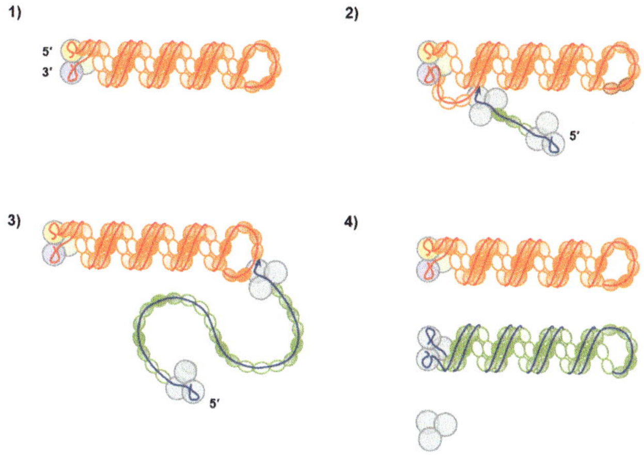

Figure 2.8 Schematic diagram of a model for RNP replication by a trans-acting polymerase. Here, newly expressed (trans-acting) trimeric viral RNA polymerase (shaded grey) carries out replication of the positive sense cRNA template (coloured red) to negative sense vRNA (coloured dark blue) which is bound by another newly expressed (assembly) viral RNA polymerase and NP (shaded green). The resident polymerase on the template is shaded in transparent colours and NP in orange. The RNA stem–loop structures represent the 5′ and 3′ terminal promoters. Although one template may theoretically be copied simultaneously by multiple trans-acting polymerases, only a single replication event is shown for simplicity. The model does not attempt to address the extent or mechanism of template and product RNP unfolding or (re)folding; the intermediate conformations shown here are speculative.

in the parental RNP would be responsible for carrying out replication in trans and that a further non-resident soluble polymerase distinct from that performing replication would become incorporated into the progeny RNP by binding the 5′ end of the nascent RNA sequence-specifically. This would trigger the addition of the first NP adjacent to the bound polymerase and initiate encapsidation of cRNA in a 5′ to 3′ direction. Thus, both newly synthesized viral polymerase and NP would be required for replication. It was not possible in these experiments to distinguish vRNA-templated from cRNA-templated replication. However, it was proposed that the cRNP to vRNP, but not the vRNP to cRNP, phase of replication may involve a *trans*-acting polymerase based on the earlier data regarding the stabilization of newly synthesized cRNA by an inactive pre-expressed polymerase and NP which demonstrated that vRNPs of infecting virions are able to synthesize cRNA *in cis* (Vreede *et al.*, 2004). This differential mode of vRNA- and cRNA-templated replication would be in line with biochemical and genetic evidence suggesting that distinct regions of the polymerase interact with vRNA and cRNA promoter regions (González and Ortín, 1999b) and with the proposal that initiation of *de novo* replication on vRNA and cRNA templates occurs at different positions (Deng *et al.*, 2006). Whereas the initiation of cRNA synthesis is directed by the 3′-terminal residues of the vRNA template, the synthesis of vRNA is initiated internally, directed by positions 4 and 5 at the 3′ end of the cRNA promoter. The resultant pppApG dinucleotide is then realigned to the 3′-terminal residues 1 and 2 for subsequent elongation and synthesis of full length vRNA. Finally, this would also provide a plausible explanation for the differing capacity of vRNPs and cRNPs to perform cap-snatching.

In support of the trans-model of replication, recent examination of negative stain EM micrographs of reconstituted RNP complexes purified from transfected cells revealed approximately one out of four RNPs with a branched arrangement in which a smaller putative nascent RNP appears to bud from a larger full-length RNP (Moeller *et al.*, 2012). Additionally, a polymerase residing at the junction of the smaller RNA with the full-length RNP was observed, consistent with the putative identification of these branched RNPs as replication intermediates in which replication is being carried out by a *trans*-acting polymerase. Once again, it was not possible in this study to distinguish vRNP from cRNP molecules. However, the recent development of an RNA-based affinity purification strategy for the isolation of RNPs from infected cells enabled the separate functional characterization of cRNPs and vRNPs (York *et al.*, 2013). It was shown once again that purified vRNPs are able to carry out both *de novo* initiated replication and globin mRNA primed transcription *in vitro*. However, it was found that cRNPs showed *in vitro* (ApG-primed) activity only in the presence of added viral RNA polymerase. Intriguingly, a replication-inactive RNA polymerase was also able to activate cRNP-templated vRNA synthesis. Therefore, it was suggested that RNP replication is performed by a *cis*-acting resident polymerase, but that a *trans*-activating polymerase is required for the activation of vRNA synthesis from a cRNP complex.

It has been proposed that the viral NEP is involved in the regulation of viral RNA synthesis (Robb *et al.*, 2009). Specifically, NEP was found to up-regulate the accumulation of replication products, especially cRNA, while down-regulating the accumulation of transcription products in RNP reconstitution assays *in vivo*. The involvement of NEP in the regulation of viral RNA synthesis gained further support when it was found that adaptive mutations in NEP can compensate for defective replication by partially or non-adapted RNA polymerase from an H5N1 avian influenza virus in mammalian cells, possibly by directly interacting with the RNA polymerase (Manz *et al.*, 2012). Another study suggested that NEP could regulate viral RNA synthesis by promoting the synthesis of small viral RNAs (svRNAs) from cRNA templates (Perez *et al*, 2010, 2012). svRNAs of 22–27 nucleotides in length, corresponding to the 5′ end of each of the vRNA segments, were found to be expressed at high levels in infected cells (Perez *et al*, 2010; Umbach *et al*, 2010). Their expression correlates with the accumulation of vRNA and a bias in RNA polymerase activity from transcription towards genome replication. Consequently, it was proposed that svRNA promotes replication, possibly through an interaction with a novel RNA-binding channel of the polymerase PA subunit (Perez *et al.*, 2012). It is plausible that svRNAs might promote the second stage of replication (cRNA to vRNA) by associating with a *trans*-acting or -activating RNA polymerase.

Role of host factors

As influenza A virus is an small obligate intracellular pathogen with limited coding capacity, it relies heavily on the host cellular factors, structures and pathways for its life cycle, as demonstrated by various genome-wide screens (reviewed in Watanabe *et al.*, 2010). Some of these factors, e.g. MxA, DDX17 and α-importins (see below), have been shown to be important determinants of host range, governing the host adaptation or cell tropism of influenza A virus, and thus have important implications for pathogenicity and cross-species transmission. However, a number of 'basal' factors have been identified that act as regulators of the activities of the viral polymerase.

Transcription

As indicated above, viral transcription is dependent on cellular RNA polymerase II (Pol II) activity for the 5′ capped RNA primers which are derived from host pre-mRNAs. Indeed, inhibitors of Pol II, e.g. alpha-amanitin, were found to specifically inhibit viral transcription (Chan *et al*, 2006; Mark *et al*, 1979). The viral polymerase was found to associate with the hyperphosphorylated C-terminal domain (CTD) of initiating Pol II and it was proposed that this association might facilitate the access of the viral polymerase to the 5′ cap of host nascent pre-mRNAs (Engelhardt *et al.*, 2005). It has also been proposed that the reduction in viral mRNA synthesis after its peak at about 4 to 6 hours post infection may be caused by a reduction in the availability of the cap donor host mRNAs due to host shut-off and/or inhibition and degradation of Pol II induced by viral infection (reviewed in Vreede and Fodor, 2010).

The initiation of viral mRNA transcription also depends on other accessory factors. Thus, it has been demonstrated that the positive transcription elongation factor b (pTEFb) interacts with influenza viral RNA polymerase complex (Zhang *et al.*, 2010). pTEFb is composed of cyclin-dependent kinase 9 (CDK9) and the cyclin T1 complex and promotes the switch from initiation to elongation during cellular transcription by phosphorylating the CTD of Pol II at serine 5. It was proposed that pTEFb might function as an adaptor to facilitate the association between viral RNA polymerase and cellular Pol II, thereby promoting viral transcription. Similarly, hCLE, a positive modulator of Pol II activity, has been shown to interact with the PA subunit of the viral polymerase and be required for viral transcription and, intriguingly, replication (Huarte *et al.*, 2001; Perez-Gonzalez *et al.*, 2006; Rodriguez *et al.*, 2011).

Another cellular protein which was found associated with the viral polymerase and shown to play a role in influenza virus transcription is the splicing-factor related protein SFPQ/PSF (Landeras-Bueno *et al.*, 2011). SFPQ/PSF is an RNA-binding protein that was shown to be essential for influenza virus transcription, increasing the efficiency of viral mRNA polyadenylation. It was speculated that SFPQ/PSF could interact both with the viral polymerase and with the viral polyadenylation signal within the RNP to promote polymerase stuttering at the site.

Replication

In contrast to transcription, replication initiates de novo with host cell rNTPs but without the requirement for a primer. However, it has been proposed that in order to escape the promoter and to facilitate the transition from initiating to elongating form, the viral replication complex is stabilized by the host's minichromosome maintenance (MCM) complex, a DNA replicative helicase (Kawaguchi and Nagata, 2007). It was proposed that MCM functions as a scaffold between the viral polymerase and the nascent RNA chain or the viral promoter through interaction with the PA subunit. In addition, two further host factors, RAF-2p48/NPI-5/UAP56 and Tat-SF1, have been reported to function as molecular chaperones to facilitate coreplicational assembly of the nascent RNA by NP during the subsequent elongation phase (Kawaguchi *et al*, 2011; Momose *et al*, 2001; Naito *et al*, 2007a).

In addition to the above, a number of cellular factors which associate with different components of the RNP complex and are proposed to play a role in its accumulation and/or functionality have been identified. Among them are molecular transport or chaperone proteins such as RanBP5, α-importins, HMGB1, the cytosolic chaperonin containing TCP-1 (CCT) and hsp90 which have all been shown to be required for normal RNP assembly or function; on the other hand, hsp70 and cyclophilin E are restrictive factors that interfere with the integrity of the RNP (Deng *et al*, 2006a; Fislova *et al*, 2010; Hutchinson *et al*, 2011; Li *et al*, 2011; Moisy *et al*, 2012; Naito *et al*, 2007b; Resa-Infante *et al*, 2008; Wang *et al*, 2011). Similarly, RNA-binding or processing factors such as NPM1 and the helicases DDX17 have been shown to promote RNP activity, whereas NF90 has been shown to negatively regulate viral replication and transcription during the early phase of infection by directly interacting with NP (Bortz *et al*, 2011; Mayer *et al*, 2007). USP11 is a cellular deubiquitinase that has been identified to interact with PB2, PA and NP and be responsible for the deubiquitination of NP, thereby restricting viral replication (Liao *et al.*, 2010). It was proposed that influenza A viral genome replication might be regulated by the ubiquitination and deubiquitination of NP. The chromatin remodeller CHD6 (chromodomain-helicase DNA binding protein 6) has also been reported to be involved in the cellular repression of influenza virus replication through interaction with the PA subunit of the polymerase and to be specifically degraded in infected cells (Alfonso *et al.*, 2011, 2013).

It is not always clear whether inhibitory host factors play a regulatory role in the infection or are an aspect of the cellular antiviral response. However, influenza viral infection has been shown to induce expression of the host protein Ebp1 (ErbB3-binding protein 1), which has been shown to bind PB1 and inhibit viral replication (Ejima *et al.*, 2011; Honda *et al.*, 2007). MxA, an interferon-induced dynamin-like GTPase, is another host restriction factor expressed in response to viral infection (Krug *et al.*, 1985). MxA plays a crucial role in preventing *trans*-species transmission by blocking the function of incoming viral RNPs through strain-specific interactions with NP (Haller *et al.*, 2010; Manz *et al.*, 2013).

Acknowledgements

Work carried out in the authors' laboratories was funded by grants BFU2010–17540/BMC (Spanish Ministry of Science), FP7–259751 (European Union) (JO); BFU2011-25090/BMC (Spanish Ministry of Science) (JM-B) and G1100138 (UK Medical Research Council) (FV).

References

Alfonso, R., Lutz, T., Rodriguez, A., Chavez, J.P., Rodriguez, P., Gutierrez, S., and Nieto, A. (2011). CHD6 chromatin remodeler is a negative modulator of influenza virus replication that relocates to inactive chromatin upon infection. Cell Microbiol. *13*, 1894–1906.

Alfonso, R., Rodriguez, A., Rodriguez, P., Lutz, T., and Nieto, A. (2013). CHD6, a cellular repressor of influenza virus replication, is degraded in human alveolar epithelial cells and mice lungs during infection. J. Virol. *87*, 4534–4544.

Amorim, M.J., Bruce, E.A., Read, E.K., Foeglein, A., Mahen, R., Stuart, A.D., and Digard, P. (2011). A Rab11- and microtubule-dependent mechanism for cytoplasmic transport of influenza A virus viral RNA. J. Virol. *85*, 4143–4156.

Area, E., Martín-Benito, J., Gastaminza, P., Torreira, E., Valpuesta, J.M., Carrascosa, J.L., and Ortín, J. (2004). Three-dimensional structure of the influenza virus RNA polymerase: localization of subunit domains. Proc. Natl. Acad. Sci. U.S.A. *101*, 308–313.

Arranz, R., Coloma, R., Chichon, F.J., Conesa, J.J., Carrascosa, J.L., Valpuesta, J.M., Ortin, J., and Martin-Benito, J. (2012). The structure of native influenza virion ribonucleoproteins. Science *338*, 1634–1637.

Avilov, S.V., Moisy, D., Naffakh, N., and Cusack, S. (2012). Influenza A virus progeny vRNP trafficking in live infected cells studied with the virus-encoded fluorescently tagged PB2 protein. Vaccine *30*, 7411–7417.

Bae, S.H., Cheong, H.K., Lee, J.H., Cheong, C., Kainosho, M., and Choi, B.S. (2001). Structural features of an influenza virus promoter and their implications for viral RNA synthesis. Proc. Natl. Acad. Sci. U.S.A. *98*, 10602–10607.

Baigent, S.J., and McCauley, J.W. (2003). Influenza type A in humans, mammals and birds: determinants of virus virulence, host-range and interspecies transmission. Bioessays *25*, 657–671.

Baudin, F., Bach, C., Cusack, S., and Ruigrok, R.W. (1994). Structure of influenza virus RNP. I. Influenza virus nucleoprotein melts secondary structure in panhandle RNA and exposes the bases to the solvent. EMBO J. *13*, 3158–3165.

Baughman, B.M., Jake Slavish, P., DuBois, R.M., Boyd, V.A., White, S.W., and Webb, T.R. (2012). Identification of influenza endonuclease inhibitors using a novel fluorescence polarization assay. ACS Chem. Biol. *7*, 526–534.

Bean, W.J., Jr., and Simpson, R.W. (1973). Primary transcription of the influenza virus genome in permissive cells. Virology *56*, 646–651.

Beaton, A.R., and Krug, R.M. (1986). Transcription antitermination during influenza viral template RNA synthesis requires the nucleocapsid protein and the absence of a 5′ capped end. Proc. Natl. Acad. Sci. U.S.A. *83*, 6282–6286.

Biswas, S.K., and Nayak, D.P. (1994). Mutational analysis of the conserved motifs of influenza A virus polymerase basic protein 1. J. Virol. *68*, 1819–1826.

Boulo, S., Akarsu, H., Ruigrok, R.W., and Baudin, F. (2007). Nuclear traffic of influenza virus proteins and ribonucleoprotein complexes. Virus Res. *124*, 12–21.

Bouloy, M., Plotch, S.J., and Krug, R.M. (1978). Globin mRNAs are primers for the transcription of influenza viral RNA in vitro. Proc. Natl. Acad. Sci. U.S.A. *75*, 4886–4890.

Chou, Y.Y., Heaton, N.S., Gao, Q., Palese, P., Singer, R., and Lionnet, T. (2013). Colocalization of different influenza viral RNA segments in the cytoplasm before viral budding as shown by single-molecule sensitivity FISH analysis. PLoS Pathog. *9*, e1003358.

Coloma, R., Valpuesta, J.M., Arranz, R., Carrascosa, J.L., Ortin, J., and Martin-Benito, J. (2009). The structure of a biologically active influenza virus ribonucleoprotein complex. PLoS Pathog. *5*, e1000491.

Compans, R.W., Content, J., and Duesberg, P.H. (1972). Structure of the ribonucleoprotein of influenza virus. J. Virol. *4*, 795–800.

de Vries, E., Tscherne, D.M., Wienholts, M.J., Cobos-Jimenez, V., Scholte, F., Garcia-Sastre, A., Rottier, P.J., and de Haan, C.A. (2011). Dissection of the influenza A virus endocytic routes reveals macropinocytosis as an alternative entry pathway. PLoS Pathog. *7*, e1001329.

Deng, T., Vreede, F.T., and Brownlee, G.G. (2006). Different de novo initiation strategies are used by influenza virus RNA polymerase on its cRNA and viral RNA promoters during viral RNA replication. J. Virol. *80*, 2337–2348.

Desselberger, U., Raccaniello, V.R., Zazra, J.J., and Palese, P. (1980). The 3′ and 5′-end terminal sequences of influenza A, B and C virus RNA segments are highly conserved and show partial inverted complementarity. Gene *8*, 315–328.

Detjen, B.M., St Angelo, C., Katze, M.G., and Krug, R.M. (1987). The three influenza virus polymerase (P) proteins not associated with viral nucleocapsids in the infected cell are in the form of a complex. J. Virol. *61*, 16–22.

Digard, P., Blok, V.C., and Inglis, S.C. (1989). Complex formation between influenza virus polymerase proteins expressed in Xenopus oocytes. Virology *171*, 162–169.

DuBois, R.M., Slavish, P.J., Baughman, B.M., Yun, M.K., Bao, J., Webby, R.J., Webb, T.R., and White, S.W. (2012). Structural and biochemical basis for development of influenza virus inhibitors targeting the PA endonuclease. PLoS Pathog. *8*, e1002830.

Eisfeld, A.J., Kawakami, E., Watanabe, T., Neumann, G., and Kawaoka, Y. (2011). RAB11A is essential for transport of the influenza virus genome to the plasma membrane. J. Virol. *85*, 6117–6126.

Ejima, M., Kadoi, K., and Honda, A. (2011). Influenza virus infection induces cellular Ebp1 gene expression. Genes Cells *16*, 927–937.

Elton, D., Digard, P., Tiley, L., and Ortín, J. (2005). Structure and function of the influenza virus RNP. In Current Topics in Influenza Virology, Kawaoka, Y. ed. (Norfolk, Horizon Scientific Press), pp. 1–92.

Elton, D., Simpson, H.M., Archer, K., Medcalf, L., Hallam, R., McCauley, J., and Digard, P. (2001). Interaction of the influenza virus nucleoprotein with the cellular CRM1-mediated nuclear export pathway. J. Virol. *75*, 408–419.
Engelhardt, O.G., Smith, M., and Fodor, E. (2005). Association of the influenza A virus RNA-dependent RNA polymerase with cellular RNA polymerase II. J. Virol. *79*, 5812–5818.
Fechter, P., and Brownlee, G.G. (2005). Recognition of mRNA cap structures by viral and cellular proteins. J. Gen. Virol. *86*, 1239–1249.
Fechter, P., Mingay, L., Sharps, J., Chambers, A., Fodor, E., and Brownlee, G.G. (2003). Two aromatic residues in the PB2 subunit of influenza A RNA polymerase are crucial for cap binding. J. Biol. Chem. *278*, 20381–20388.
Flick, R., Neumann, G., Hoffmann, E., Neumeier, E., and Hobom, G. (1996). Promoter elements in the influenza vRNA terminal structure. RNA *2*, 1046–1057.
Fodor, E. (2013). The RNA polymerase of influenza a virus: mechanisms of viral transcription and replication. Acta Virol. *57*, 113–122.
Gastaminza, P., Perales, B., Falcón, A.M., and Ortín, J. (2003). Influenza virus mutants in the N-terminal region of PB2 protein are affected in virus RNA replication but not transcription. J. Virol. *76*, 5098–5108.
Gerritz, S.W., Cianci, C., Kim, S., Pearce, B.C., Deminie, C., Discotto, L., McAuliffe, B., Minassian, B.F., Shi, S., Zhu, S., *et al.* (2011). Inhibition of influenza virus replication via small molecules that induce the formation of higher-order nucleoprotein oligomers. Proc. Natl. Acad. Sci. U.S.A. *108*, 15366–15371.
González, S., and Ortín, J. (1999a). Characterization of the influenza virus PB1 protein binding to vRNA: Two separate regions of the protein contribute to the interaction domain. J. Virol. *73*, 631–637.
González, S., and Ortín, J. (1999b). Distinct regions of influenza virus PB1 polymerase subunit recognize vRNA and cRNA templates. EMBO J. *18*, 3767–3775.
Guilligay, D., Tarendeau, F., Resa-Infante, P., Coloma, R., Crepin, T., Sehr, P., Lewis, J., Ruigrok, R.W., Ortin, J., Hart, D.J., *et al.* (2008). The structural basis for cap binding by influenza virus polymerase subunit PB2. Nat. Struct. Mol. Biol. *15*, 500–506.
Guu, T.S., Dong, L., Wittung-Stafshede, P., and Tao, Y.J. (2008). Mapping the domain structure of the influenza A virus polymerase acidic protein (PA) and its interaction with the basic protein 1 (PB1) subunit. Virology *379*, 135–142.
Haller, O., Gao, S., von der Malsburg, A., Daumke, O., and Kochs, G. (2010). Dynamin-like MxA GTPase: structural insights into oligomerization and implications for antiviral activity. J. Biol. Chem. *285*, 28419–28424.
Hara, K., Shiota, M., Kido, H., Ohtsu, Y., Kashiwagi, T., Iwahashi, J., Hamada, N., Mizoue, K., Tsumura, N., Kato, H., *et al.* (2001). Influenza virus RNA polymerase PA subunit is a novel serine protease with Ser624 at the active site. Genes Cells *6*, 87–97.
Hay, A.J., Lomniczi, B., Bellamy, A.R., and Skehel, J.J. (1977). Transcription of the influenza virus genome. Virology *83*, 337–355.
Hay, A.J., Skehel, J.J., and McCauley, J. (1980). Structure and synthesis of influenza virus complementary RNAs. Philos. Trans. R. Soc. Lond. *288*, 341–348.
He, X., Zhou, J., Bartlam, M., Zhang, R., Ma, J., Lou, Z., Li, X., Li, J., Joachimiak, A., Zeng, Z., *et al.* (2008). Crystal structure of the polymerase PA(C)-PB1(N) complex from an avian influenza H5N1 virus. Nature *454*, 1123–1126.
Herz, C., Stavnezer, E., Krug, R.M., and Gurney, T. (1981). Influenza virus, an RNA virus, synthesizes its messenger RNA in the nucleus of infected cells. Cell *26*, 391–400.
Honda, A., Mizumoto, K., and Ishihama, A. (1999). Two separate sequences of PB2 subunit constitute the RNA cap-binding site of influenza virus RNA polymerase. Genes Cells *4*, 475–485.
Honda, A., Okamoto, T., and Ishihama, A. (2007). Host factor Ebp1: selective inhibitor of influenza virus transcriptase. Genes Cells *12*, 133–142.
Horimoto, T., and Kawaoka, Y. (2005). Influenza: lessons from past pandemics, warnings from current incidents. Nat. Rev. Microbiol. 3, 591–600.
Hsu, M.T., Parvin, J.D., Gupta, S., Krystal, M., and Palese, P. (1987). Genomic RNAs of influenza viruses are held in a circular conformation in virions and in infected cells by a terminal panhandle. Proc. Natl. Acad. Sci. U.S.A. *84*, 8140–8144.
Huang, T.S., Palese, P., and Krystal, M. (1990). Determination of influenza virus proteins required for genome replication. J. Virol. *64*, 5669–5673.
Huarte, M., Sanz-Ezquerro, J.J., Roncal, F., Ortin, J., and Nieto, A. (2001). PA subunit from influenza virus polymerase complex interacts with a cellular protein with homology to a family of transcriptional activators. J. Virol. *75*, 8597–8604.

Jorba, N., Coloma, R., and Ortin, J. (2009). Genetic trans-complementation establishes a new model for influenza virus RNA transcription and replication. PLoS Pathog. *5*, e1000462.

Kawaguchi, A., and Nagata, K. (2007). De novo replication of the influenza virus RNA genome is regulated by DNA replicative helicase, MCM. EMBO J. *26*, 4566–4575.

Klumpp, K., Ruigrok, R.W., and Baudin, F. (1997). Roles of the influenza virus polymerase and nucleoprotein in forming a functional RNP structure. EMBO J. *16*, 1248–1257.

Kowalinski, E., Zubieta, C., Wolkerstorfer, A., Szolar, O.H., Ruigrok, R.W., and Cusack, S. (2012). Structural analysis of specific metal chelating inhibitor binding to the endonuclease domain of influenza pH1N1 (2009). polymerase. PLoS Pathog. *8*, e1002831.

Krug, R.M., Shaw, M., Broni, B., Shapiro, G., and Haller, O. (1985). Inhibition of influenza viral mRNA synthesis in cells expressing the interferon-induced Mx gene product. J. Virol. *56*, 201–206.

Lamb, R.A., and Choppin, P.W. (1977). Synthesis of influenza virus polypeptides in cells resistant to alpha-amanitin: evidence for the involvement of cellular RNA polymerase II in virus replication. J. Virol. *23*, 816–819.

Landeras-Bueno, S., Jorba, N., Pérez-Cidoncha, M., and Ortín, J. (2011). The splicing factor proline-glutamine rich (SFPQ/PSF) is involved in influenza virus transcription. PLoS Pathog. *7*, e1002397.

Leahy, M.B., Dobbyn, H.C., and Brownlee, G.G. (2001a). Hairpin loop structure in the 3′ arm of the influenza A virus virion RNA promoter is required for endonuclease activity. J. Virol. *75*, 7042–7049.

Leahy, M.B., Pritlove, D.C., Poon, L.L., and Brownlee, G.G. (2001b). Mutagenic analysis of the 5′ arm of the influenza A virus virion RNA promoter defines the sequence requirements for endonuclease activity. J. Virol. *75*, 134–142.

Li, M.L., Rao, P., and Krug, R.M. (2001). The active sites of the influenza cap-dependent endonuclease are on different polymerase subunits. EMBO J. *20*, 2078–2086.

Liao, T.L., Wu, C.Y., Su, W.C., Jeng, K.S., and Lai, M.M. (2010). Ubiquitination and deubiquitination of NP protein regulates influenza A virus RNA replication. EMBO J. *29*, 3879–3890.

Maier, H.J., Kashiwagi, T., Hara, K., and Brownlee, G.G. (2008). Differential role of the influenza A virus polymerase PA subunit for vRNA and cRNA promoter binding. Virology *370*, 194–204.

Manz, B., Brunotte, L., Reuther, P., and Schwemmle, M. (2012). Adaptive mutations in NEP compensate for defective H5N1 RNA replication in cultured human cells. Nat. Commun. *3*, 802.

Manz, B., Dornfeld, D., Gotz, V., Zell, R., Zimmermann, P., Haller, O., Kochs, G., and Schwemmle, M. (2013). Pandemic influenza A viruses escape from restriction by human MxA through adaptive mutations in the nucleoprotein. PLoS Pathog. *9*, e1003279.

Mark, G.E., Taylor, J.M., Broni, B., and Krug, R.M. (1979). Nuclear accumulation of influenza viral RNA transcripts and the effects of cycloheximide, actinomycin D, and alpha-amanitin. J. Virol. *29*, 744–752.

Martín-Benito, J., Area, E., Ortega, J., Llorca, O., Valpuesta, J.M., Carrascosa, J.L., and Ortín, J. (2001). Three dimensional reconstruction of a recombinant influenza virus ribonucleoprotein particle. EMBO Rep. *2*, 313–317.

Martin-Benito, J., and Ortin, J. (2013). Influenza virus transcription and replication. Adv. Virus Res. *87*, 113–137.

Mena, I., Jambrina, E., Albo, C., Perales, B., Ortin, J., Arrese, M., Vallejo, D., and Portela, A. (1999). Mutational analysis of influenza A virus nucleoprotein: identification of mutations that affect RNA replication. J. Virol. *73*, 1186–1194.

Moeller, A., Kirchdoerfer, R.N., Potter, C.S., Carragher, B., and Wilson, I.A. (2012). Organization of the influenza virus replication machinery. Science *338*, 1631–1634.

Neumann, G., Brownlee, G.G., Fodor, E., and Kawaoka, Y. (2004). Orthomyxovirus replication, transcription, and polyadenylation. Curr. Top. Microbiol. Immunol. *283*, 121–143.

Neumann, G., Castrucci, M.R., and Kawaoka, Y. (1997). Nuclear import and export of influenza virus nucleoprotein. J. Virol. *71*, 9690–9700.

Neumann, G., and Kawaoka, Y. (2011). The first influenza pandemic of the new millennium. Influenza Other Respir. Viruses *5*, 157–166.

Newcomb, L.L., Kuo, R.L., Ye, Q., Jiang, Y., Tao, Y.J., and Krug, R.M. (2009). Interaction of the influenza a virus nucleocapsid protein with the viral RNA polymerase potentiates unprimed viral RNA replication. J. Virol. *83*, 29–36.

Ng, A.K., Lam, M.K., Zhang, H., Liu, J., Au, S.W., Chan, P.K., Wang, J., and Shaw, P.C. (2012). Structural basis for RNA binding and homo-oligomer formation by influenza B virus nucleoprotein. J. Virol. *86*, 6758–6767.

Noble, E., Mathews, D.H., Chen, J.L., Turner, D.H., Takimoto, T., and Kim, B. (2011). Biophysical analysis of influenza A virus RNA promoter at physiological temperatures. J. Biol. Chem. *286*, 22965–22970.

Noda, T., and Kawaoka, Y. (2010). Structure of influenza virus ribonucleoprotein complexes and their packaging into virions. Rev. Med. Virol. *20*, 380–391.

Noton, S.L., Medcalf, E., Fisher, D., Mullin, A.E., Elton, D., and Digard, P. (2007). Identification of the domains of the influenza A virus M1 matrix protein required for NP binding, oligomerization and incorporation into virions. J. Gen. Virol. *88*, 2280–2290.

Ortega, J., Martín-Benito, J., Zürcher, T., Valpuesta, J.M., Carrascosa, J.L., and Ortín, J. (2000). Ultrastructural and functional analyses of recombinant influenza virus ribonucleoproteins suggest dimerization of nucleoprotein during virus amplification. J. Virol. *74*, 156–163.

Perales, B., Sanz-Ezquerro, J.J., Gastaminza, P., Ortega, J., Fernández-Santarén, J., Ortín, J., and Nieto, A. (2000). The replication activity of influenza virus polymerase is linked to the capacity of the PA subunit to induce proteolysis. J. Virol. *74*, 1307–1312.

Perez, J.T., Zlatev, I., Aggarwal, S., Subramanian, S., Sachidanandam, R., Kim, B., Manoharan, M., and Tenoever, B.R. (2012). A small-RNA enhancer of viral polymerase activity. J. Virol. *86*, 13475–13485.

Perez-Gonzalez, A., Rodriguez, A., Huarte, M., Salanueva, I.J., and Nieto, A. (2006). hCLE/CGI-99, a human protein that interacts with the influenza virus polymerase, is a mRNA transcription modulator. J. Mol. Biol. *362*, 887–900.

Pinto, L.H., and Lamb, R.A. (2006). The M2 proton channels of influenza A and B viruses. J. Biol. Chem. *281*, 8997–9000.

Pons, M.W. (1973). The inhibition of influenza virus RNA synthesis by actinomycin D and cycloheximide. Virology *51*, 120–128.

Portela, A., and Digard, P. (2002). The influenza virus nucleoprotein: a multifunctional RNA-binding protein pivotal to virus replication. J. Gen. Virol. *83*, 723–734.

Pritlove, D.C., Poon, L.L.M., Devenish, L.J., Leahy, M.B., and Brownlee, G.G. (1999). A hairpin loop at the 5′ end of influenza A virus virion RNA is required for synthesis of poly(A)+ mRNA in vitro. J. Virol. *73*, 2109–2114.

Regan, J.F., Liang, Y., and Parslow, T.G. (2006). Defective assembly of influenza A virus due to a mutation in the polymerase subunit PA. J. Virol. *80*, 252–261.

Resa-Infante, P., Jorba, N., Coloma, R., and Ortín, J. (2011). The influenza virus RNA synthesis machine: Advances in its structure and function. RNA Biol. *8*, 1–9.

Resa-Infante, P., Recuero-Checa, M.A., Zamarreño, N., Llorca, O., and Ortín, J. (2010). Structural and functional characterization of an influenza virus RNA polymerase-genomic RNA complex. J. Virol. *84*, 10477–10487.

Robb, N.C., Smith, M., Vreede, F.T., and Fodor, E. (2009). NS2/NEP protein regulates transcription and replication of the influenza virus RNA genome. J. Gen. Virol. *90*, 1398–1407.

Robertson, J.S. (1979). 5′ and 3′ terminal nucleotide sequences of the RNA genome segments of influenza virus. Nucleic Acid Res. *6*, 3745–3757.

Rodriguez, A., Perez-Gonzalez, A., and Nieto, A. (2007). Influenza virus infection causes the specific degradation of the largest subunit of cellular RNA polymerase II. J. Virol. *81*, 5315–5324.

Rodriguez, A., Perez-Gonzalez, A., and Nieto, A. (2011). Cellular human CLE/C14orf166 protein interacts with influenza virus polymerase and is required for viral replication. J. Virol. *85*, 12062–12066.

Rossman, J.S., and Lamb, R.A. (2011). Influenza virus assembly and budding. Virology *411*, 229–236.

Rossman, J.S., Leser, G.P., and Lamb, R.A. (2012). Filamentous influenza virus enters cells via macropinocytosis. J. Virol. *86*, 10950–10960.

Rott, R., and Scholtissek, C. (1970). Specific inhibition of influenza replication by alpha-amanitin. Nature *228*, 56.

Ruigrok, R.W., and Baudin, F. (1995). Structure of influenza virus ribonucleoprotein particles. II. Purified RNA-free influenza virus ribonucleoprotein forms structures that are indistinguishable from the intact influenza virus ribonucleoprotein particles. J. Gen. Virol. *76*, 1009–1014.

Sanz-Ezquerro, J.J., Zürcher, T., de la Luna, S., Ortin, J., and Nieto, A. (1996). The amino-terminal one-third of the influenza virus PA protein is responsible for the induction of proteolysis. J. Virol. *70*, 1905–1911.

Shapiro, G.I., Gurney, T.J., and Krug, R.M. (1987). Influenza virus gene expression: control mechanisms at early and late times of infection and nuclear-cytoplasmic transport of virus-specific RNAs. J. Virol. *61*, 764–773.

Shapiro, G.I., and Krug, R.M. (1988). Influenza virus RNA replication in vitro: synthesis of viral template RNAs and virion RNAs in the absence of an added primer. J. Virol. *62*, 2285–2290.

Shaw, M., and Palese, P. (2013). Orthomyxoviridae. In Fields Virology, 6th edn, Knipe, D.M., and Howley, P. eds. (Philadelphia, Lippincott, Williams and Wilkins), pp. 1151–1185.
Skehel, J.J., and Wiley, D.C. (2000). Receptor binding and membrane fusion in virus entry: the influenza hemagglutinin. Annu. Rev. Biochem. *69*, 531–569.
Subbarao, E.K., London, W., and Murphy, B.R. (1993). A single amino acid in the PB2 gene of influenza A virus is a determinant of host range. J. Virol. *67*, 1761–1764.
Sugiyama, K., Obayashi, E., Kawaguchi, A., Suzuki, Y., Tame, J.R., Nagata, K., and Park, S.Y. (2009). Structural insight into the essential PB1-PB2 subunit contact of the influenza virus RNA polymerase. EMBO J. *28*, 1803–1811.
Tarendeau, F., Boudet, J., Guilligay, D., Mas, P.J., Bougault, C.M., Boulo, S., Baudin, F., Ruigrok, R.W., Daigle, N., Ellenberg, J., *et al.* (2007). Structure and nuclear import function of the C-terminal domain of influenza virus polymerase PB2 subunit. Nat. Struct. Mol. Biol. *14*, 229–233.
Tarendeau, F., Crepin, T., Guilligay, D., Ruigrok, R.W., Cusack, S., and Hart, D.J. (2008). Host determinant residue lysine 627 lies on the surface of a discrete, folded domain of influenza virus polymerase PB2 subunit. PLoS Pathog. *4*, e1000136.
Taubenberger, J.K., Reid, A.H., Janczewski, T.A., and Fanning, T.G. (2001). Integrating historical, clinical and molecular genetic data in order to explain the origin and virulence of the 1918 Spanish influenza virus. Philos. Trans. R. Soc. Lond. *356*, 1829–1839.
Tiley, L.S., Hagen, M., Mathews, J.T., and Krystal, M. (1994). Sequence-specific binding of the influenza virus RNA polymerase to sequences located at the 5′-end of the viral RNAs. J. Virol. *68*, 5108–5116.
Torreira, E., Schoehn, G., Fernandez, Y., Jorba, N., Ruigrok, R.W., Cusack, S., Ortin, J., and Llorca, O. (2007). Three-dimensional model for the isolated recombinant influenza virus polymerase heterotrimer. Nucleic Acids Res. *35*, 3774–3783.
Turrell, L., Lyall, J.W., Tiley, L.S., Fodor, E., and Vreede, F.T. (2013). The role and assembly mechanism of nucleoprotein in influenza A virus ribonucleoprotein complexes. Nat. Commun. *4*, 1591.
Vreede, F.T., and Brownlee, G.G. (2007). Influenza virion-derived viral ribonucleoproteins synthesize both mRNA and cRNA in vitro. J. Virol. *81*, 2196–2204.
Vreede, F.T., and Fodor, E. (2010). The role of the influenza virus RNA polymerase in host shut-off. Virulence *1*, 436–439.
Vreede, F.T., Jung, T.E., and Brownlee, G.G. (2004). Model suggesting that replication of influenza virus is regulated by stabilization of replicative intermediates. J. Virol. *78*, 9568–9572.
Wang, P., Palese, P., and O'Neill, R.E. (1997). The NPI-1/NPI-3 (karyopherin alpha) binding site on the influenza a virus nucleoprotein NP is a nonconventional nuclear localization signal. J. Virol. *71*, 1850–1856.
Watanabe, T., and Kawaoka, Y. (2011). Pathogenesis of the 1918 pandemic influenza virus. PLoS Pathog. *7*, e1001218.
Watanabe, T., Watanabe, S., and Kawaoka, Y. (2010). Cellular networks involved in the influenza virus life cycle. Cell Host Microbe 7, 427–439.
Ye, Q., Krug, R.M., and Tao, Y.J. (2006). The mechanism by which influenza A virus nucleoprotein forms oligomers and binds RNA. Nature *444*, 1078–1082.
York, A., Hengrung, N., Vreede, F.T., Huiskonen, J.T., and Fodor, E. (2013). Isolation and characterization of the positive-sense replicative intermediate of a negative-strand RNA virus. Proc. Natl. Acad. Sci. U.S.A. *110*, E4238–4245.
Yu, M., Liu, X., Cao, S., Zhao, Z., Zhang, K., Xie, Q., Chen, C., Gao, S., Bi, Y., Sun, L., *et al.* (2012). Identification and characterization of three novel nuclear export signals in the influenza A virus nucleoprotein. J. Virol. *86*, 4970–4980.
Zhang, J., Li, G., and Ye, X. (2010). Cyclin T1/CDK9 interacts with influenza A virus polymerase and facilitates its association with cellular RNA polymerase II. J. Virol. *84*, 12619–12627.
Zheng, W., and Tao, Y.J. (2013). Structure and assembly of the influenza A virus ribonucleoprotein complex. FEBS Lett. *587*, 1206–1214.

Recent Progress in Understanding Influenza B Virus Haemagglutinin

3

Fengyun Ni and Qinghua Wang

Abstract

This chapter focuses on recent progress in understanding influenza B virus haemagglutinin (HA) in three aspects: the roles of Phe-95 in receptor binding and host tropism, the structural basis of the divergent evolution, and the membrane fusion mechanisms as compared to influenza A virus HAs.

Introduction

Influenza A and B viruses remain a major cause of human morbidity and mortality in seasonal flu epidemics. Influenza B virus has two co-circulating lineages, Yamagata lineage and Victoria lineage, which diverged from each other in early 1970 (Chen *et al.*, 2007; Shen *et al.*, 2009). Different from influenza A virus, influenza B virus has a very limited host range, circulating almost exclusively among humans and seals (Osterhaus *et al.*, 2000). In addition, influenza B viruses were found to have overall lower receptor-binding affinities than influenza A viruses (Matrosovich *et al.*, 1993). Our group has made significant progress in understanding influenza B virus HA in three aspects: the roles of Phe-95 in receptor binding and host tropism (Ni *et al.*, 2014b), the structural basis of the divergent evolution of the two lineages (Ni *et al.*, 2013), and the membrane-fusion mechanisms as compared to influenza A virus HAs (Ni *et al.*, 2014a), which will be the main focus of this chapter.

The roles of Phe-95 in receptor binding and host tropism

In marked contrast to influenza A/H1~H15 HAs, which have Tyr-98 at the base of the receptor-binding site, influenza B virus HA has Phe-95 instead (based on the numbering of influenza B/Hong Kong/8/73 (B/HK/73) HA) (Wang *et al.*, 2007, 2008, 2010). This is similar to the Phe-98 residue observed in influenza A/H16~H17 HA proteins (Fouchier *et al.*, 2005; Sun *et al.*, 2013; Tong *et al.*, 2012; Zhu *et al.*, 2013). When Tyr-98 is present, the hydroxyl group on its side chain makes one hydrogen bond with His-183 to stabilize the base of the receptor-binding site and two additional hydrogen bonds with the Sia-1 moiety of the bound receptors (Weis *et al.*, 1988). The absence of the hydroxyl group on the side chain of Phe-95 in influenza B virus HA results in the loss of all three hydrogen bonds (Wang *et al.*, 2007), and is probably responsible for the low binding affinity of influenza B virus (Matrosovich *et al.*, 1993). Since the glycosylation site at Asn194 on the 190-helix that forms the upper edge of the receptor-binding site is frequently lost in egg-adapted variants and sporadic field isolates, we tested the mutation Phe95→Tyr on influenza B virus HA with a glycosylation at 194 (wild type) or without (Asn194→Asp). Our study showed that the Phe95→Tyr mutation restored all three hydrogen bonds and enhanced the receptor-binding affinity to a similar level as influenza A virus HAs (Ni *et al.*, 2014b). However, the stronger receptor-binding affinity of the Phe95→Tyr mutant did not bestow a higher viral replication rate in mice, suggesting that a delicate balance between HA and NA activities is a key for virus fitness.

The Phe95→Tyr mutation enhanced receptor-binding affinity of influenza B/Yamagata/73 and B/Lee/40 HAs

In dose-dependent glycan binding assays using an avian-like Neu5Acα(2,3)Gal receptor analogue (3′SLN-LN) and a human-like Neu5Acα(2,6)Gal receptor analogue (6′SLN-LN), the wild-type and Phe95→Tyr B/Yamagata/73 HA had an apparent dissociation constants of 5.8×10^{-3} M and 3.5×10^{-6} M for the 3′SLN-LN, 2.3×10^{-4} M and 1.6×10^{-11} M for the 6′SLN-LN, respectively. Thus, the mutation Phe95→Tyr resulted in an almost 10^7 higher binding affinity for 6′SLN-LN (Table 3.1).

The apparent dissociation constants for the mutation Asn194→Asp were 4.5×10^{-12} M for 3′SLN-LN and 7.5×10^{-5} M for 6′SLN-LN. The ~10^9 times higher affinity of the Asn194→Asp mutant for 3′SLN-LN than the wild-type HA helped explain why, in order to adapt to the Neu5Acα(2,3)Gal-enriched environment in eggs, it is advantageous to lose the glycosylation at HA_1 194–196, which is frequently observed in egg-adapted variants.

Similar to the single mutant Phe95→Tyr, the double mutant Phe95→Tyr/Asn194→Asp improved the binding for 6′SLN-LN receptors by about 10^7 times compared with Asn194→Asp (Table 3.1). Clearly, regardless of whether or not there is a glycosylation at HA_1 194, the mutation Phe95→Tyr consistently significantly enhanced the binding of HA for 6′SLN-LN receptors. In contrast, while the loss of the glycosylation at HA_1 194

Table 3.1 Equilibrium dissociation constants of recombinant wild-type influenza B virus HA proteins and their mutants in binding to Neu5Acα(2,3)Gal and Neu5Acα(2,6)Gal receptor analogues

	3′SLN-LN*		6′SLN-LN*	
HA	K_d'	R^2	K_d'	R^2
B/Yamagata/73				
Wild type	$5.8 \pm 4.7 \times 10^{-3}$ M	0.97 ± 0.01	$2.3 \pm 0.2 \times 10^{-4}$ M	0.97 ± 0.01
Phe95→Tyr	$3.5 \pm 3.1 \times 10^{-6}$ M	0.991 ± 0.006	$1.6 \pm 1.0 \times 10^{-11}$ M	0.995 ± 0.001
Asn194→Asp	$4.5 \pm 1.7 \times 10^{-12}$ M	0.997 ± 0.001	$7.5 \pm 1.1 \times 10^{-5}$ M	0.987 ± 0.001
Phe95→Tyr/Asn194→Asp	$1.1 \pm 0.1 \times 10^{-11}$ M	0.994 ± 0.001	$3.3 \pm 1.8 \times 10^{-12}$ M	0.971 ± 0.002
B/Lee/40				
Asn194→Asp	$8.7 \pm 5.5 \times 10^{-11}$ M	0.98 ± 0.01	$4.74 \pm 0.01 \times 10^{-6}$ M	0.978 ± 0.001
Phe95→Tyr/Asn194→Asp	$2.4 \pm 1.7 \times 10^{-8}$ M	0.989 ± 0.006	$2.4 \pm 0.4 \times 10^{-9}$ M	0.99 ± 0.01

*The apparent dissociation constant (K_d') and the *R*-square (R^2) were obtained by fitting the data to the linearized Hill equation in order to quantitatively determine the relative binding affinities of HA and its mutants. Their absolute values should be compared only in this context.

increased the affinity for 3′SLN-LN by 10^9 times (comparing Asn194→Asp and wild type), no further increase was observed for Phe95→Tyr/Asn194→Asp. Thus, in the double mutant Phe95→Tyr/Asn194→Asp, the enhanced binding for 3′SLN-LN is likely from Asn194→Asp, while the tighter binding for 6′SLN-LN is from Phe95→Tyr.

Similarly, the Asn194→Asp mutation in B/Lee/40 HA resulted ~10^5 times stronger binding for 3′SLN-LN than for 6′SLN-LN. However, the introduction of Phe95→Tyr into B/Lee/40 HA containing the Asn194→Asp mutation enhanced the binding affinity for 6′SLN-LN by ~2000 times, but at the same time decreased the binding for 3′SLN-LN by ~300-fold (Table 3.1).

The B/Yamagata/73 HA Phe95→Tyr mutant competitively blocks the binding and infection of influenza A virus

While the Phe95→Tyr mutation significantly enhanced the binding affinity of influenza B virus HA to a level that is comparable to those of influenza A virus (dissociation constants at picomolar range) (Jayaraman *et al.*, 2011; Pappas *et al.*, 2010; Srinivasan *et al.*, 2008; Viswanathan *et al.*, 2010), can they efficiently compete against the binding and infection by influenza A virus? With 400 μg recombinant influenza B/Yamagata/73 HA protein, the wild-type HA had about 2-fold inhibition against human influenza A/H3N2 virus, and the Phe95→Tyr mutant displayed 8-fold inhibition. Most strikingly, while the Asn194→Asp single mutant exhibited very weak inhibition against influenza A/H3N2 virus, the mutant Phe95→Tyr/Asn194→Asp completely blocked the infection of influenza A virus with 400 μg, 200 μg or even as low as 100 μg recombinant protein. Clearly, the higher binding affinity of the Phe95→Tyr and Phe95→Tyr/Asn194→Asp mutants for sialic acid receptors endorsed a much stronger competition against influenza A/H3N2 virus infection.

Agglutination of erythrocytes by recombinant B/Lee/40 viruses

Consistent with the high binding affinity of the recombinant Asn194→Asp HA protein for 3′SLN-LN receptors, the recombinant/Lee/40 virus containing Asn194→Asp virus bound more strongly for chicken, turkey and guinea pig erythrocytes (containing mixed Neu5Acα(2,3)Gal and Neu5Acα(2,6)Gal receptors) than for sheep, horse and bovine erythrocytes (containing predominantly Neu5Aca(2,6)Gal receptors) (Ito *et al.*, 1997a; Medeiros *et al.*, 2001; Takemae *et al.*, 2010). Its binding to horse erythrocytes was particularly poor, consistent with the 100% Neu5Gc sialic acids on horse erythrocytes (Suzuki *et al.*, 1985) that can not be recognized by the Asn194→Asp protein on B/Yamagata/73 HA (Ni *et al.*, 2014b). In marked contrast, the Phe95→Tyr/Asn194→Asp virus bound at a higher titre to sheep, horse and bovine erythrocytes, agreeing with the stronger binding of the Phe95→Tyr/Asn194→Asp HA protein for Neu5Acα(2,6)Gal receptors (for sheep and bovine erythrocytes) and for Neu5Gc-containing sialic acids (for horse erythrocytes). In addition, incubating the virus–erythrocyte mixtures at 37°C for 2 hours to allow the cleavage of sialic acids by viral NA protein released the majority of Asn194→Asp virus but not the Phe95→Tyr/Asn194→Asp virus. Only after overnight incubation at 37°C, was the Phe95→Tyr/Asn194→Asp virus eluted from most erythrocytes but remained bound to guinea pig and horse erythrocytes at a significant level. These data suggest a potential activity mismatch between the native NA and the Phe95→Tyr/Asn194→Asp HA mutant, thus a longer incubation time is needed.

Replication of recombinant B/Lee/40 viruses in MDCK cells and mice

In marked contrast to the stronger binding affinity for sialic acid receptors, the virus harbouring the Phe95→Tyr/Asn194→Asp mutant replicated to a similar titre as the Asn194→Asp virus in MDCK cell line that is known to contain both Neu5Acα(2,3)Gal and Neu5Acα(2,6)Gal receptors (Govorkova *et al.*, 1996; Ito *et al.*, 1997b). Most strikingly, in viral replication study in mice, the Phe95→Tyr/Asn194→Asp virus had an average titre of 2.2×10^2 pfu/ml, much lower than the average titre of 2.7×10^5 pfu/ml for the Asn194→Asp virus. This ~1000-fold attenuation is likely the results of two facts: (a) the ~300 times lower binding affinity of the Phe95→Tyr/Asn194→Asp protein, compared with Asn194→Asp, for Neu5Acα(2,3)Gal receptors (Ni *et al.*, 2014b) that are almost exclusively found in mouse airway epithelial cells (Tang and Chong, 2009); and (b) the potential mismatch between the augmented HA binding affinity and the relatively low activity of the native NA that may hinder the timely release and re-infection by the Phe95→Tyr/Asn194→Asp virus.

Structural basis for the effects of Phe95→Tyr on binding to receptors

The crystal structures of B/Lee/40 HA containing Phe95→Tyr/Asn194→Asp and its complexes with human-like LSTc and avian-like LSTa receptor analogues provided a structural basis for the effects of the Phe95→Tyr mutation on binding to receptors. As expected, the extra hydroxyl group of the introduced Tyr-95 mediated an extra hydrogen bond with His-191, one of the three key residues constituting the base of the receptor-binding site of influenza B virus HA (Ni *et al.*, 2014b). Furthermore, two additional hydrogen bonds between the Sia-1 moiety and the hydroxyl group of Tyr-95 strengthened the interaction with the bound receptor analogues, LSTc and LSTa. Thus, the mutation Phe95→Tyr restored all three hydrogen bonds that the hydroxyl group of Tyr-98 makes in influenza A/H3 HA (Weis *et al.*, 1988).

Different from the higher position of the Sia-1 moiety in the receptor-binding site of B/Yamanashi/98 HA (containing Phe-95), Tyr-95 pulled the Sia-1 moiety deeper into the receptor-binding site with a rotation of ~18°. This lower sitting position of Sia-1 in Phe95→Tyr resulted in a closer spatial location of the terminal sugar rings of LSTa with the glycosylation at HA_1 230 that is unique to B/Lee/40 HA. This closer proximity may be responsible for the reduced binding affinity for 3′SLN-LN when Phe95→Tyr was introduced into the B/Lee/40 HA Asn194→Asp background.

The roles of receptor binding of HA in influenza B virus pathogenicity

Luckily for us, the lack of major reservoirs for influenza B virus outside the human population is believed to be one of the main reasons that influenza B virus does not cause human pandemics as influenza A virus (Gamblin and Skehel, 2010; Skehel and Wiley, 2000; Steinhauer, 2010; Wang, 2010; Wiley and Skehel, 1987). However, it remained an enigma whether there exists a correlation between the limited host range and the lower receptor binding affinity of HA of naturally occurring influenza B virus. A recent study by Palese and co-workers suggested that this is indeed possible: when influenza B virus HA was replaced with an influenza A/H1 HA in the background of influenza B virus, the chimeric influenza B virus resulted in significant weight loss in infected mice (Hai *et al.*, 2011). Thus it is striking that the single Phe95→Tyr mutation at the receptor-binding site was able to promote the binding affinity of influenza B/Yamagata/73 HA to a comparable level as that of influenza A virus HA, regardless of human or avian-like receptors (Ni *et al.*, 2014b). The enhanced receptor-binding affinities enabled its efficient binding to three cultured cell lines containing a varied range of glycan composition for which the wild-type B/Yamagata/73 HA bound very poorly. While it is not known when, how and why influenza B virus HA acquired the Tyr95→Phe mutation in the course of evolution, it is likely that some or all of the other viral proteins of influenza B virus have undergone concomitant changes, including a delicate balance between HA and NA (Mitnaul *et al.*, 2000). The significantly enhanced receptor-binding affinity of the Phe95→Tyr mutant may create an imbalance in the equation, thus compromising the replication efficiency of the recombinant virus in mice (Ni *et al.*, 2014b).

Structural basis for the divergent evolution

Influenza B virus contains two co-circulating lineages – the B/Victoria and B/Yamagata lineage – that diverged from each other in early 1970s. However, a mechanistic understanding of their divergent evolution was still lacking. Structural and sequence analysis of undiverged and diverged influenza B virus HAs revealed the molecular basis for the divergent evolution (Ni *et al.*, 2013). Furthermore, HAs of recent influenza B virus strains display much stronger molecular interactions with terminal sialic acid of bound receptors, which may allow for a broader tissue tropism for which further investigation is urgently needed.

Antigenic structure of influenza B virus HAs

We compared known influenza B virus HA structures: B/HK/73 representing undiverged early strains (PDB codes: 3BT6, 2RFT and 2RFU) (Wang *et al.*, 2007, 2008), B/Brisbane/08 of the B/Victoria lineage (PDB code: 4FQM) (Dreyfus *et al.*, 2012), B/Florida/06 (in the region of HA_1 33–324, PDB code: 4FQJ) (Dreyfus *et al.*, 2012) and B/Yamanashi/98 of the B/Yamagata lineage (PDB code: 4M40) (Ni *et al.*, 2013). Despite overall structural similarities, regions with large structural variations were observed when using the unliganded structure of B/HK/73 HA as a reference (PDB code: 3BT6). These regions were always at the 120-loop, 150-loop, 160-loop and 190-helix. Interestingly, the structural differences in the 150-loop region of B/Yamagata lineage HAs are much more eminent than that of B/Victoria lineage, agreeing with the observation that the 150-loop region is a particularly strong neutralizing epitope for B/Yamagata lineage strains in recent isolates (Nakagawa *et al.*, 2003; Shen *et al.*, 2009).

There is a strikingly large structural rearrangement in the region of HA_1 235–240 for all recent strains compared to B/HK/73 HA. The residue Glu-235 in B/HK/73 HA is replaced by Gly-235 in 100% B/Victoria lineage and 99% B/Yamagata lineage strains (Ni *et al.*, 2013, 2014b). Gly-235 led to a more extended 240-loop and one-residue shift in side-chain orientation. Specifically, the side chain of Pro-238 in B/Yamanashi/98 and B/Brisbane/08 HAs was placed at a similar location to that of Leu-237 in B/HK/73 HA. Thus, the side chain of Gln-239 in all other influenza B virus HA structures was at the same location as that of Pro-238 in B/HK/73 HA, pointing towards the receptor binding site. The structural changes in this region could profoundly change the antigenic and receptor-binding properties of the protein.

Four major epitopes have been assigned on the structure of B/HK/73 HA: the 120-loop, 150-loop, 160-loop and 190-helix and their respective surrounding regions in previous studies (Berton *et al.*, 1984; Berton and Webster, 1985; Hovanec and Air, 1984; Rivera *et al.*, 1995; Wang, 2010; Wang *et al.*, 2008; Webster and Berton, 1981). Analysis of 278

HA sequences from B/Victoria lineage and 282 HA sequences from B/Yamagata lineage confirmed that amino acid substitutions in the sequences are concentrated on these four epitope regions. The high amino acid substitution frequency and the large structural variations of these regions are probably interconnected: the high structural flexibility of these regions makes them easily to accommodate drifting mutations without compromising the structural integrity of influenza B virus HA, and the drifting mutations introduced therein could easily cause structural changes that are large enough to evade recognition by neutralizing antibodies.

Importantly, among the four major epitopes of influenza B virus HAs, differential selection pressures appeared to operate on B/Victoria or B/Yamagata lineage strains. For example, 150-loop was under stronger positive selection pressure in the B/Yamagata lineage than in the B/Victoria lineage. In contrast, the 160-loop that was once specific for the B/Victoria lineage is now also being used by the B/Yamagata lineage in recent years. Furthermore, the 150-loop, 160-loop and 190-helix likely constitute a large continuous antigenic site for their close spatial locations and the facts that neutralizing antibodies recognizing the 150- and 160-loops, and the 190-helix competed with each other (Berton and Webster, 1985; Hovanec and Air, 1984) and that they all interacted with neutralizing antibody CR8033 (Dreyfus *et al.*, 2012). On the other hand, the lack of cross-reactivity between the antibodies recognizing the 120-loop region and the 160-loop/190-helix (Berton and Webster, 1985; Hovanec and Air, 1984) and the fact that the footprint of the antibody CR8071 was limited to the 120-loop (Dreyfus *et al.*, 2012) suggest that the 120-loop is a separate antigenic site.

The receptor binding site and the B/Yamanashi/98 HA–LSTa complex

In B/HK/73 HA (Wang *et al.*, 2007), the receptor-binding site was stabilized by π-stacking interactions among aromatic residues and three additional hydrogen bonds between Tyr-202 and His-191, Ser-140 and Trp-158, Pro-238 and Ser-240. In B/Yamanashi/98 HA, the π-stacking interactions were conserved. Although a rotation of the side chain of Trp-158 broke the hydrogen bond with Ser-140, a new hydrogen bond was formed between Trp-158 and Tyr-202. Moreover, the large structural rearrangement in the 240-loop caused the loss of the interaction between Pro-238 and Ser-240, however a hydrogen bond was gained between the side chains of Gln-239 and Ser-140. Thus, similar π-stacking interactions and the same number of hydrogen bonds were observed in the receptor-binding site of both B/HK/73 and B/Yamanashi/98 HAs.

In the complex structure of B/Yamanashi/98 HA-LSTa, the first four sugar rings, Sia-1, Gal-2, GlcNAc-3 and Gal-4, were clearly visible. The Sia-1 moiety made extensive hydrogen bonding interactions within the receptor-binding site, including one each with Gly-141, Ser-140, Asp-193 and Ser-240. These four hydrogen bonds were also found between LSTa and B/HK/73 HA. In addition, B/Yamanashi/98 HA made five new hydrogen bonds that were not seen in B/HK/73 HA: one by the side chain of Arg-136, two by the main-chain carbonyl of Thr-139 and two by the side chain of Gln-239.

The additional hydrogen bonds with Thr-139 appeared to be due to the ~0.9 Å lower sitting position of the bound LSTa Sia-1 in the receptor-binding site, thus closer to HA_1 139–141 in B/Yamanashi/98 HA. As a result of the ~1.2-Å left shift of HA_1 139~141 in the receptor binding site of B/Yamanashi/98 HA compared with B/HK/73 HA, the bound Sia-1 was similarly left-shifted.

The new hydrogen bond with $HA_1$136 was due to the substitution Ile-136→Arg. This substitution was found in 98% B/Yamagata strains and 1% B/Victoria strains. However, a similar substitution Ile-136→Lys was found in 1% B/Yamagata strains and 97% B/Victoria strains. The side chains of Arg-136 in B/Yamanashi/98 HA and Lys-136 in B/Brisbane/08 HA were located at a similar position. Therefore, the hydrogen bond between the side-chain of Arg-136 and Sia-1 is expected to be present in all these B/Yamagata and B/Victoria strains.

The additional two hydrogen bonds with Gln-239 were probably the consequence of the large structural rearrangement in the 240-loop due to Gly-235. This new conformation of the 240-loop is common for B/Yamanashi/98 and B/Brisbane/08 HA structures and the residue Gly-235 was observed in 100% of B/Victoria lineage and 99% of B/Yamagata lineage strains. Therefore, these two hydrogen bonds with Gln-239 are probably preserved in almost all recent influenza B virus HAs.

Altogether, these five new hydrogen bonds observed between B/Yamanashi/98 HA and LSTa Sia-1 are expected to be present in HAs of almost all currently circulating influenza B virus strains in binding to both human-like and avian-like receptors that share the Sia-1 moiety. Therefore, current influenza B virus of both lineages has evolved a receptor-binding site that is capable of binding to Sia-1 with a much higher affinity than B/HK/73 HA. A stronger binding with receptors might allow for a different tissue tropism of these recent influenza B virus strains, for which further investigation is required.

Structural insights into membrane-fusion mechanism mediated by influenza virus haemagglutinin

The merger of influenza viral envelope with host endosomal membrane is accompanied by a large-scale structural rearrangement of HA in transitioning from pre-fusion to post-fusion states. The structural rearrangements include (a) the dissociation of HA_1–HA_1 monomers, (b) the folding of region B from a loop in pre-fusion state to a helical conformation in post-fusion state, (c) the delivery of the fusion peptide to target membrane and (d) the folding-back of helix E to deliver the C-terminal transmembrane domain to the same end of the molecule as the fusion peptide (Bullough *et al.*, 1994; Chen *et al.*, 1999). A recent study of an early fusion intermediate of influenza A/H2 HA suggested that steps (a) and (b) probably precede step (c) (Xu and Wilson, 2011), while a study on single influenza virions indicated that step c) is a rate-limiting step for hemifusion (Ivanovic *et al.*, 2013). The newly determined structure of influenza B virus HA_2 in post-fusion state allowed a structural and mechanistic look into this process (Ni *et al.*, 2014a).

The overall structure of influenza B virus HA_2

Influenza A/H3N2 and B virus HA_2 share a very low sequence identity of ~29%. The most conserved regions included the N-terminal region containing a part of the N-cap and region A, while region B and the C-terminal fragment were the most variable. However, both HA_2 folded into the same hairpin-like structures. The central long three-helical coiled coil was assembled from three segments – helix A (residues 38–55), helix B (residues 56–75) and helix C (residues 76–105) – forming, respectively, a short a-helix, a loop and a part of the long helix in the pre-fusion state. The N-cap domain (residues 31–37) stopped the extension of the central three-helical coiled coil. The long central helix was followed by loop D (residues 106–111) that was a part of a long central helix in the pre-fusion state. Following this loop was helix E (residues 112–125) that packed against the long central helix to form a six-helical bundle. Loop F (residues 126–145) and helix G (residues 146–153) had relatively weaker electron densities and higher *B*-factors, suggesting a greater structural flexibility. Consistent with this observation, for the reported influenza A/H3N2 virus HA_2 structure (PDB accession code: 1QU1) where there were two trimers in the asymmetric unit, this region displayed different conformations, including α-helix, β-sheet or random coil, in different chains (Chen *et al.*, 1999). The C-terminal fragment (residues 154–181) bound along the groove formed by two neighbouring central helices and interacted with the N-cap domain at the end of the molecule.

The protein hydrophobic core

For the central three-helical coiled coil in the post-fusion structures, helices A and C, but not helix B, were superimposed very well between influenza A/H3N2 and B virus HA_2, which agreed well with the high sequence variability in this region. Within the protein hydrophobic core, the residues were either identical (in helix A and N- and C-termini of helix C) or highly conserved in hydrophobicity (in helix B and the middle of helix C). The only exception was a buried Glu-59 in influenza B virus HA_2 where the corresponding residue in influenza A/H3N2 HA_2 was Thr-59. The side-chain of Glu-59 pointed towards the 3-fold axis and was surrounded by two large hydrophobic residues, Leu-63 and Leu-164, and a hydrophilic residue, Asn-62. It has been shown in Marburg virus glycoprotein GP2 that buried Glu residues led to a higher stability at low pH, thus favouring the formation of the post-fusion structure (Harrison *et al.*, 2012; Koellhoffer *et al.*, 2012). Indeed, influenza B virus HA_2 was more stable at low pH, with an approximate melting temperature of 42°C at pH 7.2 and 60°C at pH 5.2 (Ni *et al.*, 2014a).

The N-cap domain

In influenza B virus HA_2, the N-terminal residues 34–37 formed the N-cap domain to stop the extension of the central three-helical coiled coil. The side chains of the highly conserved Asp-37 contributed hydrogen bonds with the main-chain amide groups of Leu-38 and Ser-40 on the same subunit. In addition, the carbonyl group of Asp-37 made two hydrogen bonds with Thr-41.

As the N-cap domain extended towards a neighbouring subunit, one hydrogen bond was formed between the carbonyl group of Val-34 and the amide group of Leu-38. In addition, the three N-caps interacted with each other at the threefold axis by forming two layers of hydrophobic interactions, among three Ala-36 and three Ala-35, and making three hydrogen bonds between the carbonyl group of Ala-36 with the amide group of the same residue on the neighbouring subunit. The N-cap also interacted with the C-terminal fragment through one hydrogen bond between Asp-37 and Thr-174. Collectively, these interactions stabilized the N-cap domain and stopped the central coiled coil structure from extending further.

The interactions between the central helices and the C-terminal fragment

The docking of the C-terminal fragment into the groove formed by neighbouring central helices is the key to bring together the C-terminal transmembrane domain and the N-terminal fusion peptide for membrane fusion. We found that, the binding of each C-terminal fragment with the central helices resulted in a total buried surface area of 2315.5 $Å^2$ for influenza

B virus HA_2, which was a bit smaller than the interface in influenza A/H3N2 virus HA_2 (at 2550.1 $Å^2$). The interface in influenza B virus HA_2 was predominantly hydrophobic, containing a polar area of 591.6 $Å^2$ and an apolar area of 1723.9 $Å^2$. In contrast, influenza A/H3N2 HA_2 had the polar and apolar interface areas of 1020.3 $Å^2$ and 1529.8 $Å^2$, respectively. Thus, the polar interface between the central helices and C-terminal fragment in influenza A/H3N2 HA_2 was almost twice as large as that of influenza B virus HA_2. The slightly larger interface in influenza A/H3N2 virus HA_2 may compensate for the more polar nature of the interface.

Comparisons of the structures at the pre-fusion state

The pre-fusion structures of HA are the starting point for the large-scale conformational change in low-pH-mediated membrane fusion. Interestingly, a large internal cavity beneath the HA_1 subunits and just atop of the C-terminus of the B-loop was constantly found in influenza A virus HAs, but not in influenza B virus HAs (Ni *et al.*, 2014a). These internal cavities were directly connected to outside aqueous solution, indicating that protons could more easily diffuse into the interior of influenza A virus HA molecules than into influenza B virus HA.

On the other hand, in influenza B virus HA, the fusion peptide pointed away from its own helix A and helix B to interact with those of a neighbouring subunit via residues Phe-2 and Phe-3 and adopted a lower position in the structure, thus losing most of the polar interactions with Asn-109 and Asp-112. It has been previously shown that compromised interactions between the fusion peptide and Asp-112 destabilized the pre-fusion state, raised the fusion pH and accelerated the kinetics of membrane fusion (Daniels *et al.*, 1985, 1987; Ivanovic *et al.*, 2013). In sharp contrast, the fusion peptide of influenza A virus HA was located near the threefold symmetry axis of the molecule and makes a total of six hydrogen bonds with Asp-112 and one hydrogen bond with Asp-109. Thus, the fusion peptide and its interacting residues were more exposed in influenza B virus HA (Wang *et al.*, 2008) than in influenza A virus HA.

The mechanism of low-pH induced large-scale conformational change of HA

The wealth information of pre-fusion structures of influenza A and B virus HAs has revealed similar ionic residue clusters that are strategically placed in pre-fusion structures and similar pathways for the large-scale conformational change (Ni *et al.*, 2014a; Wang, 2010; Wang *et al.*, 2008). However, the detailed mechanisms used by influenza A and B virus HA proteins probably differ. For instance, influenza A virus HA constantly have much loosely packed HA_1–HA_1 interfaces, and contain B-loops that are more exposed than in influenza B virus HA (Ni *et al.*, 2014a). These structural features of influenza A virus HAs might lead to a high sensitivity to pH changes. On the other hand, the less buried position of the fusion peptide in influenza B virus HAs and its weakened interactions with Asp-112 and Asn-109, and the higher helical propensity of the B-loop could result in lower transition-state energy barriers (Weis *et al.*, 1990) for influenza B virus HA. Recent studies clearly indicated a role of fusion pH in pathogenicity and transmission of influenza virus (DuBois *et al.*, 2011; Galloway *et al.*, 2013; Herfst *et al.*, 2012; Imai *et al.*, 2012; Reed *et al.*, 2010). To maintain virus fitness, a delicate balance is needed between stabilizing and destabilizing forces to keep the pre-fusion HA in a suitable metastable state. Now with the newly determined crystal structure of influenza B virus HA_2 in post-fusion state (Ni *et al.*, 2014a), it is now possible to systematically investigate the key chemical/structural elements that impact HA's fusion pH and kinetics and their contributions to the pathogenicity and transmissibility of influenza virus.

Conclusions

In addition to causing seasonal flu epidemics, influenza A virus is also responsible for all human pandemics known to date. In marked contrast, influenza B virus only causes seasonal epidemics. Different from influenza A virus, influenza B virus has a very limited host range, circulating almost exclusively among humans and seals. The lack of reservoirs of influenza B virus outside the human population is believed to be one of the major reasons that influenza B virus does not cause human pandemics as influenza A virus. In addition, influenza B viruses were found to have overall lower receptor-binding affinities than influenza A viruses. Our earlier structural study of influenza B virus HA revealed a surprising difference within the receptor-binding site: Phe-95 in influenza B virus HA, in contrast to an absolutely conserved Tyr-98 in influenza A/H1~H15 HAs. Our most recent mutagenesis and structural study of Phe95→Tyr suggests that Phe-95 is most likely the molecular basis for the low receptor-binding affinities and the limited host range of naturally circulating influenza B viruses (Ni *et al.*, 2014b). The inability for the recombinant virus harbouring the Phe95→Tyr/Asn194→Asp mutation in B/Lee/40 background to replicate efficiently in mice indicate a delicate balance between HA and NA activities for adequate viral fitness. Importantly, recent field isolates of influenza B virus appeared to bind more strongly with avian or human-like receptors than earlier undiverged strains (Ni *et al.*, 2013). It is not known whether these recent strains have also evolved a more active NA. Influenza B virus containing HA of higher receptor-binding affinity combined with a matched NA activity might allow for an expansion of host tropism and pose a higher risk to humans. Together with the newly determined crystal structure of influenza B virus HA_2 in post-fusion state (Ni *et al.*, 2014a), a new era of systematically investigating the key chemical/structural elements that impact HA's fusion pH and kinetics and their contributions to the pathogenicity and transmissibility of influenza virus shall begin.

Acknowledgements

Q.W. thanks support from the National Institutes of Health (R01-AI067839 and R01-GM116280) and the Welch Foundation (Q-1826).

References

Berton, M.T., Naeve, C.W., and Webster, R.G. (1984). Antigenic structure of the influenza B virus hemagglutinin: nucleotide sequence analysis of antigenic variants selected with monoclonal antibodies. J. Virol. *52*, 919–927.

Berton, M.T., and Webster, R.G. (1985). The antigenic structure of the influenza B virus hemagglutinin: operational and topological mapping with monoclonal antibodies. Virology *143*, 583–594.

Bullough, P.A., Hughson, F.M., Skehel, J.J., and Wiley, D.C. (1994). Structure of influenza hemagglutinin at the pH of membrane fusion. Nature *371*, 37–43.

Chen, J., Skehel, J.J., and Wiley, D.C. (1999). N- and C-terminal residues combine in the fusion-pH influenza hemagglutinin HA(2) subunit to form an N cap that terminates the triple- stranded coiled coil. Proc. Natl. Acad. Sci. U.S.A. *96*, 8967–8972.

Chen, J.M., Guo, Y.J., Wu, K.Y., Guo, J.F., Wang, M., Dong, J., Zhang, Y., Li, Z., and Shu, Y.L. (2007). Exploration of the emergence of the Victoria lineage of influenza B virus. Arch. Virol. *152*, 415–422.

Daniels, P.S., Jeffries, S., Yates, P., Schild, G.C., Rogers, G.N., Paulson, J.C., Wharton, S.A., Douglas, A.R., Skehel, J.J., and Wiley, D.C. (1987). The receptor-binding and membrane-fusion properties of influenza virus variants selected using anti-hemagglutinin monoclonal antibodies. EMBO J. *6*, 1459–1465.

Daniels, R.S., Downie, J.C., Hay, A.J., Knossow, M., Skehel, J.J., Wang, M.L., and Wiley, D.C. (1985). Fusion mutants of the influenza virus hemagglutinin glycoprotein. Cell *40*, 431–439.

Dreyfus, C., Laursen, N.S., Kwaks, T., Zuijdgeest, D., Khayat, R., Ekiert, D.C., Lee, J.H., Metlagel, Z., Bujny, M.V., Jongeneelen, M., *et al.* (2012). Highly conserved protective epitopes on influenza B viruses. Science *337*, 1343–1348.

DuBois, R.M., Zaraket, H., Reddivari, M., Heath, R.J., White, S.W., and Russell, C.J. (2011). Acid stability of the hemagglutinin protein regulates H5N1 influenza virus pathogenicity. PLoS Pathog. *7*, e1002398.

Fouchier, R.A., Munster, V., Wallensten, A., Bestebroer, T.M., Herfst, S., Smith, D., Rimmelzwaan, G.F., Olsen, B., and Osterhaus, A.D. (2005). Characterization of a novel influenza A virus hemagglutinin subtype (H16) obtained from black-headed gulls. J. Virol. *79*, 2814–2822.

Galloway, S.E., Reed, M.L., Russell, C.J., and Steinhauer, D.A. (2013). Influenza HA subtypes demonstrate divergent phenotypes for cleavage activation and pH of fusion: implications for host range and adaptation. PLoS Pathog. *9*, e1003151.

Gamblin, S.J., and Skehel, J.J. (2010). Influenza hemagglutinin and neuraminidase membrane glycoproteins. J. Biol. Chem. *285*, 28403–28409.

Govorkova, E.A., Murti, G., Meignier, B., de Taisne, C., and Webster, R.G. (1996). African green monkey kidney (Vero) cells provide an alternative host cell system for influenza A and B viruses. J. Virol. *70*, 5519–5524.

Hai, R., Garcia-Sastre, A., Swayne, D.E., and Palese, P. (2011). A reassortment-incompetent live attenuated influenza virus vaccine for protection against pandemic virus strains. J. Virol. *85*, 6832–6843.

Harrison, J.S., Koellhoffer, J.F., Chandran, K., and Lai, J.R. (2012). Marburg virus glycoprotein GP2: pH-dependent stability of the ectodomain alpha-helical bundle. Biochemistry *51*, 2515–2525.

Herfst, S., Schrauwen, E.J., Linster, M., Chutinimitkul, S., de Wit, E., Munster, V.J., Sorrell, E.M., Bestebroer, T.M., Burke, D.F., Smith, D.J., *et al.* (2012). Airborne transmission of influenza A/H5N1 virus between ferrets. Science *336*, 1534–1541.

Hovanec, D.L., and Air, G.M. (1984). Antigenic structure of the hemagglutinin of influenza virus B/Hong Kong/8/73 as determined from gene sequence analysis of variants selected with monoclonal antibodies. Virology *139*, 384–392.

Imai, M., Watanabe, T., Hatta, M., Das, S.C., Ozawa, M., Shinya, K., Zhong, G., Hanson, A., Katsura, H., Watanabe, S., *et al.* (2012). Experimental adaptation of an influenza H5 HA confers respiratory droplet transmission to a reassortant H5 HA/H1N1 virus in ferrets. Nature *486*, 420–428.

Ito, T., Suzuki, Y., Mitnaul, L., Vines, A., Kida, H., and Kawaoka, Y. (1997a). Receptor specificity of influenza A viruses correlates with the agglutination of erythrocytes from different animal species. Virology *227*, 493–499.

Ito, T., Suzuki, Y., Takada, A., Kawamoto, A., Otsuki, K., Masuda, H., Yamada, M., Suzuki, T., Kida, H., and Kawaoka, Y. (1997b). Differences in sialic acid-galactose linkages in the chicken egg amnion and allantois influence human influenza virus receptor specificity and variant selection. J. Virol. *71*, 3357–3362.

Ivanovic, T., Choi, J.L., Whelan, S.P., van Oijen, A.M., and Harrison, S.C. (2013). Influenza-virus membrane fusion by cooperative fold-back of stochastically induced hemagglutinin intermediates. Elife 2, e00333.

Jayaraman, A., Pappas, C., Raman, R., Belser, J.A., Viswanathan, K., Shriver, Z., Tumpey, T.M., and Sasisekharan, R. (2011). A single base-pair change in 2009 H1N1 hemagglutinin increases human receptor affinity and leads to efficient airborne viral transmission in ferrets. PLoS One *6*, e17616.

Koellhoffer, J.F., Malashkevich, V.N., Harrison, J.S., Toro, R., Bhosle, R.C., Chandran, K., Almo, S.C., and Lai, J.R. (2012). Crystal structure of the Marburg virus GP2 core domain in its postfusion conformation. Biochemistry *51*, 7665–7675.

Matrosovich, M.N., Gambaryan, A.S., Tuzikov, A.B., Byramova, N.E., Mochalova, L.V., Golbraikh, A.A., Shenderovich, M.D., Finne, J., and Bovin, N.V. (1993). Probing of the receptor-binding sites of the H1 and H3 influenza A and influenza B virus hemagglutinins by synthetic and natural sialosides. Virology *196*, 111–121.

Medeiros, R., Escriou, N., Naffakh, N., Manuguerra, J.C., and van der Werf, S. (2001). Hemagglutinin residues of recent human A(H3N2) influenza viruses that contribute to the inability to agglutinate chicken erythrocytes. Virology *289*, 74–85.

Mitnaul, L.J., Matrosovich, M.N., Castrucci, M.R., Tuzikov, A.B., Bovin, N.V., Kobasa, D., and Kawaoka, Y. (2000). Balanced hemagglutinin and neuraminidase activities are critical for efficient replication of influenza A virus. J. Virol. *74*, 6015–6020.

Nakagawa, N., Kubota, R., Nakagawa, T., and Okuno, Y. (2003). Neutralizing epitopes specific for influenza B virus Yamagata group strains are in the 'loop'. J. Gen. Virol. *84*, 769–773.

Ni, F., Chen, X., Shen, J., and Wang, Q. (2014a). Structural insights into the membrane fusion mechanism mediated by influenza virus hemagglutinin. Biochemistry *53*, 846–854.

Ni, F., Kondrashkina, E., and Wang, Q. (2013). Structural basis for the divergent evolution of influenza B virus hemagglutinin. Virology *446*, 112–122.

Ni, F., Nnadi Mbawuike, I., Kondrashkina, E., and Wang, Q. (2014b). The roles of hemagglutinin Phe-95 in receptor binding and pathogenicity of influenza B virus. Virology *450–451*, 71–83.

Osterhaus, A.D., Rimmelzwaan, G.F., Martina, B.E., Bestebroer, T.M., and Fouchier, R.A. (2000). Influenza B virus in seals. Science *288*, 1051–1053.

Pappas, C., Viswanathan, K., Chandrasekaran, A., Raman, R., Katz, J.M., Sasisekharan, R., and Tumpey, T.M. (2010). Receptor specificity and transmission of H2N2 subtype viruses isolated from the pandemic of 1957. PLoS One *5*, e11158.

Reed, M.L., Bridges, O.A., Seiler, P., Kim, J.K., Yen, H.L., Salomon, R., Govorkova, E.A., Webster, R.G., and Russell, C.J. (2010). The pH of activation of the hemagglutinin protein regulates H5N1 influenza virus pathogenicity and transmissibility in ducks. J. Virol. *84*, 1527–1535.

Rivera, K., Thomas, H., Zhang, H., Bossart-Whitaker, P., Wei, X., and Air, G.M. (1995). Probing the structure of influenza B hemagglutinin using site-directed mutagenesis. Virology *206*, 787–795.

Shen, J., Kirk, B.D., Ma, J., and Wang, Q. (2009). Diversifying selective pressure on influenza B virus hemagglutinin. J. Med. Virol. *81*, 114–124.

Skehel, J.J., and Wiley, D.C. (2000). Receptor binding and membrane fusion in virus entry: the influenza hemagglutinin. Annu. Rev. Biochem. *69*, 531–569.

Srinivasan, A., Viswanathan, K., Raman, R., Chandrasekaran, A., Raguram, S., Tumpey, T.M., Sasisekharan, V., and Sasisekharan, R. (2008). Quantitative biochemical rationale for differences in transmissibility of 1918 pandemic influenza A viruses. Proc. Natl. Acad. Sci. U.S.A. *105*, 2800–2805.

Steinhauer, D. (2010). Influenza A virus hemagglutinin glycoproteins. In Influenza: Molecular Virology, Q. Wang, and Y.J. Tao, eds. (Norfolk, UK: Caister Academic Press), pp. 69–108.

Sun, X., Shi, Y., Lu, X., He, J., Gao, F., Yan, J., Qi, J., and Gao, G.F. (2013). Bat-derived influenza hemagglutinin H17 does not bind canonical avian or human receptors and most likely uses a unique entry mechanism. Cell Rep. 3, 769–778.

Suzuki, Y., Matsunaga, M., and Matsumoto, M. (1985). N-Acetylneuraminyllactosylceramide, GM3-NeuAc, a new influenza A virus receptor which mediates the adsorption-fusion process of viral infection. Binding specificity of influenza virus A/Aichi/2/68 (H3N2) to membrane-associated GM3 with different molecular species of sialic acid. J. Biol. Chem. *260*, 1362–1365.

Takemae, N., Ruttanapumma, R., Parchariyanon, S., Yoneyama, S., Hayashi, T., Hiramatsu, H., Sriwilaijaroen, N., Uchida, Y., Kondo, S., Yagi, H., *et al.* (2010). Alterations in receptor-binding properties of swine influenza viruses of the H1 subtype after isolation in embryonated chicken eggs. J. Gen. Virol. *91*, 938–948.

Tang, X., and Chong, K.T. (2009). Histopathology and growth kinetics of influenza viruses (H1N1 and H3N2) in the upper and lower airways of guinea pigs. J. Gen. Virol. *90*, 386–391.

Tong, S., Li, Y., Rivailler, P., Conrardy, C., Castillo, D.A., Chen, L.M., Recuenco, S., Ellison, J.A., Davis, C.T., York, I.A., *et al.* (2012). A distinct lineage of influenza A virus from bats. Proc. Natl. Acad. Sci. U.S.A. *109*, 4269–4274.

Viswanathan, K., Koh, X., Chandrasekaran, A., Pappas, C., Raman, R., Srinivasan, A., Shriver, Z., Tumpey, T.M., and Sasisekharan, R. (2010). Determinants of glycan receptor specificity of H2N2 influenza A virus hemagglutinin. PLoS One *5*, e13768.

Wang, Q. (2010). Influenza type B virus hemagglutinin: antigenicity, receptor binding and membrane fusion. In Influenza: Molecular Virology, Wang, Q., and Tao, Y.J. eds. (Norfolk, UK: Caister Adademic Press), pp. 29–52.

Wang, Q., Cheng, F., Lu, M., Tian, X., and Ma, J. (2008). Crystal Structure of Unliganded Influenza B Virus Hemagglutinin. J. Virol. *82*, 3011–3020.

Wang, Q., Tian, X., Chen, X., and Ma, J. (2007). Structural basis for receptor specificity of influenza B virus hemagglutinin. Proc. Natl. Acad. Sci. U.S.A. *104*, 16874–16879.

Webster, R.G., and Berton, M.T. (1981). Analysis of antigenic drift in the hemagglutinin molecule of influenza B virus with monoclonal antibodies. J. Gen. Virol. *54*, 243–251.

Weis, W., Brown, J.H., Cusack, S., Paulson, J.C., Skehel, J.J., and Wiley, D.C. (1988). Structure of the influenza virus haemagglutinin complexed with its receptor, sialic acid. Nature 333, 426–431.
Weis, W.I., Cusack, S.C., Brown, J.H., Daniels, R.S., Skehel, J.J., and Wiley, D.C. (1990). The structure of a membrane fusion mutant of the influenza virus haemagglutinin. EMBO J. *9*, 17–24.
Wiley, D.C., and Skehel, J.J. (1987). The structure and function of the hemagglutinin membrane glycoprotein of influenza virus. Annu. Rev. Biochem. *56*, 365–394.
Xu, R., and Wilson, I.A. (2011). Structural characterization of an early fusion intermediate of influenza virus hemagglutinin. J. Virol. *85*, 5172–5182.
Zhu, X., Yu, W., McBride, R., Li, Y., Chen, L.M., Donis, R.O., Tong, S., Paulson, J.C., and Wilson, I.A. (2013). Hemagglutinin homologue from H17N10 bat influenza virus exhibits divergent receptor-binding and pH-dependent fusion activities. Proc. Natl. Acad. Sci. U.S.A. *110*, 1458–1463.

Structure and Assembly of the Influenza A Virus Ribonucleoprotein Complex

4

Wenjie Zheng, Wenting Zhang, Yusong R. Guo and Yizhi Jane Tao

Abstract

The genome of the influenza A virus as well as other orthomyxoviruses comprises eight segments of single-stranded, negative-sense RNA that are encapsidated as individual rod-shaped ribonucleoprotein complexes (RNPs). Influenza A virus RNPs play critical roles during virus infection by directing viral RNA replication and transcription, intracellular trafficking of the viral RNA, gene reassortment as well as genome packaging into progeny viruses. Biochemically each RNP contains a viral RNA, a viral polymerase and multiple copies of the viral nucleoprotein (NP). Built on over 40 years of intensive research, exciting developments in recent years have substantially enhanced our understanding of the structure and function of various molecular components of RNP as well as the double-helical RNP structure itself.

Introduction

Influenza A viruses are enveloped, single-stranded, negative-sense RNA viruses (Lamb and Krug, 2001). The genome of the influenza A virus is segmented into eight RNA molecules, each folded into a rod-shaped, double-helical ribonucleoprotein complex (RNP). Each RNP contains a viral RNA, a heterotrimeric viral polymerase (consisting of PA, PB1, and PB2) and multiple copies of the viral-encoded nucleoprotein (NP) that bind viral RNA in a non-specific manner (Compans *et al.*, 1972; Heggeness *et al.*, 1982; Jennings *et al.*, 1983; Ruigrok and Baudin, 1995).

The RNPs of the influenza A virus play crucial roles during the virus infection cycle (Fig. 4.1). Influenza A virus enters the host cell by clathrin-mediated endocytosis, and after viral membrane fusion in the endosome, releases viral RNPs into the cytosol. Viral RNPs enter the host nucleus by active transport. In the nucleus, the RNPs from the infecting virus serve as active templates for the synthesis of viral mRNA as well as anti-genomic, complementary RNAs (cRNA). The cRNAs are replication intermediates that direct the synthesis of nascent virion RNAs (vRNAs). Nascent cRNAs and vRNA are both encapsidated into RNP structures by interacting with newly synthesized NP, PB1, PB2 and PA that are imported to the nucleus. After their assembly, RNPs are exported out of the nucleus in a process facilitated by two other influenza virus proteins M1 and NEP. In the cytosol, influenza virus RNPs are further transported to the cytoplasmic membrane where they become selectively packaged into budding virions.

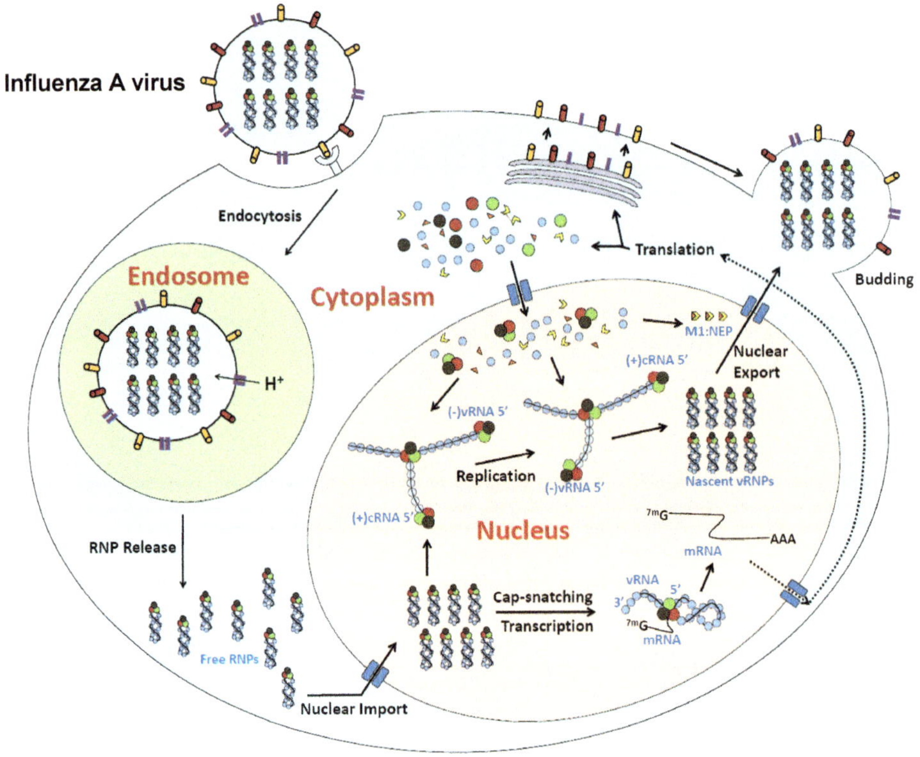

Figure 4.1 The influenza A virus life cycle. The RNPs are represented by helical hairpins, with the polymerase subunits (red, brown, and green) and NP (cyan) shown in different colours. In the nucleus, the viral transcription and replication processes are depicted according to model proposed by Jorba *et al* (Jorba *et al.*, 2009). Modified from Das *et al.* (2010).

Technical advances in recent years have enabled exciting new findings in our studies of the influenza virus RNP that have substantially elevated our understanding of its structure, function and assembly. In this chapter, we will primarily discuss new findings related to the structure of RNP and its molecular components. The assembly process of RNP and its intracellular trafficking will also be discussed. The replication and transcription aspects of the RNP are covered in Chapter 2.

Overall structure and properties of the RNP

RNPs purified from virions have been examined by electron microscopy (EM) in great detail. Back in the 60s and 70s, it was found that isolated RNPs are rod-shaped structures about 10 nm in width (Compans *et al.*, 1972; Pons *et al.*, 1969). Statistically, purified RNPs could be categorized into three length groups: 90–110 nm, 60–90 nm and 30–50 nm. Considering that RNPs have a uniform diameter, the length of an RNP likely correlates with the size of its associating vRNA. The rod-shaped RNPs are structurally flexible and appeared to adopt a right-hand, double-helical structure in negative-staining EM (Compans *et al.*, 1972). Immuno-EM indicated that the viral polymerase complex is located at one end of the helical rod (Murti *et al.*, 1988). Interestingly, RNPs are able to maintain an intact structure even in the absence of vRNA, suggesting that NP plays a major role in the overall structural organization and stabilization of the RNP (Ruigrok and Baudin, 1995).

Over the years various biochemical and biophysical techniques have been used to probe the structure of the influenza RNP. The 5′ and 3′ end of each vRNA contain partially complementary sequences that are 12–13 nt in length (Hsu *et al.*, 1987; Klumpp *et al.*, 1997). These sequences, which are highly conserved among the eight viral gene segments and supposedly form a panhandle structure, provide specific binding sites for the influenza heterotrimeric polymerase complex (Desselberger *et al.*, 1980; Hagen *et al.*, 1994; Luytjes *et al.*, 1989; Neumann *et al.*, 2004; Neumann and Hobom, 1995; Robertson, 1979; Skehel and Hay, 1978). The influenza A virus RNPs unwind under high/low salt conditions, giving rise to closed circular structures (Klumpp *et al.*, 1997). Chemical probing experiments indicated that RNA binds to NP with its phosphate backbone with nucleotide bases facing solvent (Elton *et al.*, 1999). RNAs associated with RNPs can be displaced by polyvinylsulfate (PVS), a negatively charged polymer (Goldstein and Pons, 1970). Furthermore, the vRNAs in the influenza virus RNPs were readily digested by RNase treatment (Baudin *et al.*, 1994), suggesting that very little protection was provided by the bound NP. These findings indicate that the RNPs of the influenza A virus adopt a unique structure compared with the nucleocapsids from non-segmented, negative-sense RNA viruses (see, for example, Longhi, 2009).

Structures of the RNP protein components

Owing to the inherent structural flexibility of RNPs, high-resolution structural analysis of intact RNPs is challenging. Nevertheless, atomic structures of all the RNP protein components have become available in the last few years. These structures include NP, a number of protein fragments derived from the viral polymerase complex, and the intact heterotrimeric polymerase in complex with a vRNA promoter (Pflug *et al.*, 2014; Reich *et al.*, 2014). Recently, a cryo-EM structure of the influenza virus RNA polymerase complex has also been determined at 4.3 Å resolution, which shows the formation of polymerase dimers and tetramers (Chang *et al.*, 2015).

NP

The influenza A virus NP is a multifunctional protein that has been shown to interact with a number of viral (e.g. PA, PB1, PB2, M1, etc.) and host proteins (e.g. RAF-2p48/UAP56 and Tat-SF1, etc.) (Portela and Digard, 2002). One of the NP's primary functions is to coat viral RNA to facilitate its folding into a double-helical RNP structure. To date, crystal structures of three influenza virus NPs and also an isavirus NP are available from the *Orthomyxoviridae* family (Ng *et al.*, 2008, 2012; Ye *et al.*, 2006; Zheng *et al.*, 2013), all forming ring structures in the absence of RNA. Although their oligomers vary in size, all four NP proteins assume the overall shape of a crescent with a head and a body domain (Fig. 4.2a). In between the two domains is a deep groove enriched in basic amino acid residues that may function as the RNA-binding site. It has been shown the mutation of several arginine residues from the two flexible loops within the groove resulted in dramatic reduction of the RNA-binding affinity of influenza A virus NP (Ng *et al.*, 2008). Oligomerization of the NP is mediated by an extended tail loop structure (i.e. aa 402–428 in the influenza A virus NP) located at the

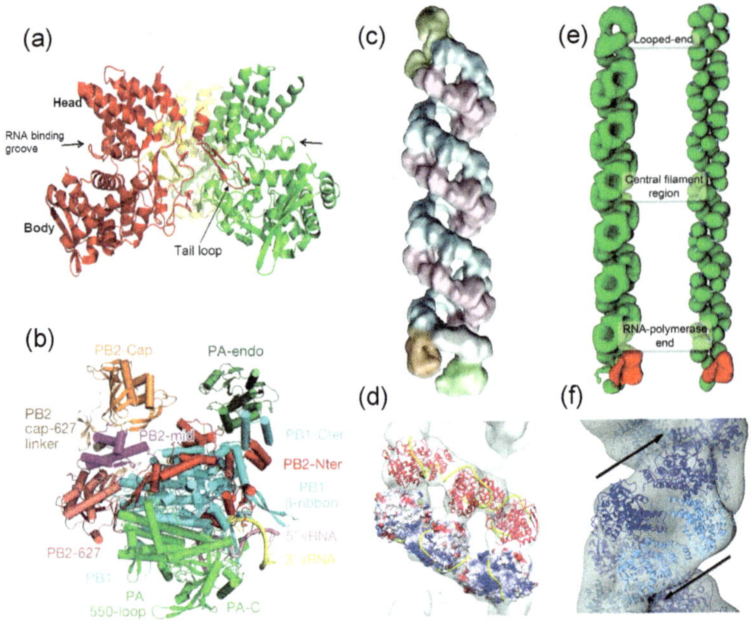

Figure 4.2 The influenza A virus RNP structure. (a) Crystal structure of the influenza A virus NP. The three subunits of the NP trimer are coloured differently (Ng *et al.*, 2008; Ye *et al.*, 2006). (b) Crystal structure of the influenza A virus polymerase trimer in complex with the viral promoter [reprinted with permission from MacMillan Publishers Ltd: Nature (Pflug *et al.*, 2014), copyright (2014)]. (c) Cryo-EM reconstruction of a double-helical RNP by Arranz *et al.* (2012). The viral polymerase complex is located at the bottom end of the RNP and is shown in green and orange. The two opposite-running NP-RNA strands are coloured differently in blue and pink. The NP-RNA turning loop on the top end of the RNP is highlighted in dark green. (d) Helical stem of the RNP from (c) fitted with NP crystal structure and modelled with RNA (in yellow) [(c) and (d) from Arranz *et al.* (2012). Reprinted with permission from AAAS.]. (e) Cryo-EM reconstruction of a RNP by Moeller *et al.* (2012). On the right is a model showing the RNP organization. The viral polymerase is highlighted in red. (f) Central filament region from (e) fitted with NP crystal structure protomers. Arrows indicate RNA polarity. [(e and f) from Moeller *et al.* (2012). Reprinted with permission from AAAS.]

back of each NP molecule (Ng *et al.*, 2008; Ye *et al.*, 2006). Loss of NP oligomerization due to amino acid substitutions in the tail loop resulted in NP mutants unable to support viral gene expression in mini-genome assays (Ye *et al.*, 2012).

In addition to NP oligomers, the structure of an influenza A virus NP monomer (i.e. the R416A mutant) has been determined (Chenavas et al., 2013b). In the NP monomer, the tail loop that protrudes to a neighbouring protomer in the trimer structure interacts with equivalent sites on the mutant monomer surface, thus avoiding polymerization. At the meantime, the C-terminus of the monomer is bound to the side of the RNA binding surface, lowering its positive charge. It was also found that serine 165 was phosphorylated and conserved in all influenza A and B viruses (Chenavas et al., 2013b). Because the S165D NP mutant displays a lowered affinity for RNA compared with wild-type monomeric NP, it was proposed that phosphorylation may regulate the polymerization state and RNA binding of NP in the infected cell.

Owing to its highly conserved structure and multifunctional nature, the influenza virus NP has attracted much attention lately as a druggable target (Chenavas *et al.*, 2013a; Cianci *et al.*, 2013; Monod *et al.*, 2015). Drug compounds that promote aberrant NP aggregation can effectively inhibit influenza A virus replication in cell cultures (Gerritz *et al.*, 2011; Kao *et al.*, 2010). Nucleozin, which stabilizes interaction between NP monomers, can also target the viral RNP and inhibit virus replication by blocking cytoplasmic trafficking of the viral genome (Amorim *et al.*, 2013). The NP tail-loop binding pocket has been suggested as another potential target for anti-influenza therapeutics, and small molecules that disrupt the formation of NP trimers are able to inhibit replication of WT and nucleozin-resistant strains (Kukol and Hughes, 2014; Shen *et al.*, 2011). Naproxen, which is an anti-inflammatory drug, was discovered to inhibit influenza A virus replication by targeting NP and stabilizing it in its monomeric form by binding in its RNA-binding groove (Lejal *et al.*, 2013; Tarus *et al.*, 2015). Recently, another antiviral structure was found to target a novel pocket within NP that is involved in the RNA binding, dimerization, and nuclear export functions of the protein (Kakisaka *et al.*, 2015).

Heterotrimeric polymerase complex

The influenza virus polymerase is a heterotrimeric complex consisting of PA, PB1 and PB2, with multiple enzymatic and ligand binding activities that allow the synthesis of capped, polyadenylated mRNAs during transcription as well as full-length genomic/anti-genomic RNAs during replication (Lamb and Krug, 2001). X-ray structures of several polypeptide fragments of the influenza A virus polymerase have been determined. These include: the 25-kDa N-terminal PA domain (PA-N) which displays the endonuclease activity needed for cap-snatching (Dias *et al.*, 2009; Yuan *et al.*, 2009), the 55-kDa C-terminal PA domain (PA-C) that mediates the PA–PB1 interaction (He *et al.*, 2008; Obayashi *et al.*, 2008), the PB2 aa 318–483 domain that binds to the 5′ pre-mRNA cap (Guilligay *et al.*, 2008; Tsurumura *et al.*, 2013), the PB2 aa 535–684 domain involved in host adaptation (Tarendeau *et al.*, 2008), and the PB2 C-terminal NLS-domain (aa 684–757) that binds cellular importin (Tarendeau *et al.*, 2007). PB1, the largest subunit of the polymerase, hosts the polymerase catalytic active site (Biswas and Nayak, 1994; Kobayashi *et al.*, 1994; Poch *et al.*, 1989) as well as specific binding sites for the conserved 5′ and 3′-vRNA termini (Fodor *et al.*, 1993). For PB1, the structures of the N-terminal fragment (aa 1–25) (He *et al.*, 2008; Obayashi *et al.*, 2008) which interacts with PA and the C-terminal fragment which forms a three helical bundle (aa 678–757) interacting with the N-terminus of PB2 (Sugiyama *et al.*, 2009) are available. The details of these structures can be found in reviews elsewhere (Das *et al.*, 2010; Resa-Infante *et al.*, 2011; Ruigrok *et al.*, 2010).

In a new exciting development, the crystal structure of the complete heterotrimeric polymerase in complex with the viral promoter was determined for a bat influenza A virus, which is evolutionarily related to human/avian A strains with ~70–80% identity for the three polymerase proteins (Pflug *et al.*, 2014) (Fig. 4.2b). The polymerase has a U-shaped structure, with the two protruding arms formed by the PA endonuclease and PB2 cap-binding domains, respectively. The body of the trimer is formed by PB1, which is decorated on one side by the N-terminal third of PB2 (PB2-N) and on the other side by the linker (PA-linker) that connects the PA endonuclease (PA-N) with PA-C. The trimer contains a large, internal, catalytic and RNA-binding cavity that is partially open at the top and accessible via two narrow side tunnels, the putative NTP and template entrance channels. The viral promoter adopts a base-paired structure in its distal region, while nucleotides 1–10 of the 5′ end form a compact stem–loop (hook) structure that binds tightly in a pocket formed at the interface between PA and PB1. It was speculated that the polymerase active site in PB1 likely becomes disordered in the absence of the viral promoter, thus explaining the role of the viral promoter as an essential cofactor of the viral polymerase (Pflug *et al.*, 2014). By comparing the structure of the influenza A virus polymerase to that of an influenza B virus polymerase (Reich *et al.*, 2014), also in complex with the viral promoter, it was suggested that cap-snatching involves *in situ* rotation of the PB2 cap-binding domain to direct the capped primer first towards the endonuclease and then into the polymerase active site. A structural model for cap-dependent priming by the influenza polymerase is proposed, which entails considerable conformational changes going from the pre-initiation state into the active initiation and elongation states (Reich *et al.*, 2014). A cryo-EM reconstruction of an influenza A virus polymerase subcomplex (comprising full-length PA and PB1 subunits and the N-terminal 130 amino acids fragment of PB2) was obtained at 4.3 Å resolution recently (Chang *et al.*, 2015). This structure shows the formation of a polymerase tetramer, which likely reflects the physiological states of the full-length influenza RdRP complex. It was proposed that the either one of the two dimer interfaces (1 and 2) may aid in the recruitment of another soluble RdRP to the RNP-bound RdRP for initiation of replication (Chang *et al.*, 2015).

The crystal structures of the influenza A virus polymerase complex and its various fragments enable structure-based design and optimization of new antiviral compounds. For instance, a structural study showed that several known endonuclease inhibitors, including four diketo compounds and a green tea catechin, bind to the endonuclease active site of the PA protein (Kowalinski *et al.*, 2012). These inhibitors chelate the two critical manganese ions in the active site of the enzyme, although some differences are noted in the overall ligand ordination of these compounds. Further optimization of such endonuclease inhibitors may lead to potent drugs targeting the cap-snatching endonuclease activity of influenza virus polymerase. Another promising approach to inhibit the influenza A virus replication is to disrupt the assembly of the viral heterotrimeric polymerase complex. It has been shown that short peptides derived from the N-termini of PB1 and PB2, which target the PA–PB1 and PB1–PB2 interaction interface, respectively, exhibited varying levels of effectiveness in blocking the viral polymerase activity and growth of the virus (Kashiwagi *et al.*, 2014; Reuther *et al.*, 2011; Wunderlich *et al.*, 2009). Antiviral inhibitors that block the PB2 cap-snatching activity of the influenza viral polymerase complex are also being developed (Byrn *et al.*, 2015; Pautus *et al.*, 2013; Sagong *et al.*, 2014). Lastly, favipiravir (T-705; 6-fluoro-3-hydroxy-2-pyrazinecarboxamide) is a promising antiviral drug active against a broad range of influenza viruses including oseltamivir-resistant strains (Furuta *et al.*, 2013; Kiso *et al.*, 2010). Favipiravir acts like purines or purine nucleosides in human cells and selectively inhibits RNA-dependent RNA polymerase of influenza viruses as well as many other RNA viruses (Furuta *et al.*, 2013; Kiso *et al.*, 2010).

RNP structure

The first three-dimensional structure of the influenza A virus RNP that came to light is that of an artificial mini-RNP (Area *et al.*, 2004; Coloma *et al.*, 2009; Martin-Benito *et al.*,

2001; Ortega *et al.*, 2000). To circumvent the structural flexibility problem, a mini-RNP was generated from *in vivo* amplification by expressing the three polymerase subunits, NP, and a 248nt model vRNA containing the highly conserved terminal sequences (Martin-Benito *et al.*, 2001). The mini-RNP is more structurally rigid compared to the native RNPs, thus allowing cryo-EM reconstruction to ~12 Å resolution. Cryo-EM reconstruction of the mini-RNP shows a closed ring structure consisting of nine NP molecules, with a copy of the viral polymerase attached to the outer edge of the otherwise symmetrical ring (Coloma *et al.*, 2009). The viral polymerase adopts a compact shape and simultaneously interacts with two adjacent NP molecules (Coloma *et al.*, 2009). Each NP molecule shows a two-domain morphology that agrees with previously determined NP crystal structures (Ng *et al.*, 2008; Ye *et al.*, 2006). vRNA cannot be readily discerned at this resolution, but it presumably constitutes some of the adjoining densities that connect neighbouring NP molecules. Due to the limited resolution, the boundaries between the three polymerase subunits were not obvious. Using engineered fusion tags and monoclonal antibodies, Area *et al* were able to map the rough location of PA, PB1 and PB2 in the polymerase complex (Area *et al.*, 2004). It was found that the polymerase contacts with the two NP monomers via the PB1 and PB2 subunits (Coloma *et al.*, 2009; Martin-Benito *et al.*, 2001), consistent with previous biochemical studies (Biswas *et al.*, 1998; Mena *et al.*, 1999). The RNP-associated polymerase shows similarities in overall structure compared to the EM reconstruction of a free polymerase (Area *et al.*, 2004; Torreira *et al.*, 2007), but it is also clear that some conformational changes have taken place upon the interaction with NP and/or the vRNA template.

With innovative image processing strategies, cryo-EM reconstructions of authentic RNPs were reported by two research groups in 2012 (Fig. 4.2c–f) (Arranz *et al.*, 2012; Moeller *et al.*, 2012). The RNP reconstruction reported by Moeller *et al* used RNPs generated by *in vitro* expression of the four RNP proteins (i.e. PA, PB1, PB2 and NP) via transient transfection of a human cell line in the presence of their respective vRNA segments (Moeller *et al.*, 2012). At ~20 Å resolution, the final model confirms that the RNP adopts a double helical structure with two anti-parallel strands leading to and away from the polymerase that is located at one end of the RNP (Fig. 4.2c and d). The double-helical stem region shows a rise between two neighbouring NP of 32.6 Å with 4.9 NP molecules per turn. The other cryo-reconstruction of the influenza A virus RNP was reported by Arranz *et al.* (2012) using native RNPs purified from virions. The structure also shows a double-helical stem with major and minor grooves (Fig. 4.2e and f). The rise step between adjacent NPs is 28.4 Å with a rotational angle of 60° and six NPs per turn on each strand. In both RNP structures, the putative RNA binding groove of the NP scaffold is exposed on the outer surface of the RNP. Assuming that the positively charged groove of NP serves as the RNA binding site, a vRNA was built into the final model. By following a contoured path, ~120–150 nucleotides of RNA are placed in each helical turn.

To help better understand the structural arrangement of the influenza A virus RNP, it is useful to draw an analogy with the double-helical DNA duplex. Similar to the DNA duplex, the RNP possesses two types of surface grooves: a major groove that is well separated, and a minor groove that is maintained by interactions between NP molecules associated with opposing RNA strands. While cohesion between the two anti-parallel strands in a DNA duplex is maintained by base pairing, the interaction between the two opposing arms of an RNP hairpin is solely mediated by the NP. Interactions between adjacent NP molecules on the same RNA strand are facilitated by the extended tail loop. The double-helical RNP was estimated to be ~15 nm wide and ~65 nm long for the second smallest gene segment (~1000 nt long) of the influenza A virus (Arranz *et al.*, 2012).

It is also important to note that the two models by Moeller *et al.* (2012) and Arranz *et al.* (2012) exhibit significant variations in helical parameters and NP orientations. Using crystal structure docking, Arranz *et al.* (2012) propose that the NP molecules from opposing strands contact each other through their body domains at a region near the disordered N-terminus of the NP structure. Moeller *et al.* (2012), however, suggest that the RNP helix is stabilized by the NP-RNA strand interacting with the opposing strand near the NP head domains. The most likely cause of the model difference is likely due to the different handedness of the two reconstructions, with Arranz *et al.* (2012) showing a left-handed helix and Moeller *et al.* (2012) showing a right-handed helix (Fig. 4.2d and f). It is expected that the modest resolution, rotational freedom of the NP molecules, and the source of RNP samples (viral particles vs. cells) may also contribute to some inter-model variations as well. It is worth mentioning that Ye *et al.* (2012) recently reported a NP dimer crystal structure with a dimer interface that does not involve the tail loop. Mutational analysis indicated that the dimer interface is biologically relevant, suggesting a possible role in RNP assembly. Comparing the NP dimer structure with the RNP reconstructions may help to interpret interactions made between the two opposing NP-RNA strands.

These two cryo-EM reconstructions of the RNP also offer a new look at the viral polymerase in the context of the RNP. Both Arranz *et al* and Moeller *et al.* (2012) located the viral polymerase at the open end of the RNP hairpin, simultaneously interacting with both the 5′ and 3′-ends of the vRNA (Arranz *et al.*, 2012; Moeller *et al.*, 2012). The close end of the RNP hairpin contains a small loop formed by a curved array of three to eight NP molecules. It was proposed by Moeller *et al.* (2012) that the PA C-terminal domain is structurally flexible and may help to feed the vRNA template into the polymerase active site, based on structural homology between the PA C-terminal domain and the N-terminal domain of the reovirus RNA polymerase (He *et al.*, 2008; Moeller *et al.*, 2012; Tao *et al.*, 2002). Arranz *et al* observed that the RNP-associated polymerase samples two alternative conformations, but higher resolution structural information is needed to address the biological relevance of this distribution and the possible implications.

In addition to vRNPs (i.e. RNP-containing vRNAs), the structure of cRNPs of the influenza A virus (i.e. complementary RNP or RNP-containing cRNAs) have also been characterized by EM. Using an RNA tag and affinity purification, replicative cRNP intermediate and vRNP were each specifically isolated from infected cells. Based on class averages of negative staining EM images, purified cRNP exhibits a filamentous double-helical organization with defined termini, containing the viral RNA-dependent RNA polymerase (RdRp) at one end and a loop structure at the other end. Such structural features are basically indistinguishable from those observed for the vRNP (York *et al.*, 2013). The presence of an RNA tag that is accessible within the vRNP and cRNP structures provides experimental evidence that sufficient flexibility exists within viral ribonucleoproteins that allows for the formation of secondary RNA structures. Indeed, RNA binding affinity and stoichiometry measurements performed for another orthomyxovirus (i.e. the infectious salmon anaemia virus) also indicated that each NP molecule only binds ~12 nt of RNA in isolation, suggesting that NP-free RNAs do exist on RNP structures (Zheng *et al.*, 2013).

RNP assembly *in vivo*

Newly synthesized NPs are imported back into the host cell nucleus to promote viral RNA replication and RNP assembly (Davey *et al.*, 1985; Honda *et al.*, 1988). As NP binds RNA non-specifically and has a strong tendency to self-polymerize, it is important to keep NP in a soluble, encapsidation-competent state prior to RNP assembly. Unlike non-segmented, negative-sense RNA viruses, the influenza A virus does not encode viral proteins that are known to stabilize NP and prevent its self-oligomerization. It has been proposed that phosphorylation may play an important role in regulating the self-polymerization and RNA binding activities of the influenza A virus NP (Arrese and Portela, 1996; Chenavas *et al.*, 2013b; Mondal *et al.*, 2015; Turrell *et al.*, 2015). A number of highly conserved serine residues (i.e. S165, S407 and S486) located at/near the tail loop interaction interface have been implicated in regulating NP oligomerization by reversible phosphorylation/dephosphorylation. Interestingly, Ye *et al.* (2012) recently reported that the self-oligomerization activity of NP is weak in the absence of RNA, but the interaction is kinetically stable once NP oligomerizes. Therefore, it is possible that NPs remain monomeric until they encounter v/c RNAs in the cell nucleus.

Additionally, a number of host factors have been found to be important for influenza virus replication and RNP assembly (Brass *et al.*, 2009; Hao *et al.*, 2008; Karlas *et al.*, 2010; Kawaguchi *et al.*, 2011; Konig *et al.*, 2010; Momose *et al.*, 1996, 2001, 2002; Naito *et al.*, 2007; Shapira *et al.*, 2009; Watanabe *et al.*, 2010; Zhou *et al.*, 2014). For example, RAF-2p48/UAP56 and Tat-SF1 assist the formation of the vRNA–NP complex, possibly by functioning as chaperones to suppress the non-specific aggregation of NP (Momose *et al.*, 2001; Naito *et al.*, 2007). It was also demonstrated that the fragile X mental retardation protein (FMRP) transiently associates with viral RNP and stimulates viral RNP assembly through RNA-mediated interaction with the nucleoprotein (Zhou *et al.*, 2014). On the other hand, the interferon-inducible protein Mx1 has been found to interfere with the influenza RNP assembly by disturbing the PB2–NP interaction (Verhelst *et al.*, 2012). It was also reported that cyclophilin E (CypE) inhibits RNP assembly by interfering with NP self-association and the NP–PB1 and NP–PB2 interactions (Wang *et al.*, 2011).

RNP assembly in host cells requires only four viral proteins: NP, PA, PB1 and PB2. As shown by Moeller *et al.* (2012), *in vivo* amplification of vRNAs with only these four proteins co-expressed in transfected cells produced rod-shaped RNPs with a regular helical symmetry. Therefore, although M1 and NEP are needed for RNP export from the nucleus (see below), they do not play major roles in either the assembly or structural maintenance of the RNP. This feature is again different from some of the non-segmented, negative-strand RNA viruses (i.e. rhabdoviruses), in which the matrix protein plays a major role in organizing the helical nucleocapsids by simultaneously interacting with N proteins from adjacent helical turns (Ge *et al.*, 2010).

It is likely that NP initiates viral RNA replication via interaction with the polymerase (possibly PB1 or PB2), during which process the RNA-binding ability of NP is not required (Biswas *et al.*, 1998; Gui *et al.*, 2014; Marklund *et al.*, 2012; Mena *et al.*, 1999; Newcomb *et al.*, 2009). Therefore, the NP–polymerase interaction should facilitate the initial recruitment of NPs to newly synthesized vRNAs. Further vRNA encapsidation is probably stimulated by cooperative NP–RNA interactions (Yamanaka *et al.*, 1990). Tarus *et al.* (2012) reported that *in vitro* NP oligomerization is a slow process that depends on the RNA length, with the oligomerization rate increasing drastically as the RNA length increases. On average, each

NP is associated with ~22–28 nt of RNA in the RNPs (Martin-Benito *et al.*, 2001; Ortega *et al.*, 2000). The viral polymerase is significant in maintaining the supercoiled RNP structure, since single-stranded RNA was observed when the polymerase was removed from the RNP (Klumpp *et al.*, 1997).

It is unclear when the polymerase–NP–RNA complex collapses into the supercoiled, double helical RNP structure during replication. The fact that mini-RNPs consisting of nine NP molecules only form circularly shaped rings suggests that the condensation of NP-RNA polymers into double-helical structures does not occur until nascent RNPs reach certain sizes. Moeller *et al* reported the observation of 'branched' RNPs and suggested that the branches are made of partially replicated, nascent RNPs budding from the full-length RNP templates (Moeller *et al.*, 2012). Using immuno-labelling, they showed that a second copy of the polymerase is located at the branching site in some RNPs. The observation of a second polymerase molecule is consistent with the notion that template RNPs are replicated *in trans* by free polymerase complexes and not by the polymerase molecule bound to the parental RNP (Jorba *et al.*, 2009). Although 'budding' RNPs sounds like an attractive interpretation for these branched RNP structures, whether they are truly replication intermediates or perhaps misfolded RNPs still awaits further verification. One potential concern is that the length of the budding RNPs does not seem to correlate well with the location of the RNP branches (Moeller *et al.*, 2012).

RNP assembly *in vitro*

In the late 1980s, it was reported that *in vitro* transcribed vRNAs, when mixed with NP and polymerase purified from infectious particles, could be replicated *in vitro* to produce full-length RNA copies (Honda *et al.*, 1990; Parvin *et al.*, 1989). Palese and colleagues showed that when these *in vitro* encapsidated vRNAs were introduced into permissive cells coinfected with a helper virus, they could be amplified, expressed, and packaged into progeny virions, thus leading to the development of the first-generation influenza A virus reverse genetics (Enami *et al.*, 1990; Luytjes *et al.*, 1989). For influenza viruses and other negative-stranded RNA viruses, free vRNA or cRNA are not infectious. The observation that those reconstituted RNPs were replicated *in vitro* and amplified *in vivo* indicates that some RNP-like structures might have formed. Additionally, attempts to assemble RNP *in vitro* by mixing RNA and recombinant NP have also been reported (Kingsbury *et al.*, 1987; Yamanaka *et al.*, 1990). However, these artificial RNPs may be a poor model to study native RNP as they do not seem to have the typical rod-shaped morphology (Kingsbury *et al.*, 1987; Yamanaka *et al.*, 1990). It would be interesting to find out whether the addition of both recombinant polymerase and NP to *in vitro* transcribed vRNA would produce RNPs that closely resemble those from infectious particles.

Nuclear import and export of RNPs

At the onset of infection, RNPs released from the infecting influenza A virus are actively transported from cytosol into nucleus. It is not clear whether all eight RNPs are imported to the nucleus as a large bundle, or if they are separately imported as individual RNPs. All RNP component proteins contain at least one nuclear localization signal (NLS) necessary for nuclear import. Two regions of the PA protein, residues 124–139, and 186–247, were found to contain NLSs (Nieto *et al.*, 1994). For PB1, a NLS was first found between residues 187–211 (Nath and Nayak, 1990), but later findings showed that the co-expression of PA was important for the efficient nuclear import of PB1 (Fodor and Smith, 2004). PB2 has a linear NLS with a sequence of $K_{736}RKR_{739}$ that was shown to interact with importin-a in a co-crystal structure (Mukaigawa and Nayak, 1991; Tarendeau *et al.*, 2007). Two NLSs have been identified in the NP sequence. One of these was a classical bipartite NLS that was found between residue 198 and 216 with a sequence of $K_{198}RX_{13}RKTR_{216}$ (Weber *et al.*, 1998). A non-conventional NLS (nNLS) with a consensus sequence of $S_3QGTKRSYXXM_{13}$ was also identified at the N-terminus of NP (Neumann *et al.*, 1997; O'Neill *et al.*, 1995; Wang *et al.*, 1997). Although all component proteins of the RNP carry their own NLSs, NP is the major contributor for RNP import (O'Neill *et al.*, 1995; Wang *et al.*, 1997; Wu *et al.*, 2007a). By dot blotting and immunogold labelling of vRNPs, Wu *et al* showed that the nNLS of the NP was much more accessible than the classical bipartite NLS, and that the labelled gold particles showed a regular periodicity which suggested a regular helical conformation of the RNP (Wu *et al.*, 2007b). In addition, Cros *et al.* (2005) reported that mutations in the nNLS completely abolished NP import, and that short peptides mimicking the nNLS competitively inhibited the nuclear import of the RNP. These findings are consistent with the crystal structure of NP (Ng *et al.*, 2008; Ye *et al.*, 2006), as the nNLS is solvent exposed, structurally disordered, and can be easily fitted into the substrate binding pocket of importin-α.

Because influenza A virus assembly occurs at the host cell membrane, newly synthesized RNPs need to be exported out of the nucleus, thus travelling in the opposite direction compared to their parental RNPs from the infecting virus. No nuclear export signal (NES) has been found in the component proteins of the RNP. For RNP export, two other influenza proteins, M1 and NEP, are required (Bui *et al.*, 2000; Neumann *et al.*, 2000; O'Neill *et al.*, 1998). The C-terminal domain of M1 is responsible for interaction with RNP (Baudin *et al.*, 2001), and M1-binding to the RNP likely helps to mask the NLSs on the RNP. SUMOylation of M1 is required for the interaction between M1 and viral RNP (vRNP) to form the M1–vRNP complex (Wu *et al.*, 2011). Meanwhile, M1 can directly interact with the viral protein NEP which possesses a NES signal (O'Neill *et al.*, 1998). The RNP–M1-NEP complex is recognized by the chromosome region maintenance 1 (CRM1) protein, which mediates the nuclear export of NES-containing protein/complexes from the nucleus (Fukuda *et al.*, 1997). The RNP-M1-NEP daisy chain was recently challenged by Brunotte *et al*, who propose that the C-terminal domain of NEP binds simultaneously to the viral polymerase and M1, whereas the N-terminal domain harbouring the NES can establish the interaction with CRM1 (Brunotte *et al.*, 2014). The nuclear export of RNP also requires viral activation of the cellular Raf/MEK/ERK [mitogen-activated protein kinase (MAPK)] signalling cascade that is activated late in the infection cycle, as block of the cascade resulted in retardation of RNP export and reduced titres of progeny virus (Pleschka *et al.*, 2001). It has been shown that membrane accumulation of the influenza A virus haemagglutinin triggers activation of the MAPK cascade and induces RNP export. This may represent an auto-regulative mechanism that coordinates the timing of RNP export with virus budding (Marjuki *et al.*, 2007). Cytoplasmic trafficking of the RNPs requires the involvement of vesicular trafficking system for them to be transported to the budding site beneath the plasma membrane (Jo *et al.*, 2010). The cellular microtubule networks are responsible for the moving of the viral RNPs from the microtubule organizing centre (MTOC) to the cell periphery at the late phase of infection (Momose *et al.*, 2007). Indeed, the host histone deacetylase 6 (HDAC6) is able to inhibit influenza virus infection by negatively regulating the trafficking of viral components to the site of influenza virus assembly via its substrate, acetylated microtubules (Husain and Cheung, 2014).

Specific RNP packaging

Early evidence of selective packaging came from the defective-interfering influenza RNAs (DI RNAs) (Duhaut and McCauley, 1996; Odagiri and Tashiro, 1997). DI RNAs were shown to interfere with the incorporation of some specific gene segments while sparing others, suggesting that each segment contains a unique packaging signal. Later, further evidence was provided by reverse genetics, which revealed that all eight gene segments possess such packaging signals that are required for efficient virion incorporation (Fujii *et al.*, 2003, 2005; Hutchinson *et al.*, 2008, 2010; Liang *et al.*, 2005, 2008; Muramoto *et al.*, 2006; Ozawa *et al.*, 2007; Watanabe *et al.*, 2003). EM studies have also provided strong evidence for selective packaging (Fig. 4.3). The observation of the distinctive '7 + 1' pattern of the eight

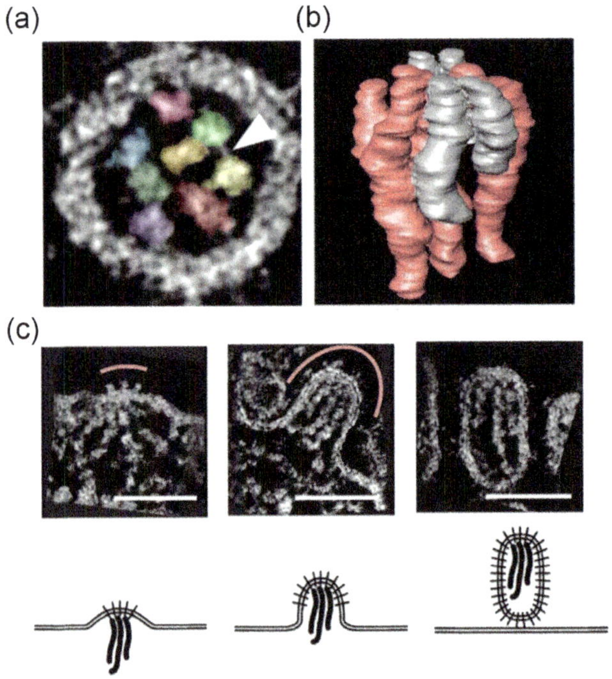

Figure 4.3 Specific packaging of the influenza A virus RNP. (a) Linkages among the eight RNPs in a virion (Noda *et al.*, 2012). A 0.5-nm-think tomogram is shown with the eight RNPs highlighted in different colours. Short string-like structures can be seen between the RNPs (arrowheads). (b) 3-D model of a multisegment RNP complex (Noda *et al.*, 2012). The four long RNPs are shown in red, while the four shorter ones are shown in grey. (c) Budding (left, middle) and mature (right) virions (Noda *et al.*, 2012). Red curves in the left and middle columns indicate the membrane region where viral spike proteins are present. Shown below are schematic diagrams of the RNP packaging process Scale bar, 100 nm. (a–c) Reprinted with permission from MacMillan Publishers Ltd: Nature [Noda *et al.*, 2012, copyright (2012)].

RNPs suggests that specific inter-RNP interactions maintain such a conformation (Noda *et al.*, 2006) (Fig. 4.3a). Recent evidence by electron tomography showed that the RNPs of the '7+1' bundle are actually different, with four longer RNPs and four shorter RNPs of significantly different lengths, consistent with the length distribution of the eight influenza RNA segments (Fournier *et al.*, 2012b; Noda *et al.*, 2012) (Fig. 4.3b). Electron tomography studies also revealed that the eight RNPs are aligned at the budding tip and interconnect with each other to form a supra-molecular assembly (Fig. 4.3c). With fluorescence *in situ* hybridization (FISH) analysis at the single-virus particle level, Chou *et al.* (2012) confirmed that the eight unique RNPs are incorporated into progeny virions by a selective packaging mechanism. Co-localization tests demonstrated that most of the virus particles have incorporated at least one of the eight RNPs. The exact copy number of each RNP was determined by comparing the photo-bleaching profiles of probes against the HA RNA segment (i.e. the RNA segment encoding the haemagglutinin protein) of the wild-type and a recombinant virus carrying two copies of the HA segments. Their results demonstrated that most virus particles contain only one copy of each of the eight RNP complexes. Furthermore, immunostaining of thin-sectioned virions showed that some RNPs are incorporated into budding virions with their polymerase-binding ends at the budding tip, whereas others align with their polymerase-binding ends at the bottom of the virion (Sugita *et al.*, 2013).

The sequence-specific signals for influenza genomic packaging have been discovered on each of the eight genomic RNAs (Hutchinson *et al.*, 2010). The 'signal regions' cover the untranslated regions (UTRs) of both termini as well as the adjacent coding sequences of the open reading frame (ORF). Many approaches have been employed to map the regions containing the packaging signals. The earliest results were obtained from experiments on DI RNAs (Duhaut and Dimmock, 1998, 2000; Duhaut and McCauley, 1996; Hughes *et al.*, 2000; Jennings *et al.*, 1983; Nayak *et al.*, 1982; Noble and Dimmock, 1995), which are shorter RNAs derived from the wild-type RNAs with certain region(s) deleted, while still maintaining the abilities to be replicated and packaged. Examination of these DI RNAs showed that the UTRs as well as the terminal coding sequences are well preserved in the DI RNAs, suggesting a significant role in genomics packaging. Later, reverse genetics experiments confirmed that all eight influenza vRNAs have bipartite packaging signals located at the 5′ and 3′ termini (Fujii *et al.*, 2003, 2005; Liang *et al.*, 2005; Marsh *et al.*, 2007; Muramoto *et al.*, 2006; Ozawa *et al.*, 2007, 2009). It was demonstrated that the UTRs together with the terminal coding regions can significantly enhance the packaging efficiency than the UTRs alone, suggesting that the coding sequences also contribute to genomic packaging (Fujii *et al.*, 2003). In addition, codons at the terminal coding regions were found to have synonymous variation rates significantly lower than expected, indicating that the RNA primary sequence is important and thus selectively preserved (Gog *et al.*, 2007). Indeed, synonymous nucleotide mutations within the packaging signal regions produce recombinant viruses with reduced replication efficiencies (Fujii *et al.*, 2005; Gog *et al.*, 2007; Hutchinson *et al.*, 2008, 2009; Liang *et al.*, 2008; Marsh *et al.*, 2007, 2008). A recent analysis using reverse genetic suggested that the packaging signal as currently defined is not necessarily essential for the packaging of the vRNA in which it resides; rather, it is required for the packaging of the full set of vRNAs (Goto *et al.*, 2013).

The localization of the packaging signals near the 5′ and 3′ termini of the vRNAs suggests that these RNA sequences should be mapped to the double-helical RNPs near the end where the viral polymerase is located. Using electron tomography 3D reconstructions,

Fournier *et al.* (2012b) show that the eight vRNPs contact each other at the budding tip of the influenza A virus particles. This contact region is thick enough to accommodate all described packaging signals. They also demonstrated that *in vitro* all vRNAs are involved in a single interaction network, with each vRNA segment interacting with at least one other vRNA partner. Fournier *et al.* (2012a) thus suggest that the RNPs are likely held together by direct base-pairings between packaging signals. When studied *in vitro*, the eight vRNAs of the influenza A virus formed a single interaction network, and the vRNA regions involved in several interactions were found to overlap with the packaging signals (Gavazzi *et al.*, 2013). Conserved RNA secondary structures have been predicted in the influenza A virus genome using comparative sequence and structure analysis (Gultyaev *et al.*, 2014). Such RNA structures are distributed over the whole segment length, including protein-coding regions. While increasing evidence point to RNA–RNA interaction as an essential determining factor in specific RNP packaging, many intriguing questions remain answered. For example, how are the packaging signals presented on the surface of the RNPs? Is vRNA completely denatured by tight wrapping around the NP scaffold, or perhaps some NP-free RNAs exist in the RNP to allow vRNA–vRNA interactions? If RNPs are incorporated into budding virions in both orientations, how would the packaging signals from different RNA segments interact with each other during the budding process to ensure specific packaging of the RNPs?

Conclusion

In the past 5 years, the progress made in our understanding of the structure and function of the influenza A virus RNP has simply been astonishing. Most importantly, the determination of the crystal structure of every protein component of the RNP has set the stage for further probing of the RNP functions at atomic level. It is expected that in the near future efforts will be made to relax the symmetry and also to improve resolution of the three-dimensional structure of the RNP, so that molecular interactions between protein–protein, protein–RNA and RNA–RNA can become available. At present, some of the most pressing questions in the influenza virus field with regard to the RNP include: (1) how RNPs rearrange their structure during viral RNA replication and transcription; (2) what is the step-by-step pathway for newly synthesized viral RNAs to interact with NP and the viral polymerase to fold into the double-helical RNP structure; (3) how RNPs interact with other viral and host proteins to get exported from the nucleus and further delivered to the cell membrane; and (4) how RNPs interact with each other to ensure specific packaging of the viral genome. It has become increasingly clear that a large number of host factors would play important regulatory or direct roles in all of the above-mentioned processes. In addition to influenza viruses, mechanistic studies of other members of the *Orthomyxoviridae* family will greatly facilitate our understanding of the RNP in general. Comparing the structure and function of the influenza virus RNP to other segmented negative-stranded RNA viruses such as bunyaviruses and non-segmented negative-stranded RNA viruses such as rhabdoviruses should provide valuable information about the evolutionary relationship among those viruses.

Acknowledgements

The authors are supported by the National Institutes of Health (AI077785) and the Robert A. Welch Foundation (C-1565).

References

Amorim, M.J., Kao, R.Y., and Digard, P. (2013). Nucleozin targets cytoplasmic trafficking of viral ribonucleoprotein-Rab11 complexes in influenza A virus infection. J. Virol. *87*, 4694–4703.

Area, E., Martin-Benito, J., Gastaminza, P., Torreira, E., Valpuesta, J.M., Carrascosa, J.L., and Ortin, J. (2004). 3D structure of the influenza virus polymerase complex: localization of subunit domains. Proc. Natl. Acad. Sci. U.S.A. *101*, 308–313.

Arranz, R., Coloma, R., Chichon, F.J., Conesa, J.J., Carrascosa, J.L., Valpuesta, J.M., Ortin, J., and Martin-Benito, J. (2012). The structure of native influenza virion ribonucleoproteins. Science *338*, 1634–1637.

Arrese, M., and Portela, A. (1996). Serine 3 is critical for phosphorylation at the N-terminal end of the nucleoprotein of influenza virus A/Victoria/3/75. J. Virol. *70*, 3385–3391.

Baudin, F., Bach, C., Cusack, S., and Ruigrok, R.W. (1994). Structure of influenza virus RNP. I. Influenza virus nucleoprotein melts secondary structure in panhandle RNA and exposes the bases to the solvent. EMBO J. *13*, 3158–3165.

Baudin, F., Petit, I., Weissenhorn, W., and Ruigrok, R.W. (2001). In vitro dissection of the membrane and RNP binding activities of influenza virus M1 protein. Virology *281*, 102–108.

Biswas, S.K., Boutz, P.L., and Nayak, D.P. (1998). Influenza virus nucleoprotein interacts with influenza virus polymerase proteins. J. Virol. *72*, 5493–5501.

Biswas, S.K., and Nayak, D.P. (1994). Mutational analysis of the conserved motifs of influenza A virus polymerase basic protein 1. J. Virol. *68*, 1819–1826.

Brass, A.L., Huang, I.C., Benita, Y., John, S.P., Krishnan, M.N., Feeley, E.M., Ryan, B.J., Weyer, J.L., van der Weyden, L., Fikrig, E., *et al.* (2009). The IFITM proteins mediate cellular resistance to influenza A H1N1 virus, West Nile virus, and dengue virus. Cell *139*, 1243–1254.

Brunotte, L., Flies, J., Bolte, H., Reuther, P., Vreede, F., and Schwemmle, M. (2014). The nuclear export protein of H5N1 influenza A viruses recruits Matrix 1 (M1) protein to the viral ribonucleoprotein to mediate nuclear export. J. Biol. Chem. *289*, 20067–20077.

Bui, M., Wills, E.G., Helenius, A., and Whittaker, G.R. (2000). Role of the influenza virus M1 protein in nuclear export of viral ribonucleoproteins. J. Virol. *74*, 1781–1786.

Byrn, R.A., Jones, S.M., Bennett, H.B., Bral, C., Clark, M.P., Jacobs, M.D., Kwong, A.D., Ledeboer, M.W., Leeman, J.R., McNeil, C.F., *et al.* (2015). Preclinical activity of VX-787, a first-in-class, orally bioavailable inhibitor of the influenza virus polymerase PB2 subunit. Antimicrob. Agents Chemother. *59*, 1569–1582.

Chang, S., Sun, D., Liang, H., Wang, J., Li, J., Guo, L., Wang, X., Guan, C., Boruah, B.M., Yuan, L., *et al.* (2015). Cryo-EM structure of influenza virus RNA polymerase complex at 4.3 A resolution. Mol. Cell *57*, 925–935.

Chenavas, S., Crepin, T., Delmas, B., Ruigrok, R.W., and Slama-Schwok, A. (2013a). Influenza virus nucleoprotein: structure, RNA binding, oligomerization and antiviral drug target. Future Microbiol. *8*, 1537–1545.

Chenavas, S., Estrozi, L.F., Slama-Schwok, A., Delmas, B., Di Primo, C., Baudin, F., Li, X., Crepin, T., and Ruigrok, R.W. (2013b). Monomeric nucleoprotein of influenza A virus. PLoS Pathog. *9*, e1003275.

Chou, Y.Y., Vafabakhsh, R., Doganay, S., Gao, Q., Ha, T., and Palese, P. (2012). One influenza virus particle packages eight unique viral RNAs as shown by FISH analysis. Proc. Natl. Acad. Sci. U.S.A. *109*, 9101–9106.

Cianci, C., Gerritz, S.W., Deminie, C., and Krystal, M. (2013). Influenza nucleoprotein: promising target for antiviral chemotherapy. Antivir. Chem. Chemother. *23*, 77–91.

Coloma, R., Valpuesta, J.M., Arranz, R., Carrascosa, J.L., Ortin, J., and Martin-Benito, J. (2009). The structure of a biologically active influenza virus ribonucleoprotein complex. PLoS Pathog. *5*, e1000491.

Compans, R.W., Content, J., and Duesberg, P.H. (1972). Structure of the ribonucleoprotein of influenza virus. J. Virol. *10*, 795–800.

Cros, J.F., Garcia-Sastre, A., and Palese, P. (2005). An unconventional NLS is critical for the nuclear import of the influenza A virus nucleoprotein and ribonucleoprotein. Traffic *6*, 205–213.

Das, K., Aramini, J.M., Ma, L.C., Krug, R.M., and Arnold, E. (2010). Structures of influenza A proteins and insights into antiviral drug targets. Nat. Struct. Mol. Biol. *17*, 530–538.
Davey, J., Dimmock, N.J., and Colman, A. (1985). Identification of the sequence responsible for the nuclear accumulation of the influenza virus nucleoprotein in Xenopus oocytes. Cell *40*, 667–675.
Desselberger, U., Racaniello, V.R., Zazra, J.J., and Palese, P. (1980). The 3′ and 5′-terminal sequences of influenza A, B and C virus RNA segments are highly conserved and show partial inverted complementarity. Gene *8*, 315–328.
Dias, A., Bouvier, D., Crepin, T., McCarthy, A.A., Hart, D.J., Baudin, F., Cusack, S., and Ruigrok, R.W. (2009). The cap-snatching endonuclease of influenza virus polymerase resides in the PA subunit. Nature *458*, 914–918.
Duhaut, S.D., and Dimmock, N.J. (1998). Heterologous protection of mice from a lethal human H1N1 influenza A virus infection by H3N8 equine defective interfering virus: comparison of defective RNA sequences isolated from the DI inoculum and mouse lung. Virology *248*, 241–253.
Duhaut, S., and Dimmock, N.J. (2000). Approximately 150 nucleotides from the 5′ end of an influenza A segment 1 defective virion RNA are needed for genome stability during passage of defective virus in infected cells. Virology *275*, 278–285.
Duhaut, S.D., and McCauley, J.W. (1996). Defective RNAs inhibit the assembly of influenza virus genome segments in a segment-specific manner. Virology *216*, 326–337.
Elton, D., Medcalf, L., Bishop, K., Harrison, D., and Digard, P. (1999). Identification of amino acid residues of influenza virus nucleoprotein essential for RNA binding. J. Virol. *73*, 7357–7367.
Enami, M., Luytjes, W., Krystal, M., and Palese, P. (1990). Introduction of site-specific mutations into the genome of influenza virus. Proc. Natl. Acad. Sci. U.S.A. *87*, 3802–3805.
Fodor, E., Seong, B.L., and Brownlee, G.G. (1993). Photochemical cross-linking of influenza A polymerase to its virion RNA promoter defines a polymerase binding site at residues 9 to 12 of the promoter. J. Gen. Virol. *74*, 1327–1333.
Fodor, E., and Smith, M. (2004). The PA subunit is required for efficient nuclear accumulation of the PB1 subunit of the influenza A virus RNA polymerase complex. J. Virol. *78*, 9144–9153.
Fournier, E., Moules, V., Essere, B., Paillart, J.C., Sirbat, J.D., Cavalier, A., Rolland, J.P., Thomas, D., Lina, B., Isel, C., *et al.* (2012a). Interaction network linking the human H3N2 influenza A virus genomic RNA segments. Vaccine *30*, 7359–7367.
Fournier, E., Moules, V., Essere, B., Paillart, J.C., Sirbat, J.D., Isel, C., Cavalier, A., Rolland, J.P., Thomas, D., Lina, B., *et al.* (2012b). A supramolecular assembly formed by influenza A virus genomic RNA segments. Nucleic Acids Res. *40*, 2197–2209.
Fujii, K., Fujii, Y., Noda, T., Muramoto, Y., Watanabe, T., Takada, A., Goto, H., Horimoto, T., and Kawaoka, Y. (2005). Importance of both the coding and the segment-specific noncoding regions of the influenza A virus NS segment for its efficient incorporation into virions. J. Virol. *79*, 3766–3774.
Fujii, Y., Goto, H., Watanabe, T., Yoshida, T., and Kawaoka, Y. (2003). Selective incorporation of influenza virus RNA segments into virions. Proc. Natl. Acad. Sci. U.S.A. *100*, 2002–2007.
Fukuda, M., Asano, S., Nakamura, T., Adachi, M., Yoshida, M., Yanagida, M., and Nishida, E. (1997). CRM1 is responsible for intracellular transport mediated by the nuclear export signal. Nature *390*, 308–311.
Furuta, Y., Gowen, B.B., Takahashi, K., Shiraki, K., Smee, D.F., and Barnard, D.L. (2013). Favipiravir (T-705), a novel viral RNA polymerase inhibitor. Antiviral Res. *100*, 446–454.
Gavazzi, C., Isel, C., Fournier, E., Moules, V., Cavalier, A., Thomas, D., Lina, B., and Marquet, R. (2013). An in vitro network of intermolecular interactions between viral RNA segments of an avian H5N2 influenza A virus: comparison with a human H3N2 virus. Nucleic Acids Res. *41*, 1241–1254.
Ge, P., Tsao, J., Schein, S., Green, T.J., Luo, M., and Zhou, Z.H. (2010). Cryo-EM model of the bullet-shaped vesicular stomatitis virus. Science *327*, 689–693.
Gerritz, S.W., Cianci, C., Kim, S., Pearce, B.C., Deminie, C., Discotto, L., McAuliffe, B., Minassian, B.F., Shi, S., Zhu, S., *et al.* (2011). Inhibition of influenza virus replication via small molecules that induce the formation of higher-order nucleoprotein oligomers. Proc. Natl. Acad. Sci. U.S.A. *108*, 15366–15371.
Gog, J.R., Afonso Edos, S., Dalton, R.M., Leclercq, I., Tiley, L., Elton, D., von Kirchbach, J.C., Naffakh, N., Escriou, N., and Digard, P. (2007). Codon conservation in the influenza A virus genome defines RNA packaging signals. Nucleic Acids Res. *35*, 1897–1907.
Goldstein, E.A., and Pons, M.W. (1970). The effect of polyvinylsulfate on the ribonucleoprotein of influenza virus. Virology *41*, 382–384.
Goto, H., Muramoto, Y., Noda, T., and Kawaoka, Y. (2013). The genome-packaging signal of the influenza A virus genome comprises a genome incorporation signal and a genome-bundling signal. J. Virol. *87*, 11316–11322.

Gui, X., Li, R., Zhang, X., Shen, C., Yu, H., Guo, X., Kang, Y., Chen, J., Chen, H., Chen, Y., *et al.* (2014). An important amino acid in nucleoprotein contributes to influenza A virus replication by interacting with polymerase PB2. Virology *464–465*, 11–20.

Guilligay, D., Tarendeau, F., Resa-Infante, P., Coloma, R., Crepin, T., Sehr, P., Lewis, J., Ruigrok, R.W., Ortin, J., Hart, D.J., *et al.* (2008). The structural basis for cap binding by influenza virus polymerase subunit PB2. Nat. Struct. Mol. Biol. *15*, 500–506.

Gultyaev, A.P., Tsyganov-Bodounov, A., Spronken, M.I., van der Kooij, S., Fouchier, R.A., and Olsthoorn, R.C. (2014). RNA structural constraints in the evolution of the influenza A virus genome NP segment. RNA Biol. *11*, 942–952.

Hagen, M., Chung, T.D., Butcher, J.A., and Krystal, M. (1994). Recombinant influenza virus polymerase: requirement of both 5′ and 3′ viral ends for endonuclease activity. J. Virol. *68*, 1509–1515.

Hao, L., Sakurai, A., Watanabe, T., Sorensen, E., Nidom, C.A., Newton, M.A., Ahlquist, P., and Kawaoka, Y. (2008). Drosophila RNAi screen identifies host genes important for influenza virus replication. Nature *454*, 890–893.

He, X., Zhou, J., Bartlam, M., Zhang, R., Ma, J., Lou, Z., Li, X., Li, J., Joachimiak, A., Zeng, Z., *et al.* (2008). Crystal structure of the polymerase PA(C)-PB1(N) complex from an avian influenza H5N1 virus. Nature *454*, 1123–1126.

Heggeness, M.H., Smith, P.R., Ulmanen, I., Krug, R.M., and Choppin, P.W. (1982). Studies on the helical nucleocapsid of influenza virus. Virology *118*, 466–470.

Honda, A., Mukaigawa, J., Yokoiyama, A., Kato, A., Ueda, S., Nagata, K., Krystal, M., Nayak, D.P., and Ishihama, A. (1990). Purification and molecular structure of RNA polymerase from influenza virus A/PR8. J. Biochem. *107*, 624–628.

Honda, A., Ueda, K., Nagata, K., and Ishihama, A. (1988). RNA polymerase of influenza virus: role of NP in RNA chain elongation. J. Biochem. *104*, 1021–1026.

Hsu, M.T., Parvin, J.D., Gupta, S., Krystal, M., and Palese, P. (1987). Genomic RNAs of influenza viruses are held in a circular conformation in virions and in infected cells by a terminal panhandle. Proc. Natl. Acad. Sci. U.S.A. *84*, 8140–8144.

Hughes, M.T., Matrosovich, M., Rodgers, M.E., McGregor, M., and Kawaoka, Y. (2000). Influenza A viruses lacking sialidase activity can undergo multiple cycles of replication in cell culture, eggs, or mice. J. Virol. *74*, 5206–5212.

Husain, M., and Cheung, C.Y. (2014). Histone deacetylase 6 inhibits influenza A virus release by downregulating the trafficking of viral components to the plasma membrane via its substrate, acetylated microtubules. J. Virol. *88*, 11229–11239.

Hutchinson, E.C., Curran, M.D., Read, E.K., Gog, J.R., and Digard, P. (2008). Mutational analysis of cis-acting RNA signals in segment 7 of influenza A virus. J. Virol. *82*, 11869–11879.

Hutchinson, E.C., von Kirchbach, J.C., Gog, J.R., and Digard, P. (2010). Genome packaging in influenza A virus. J. Gen. Virol. *91*, 313–328.

Hutchinson, E.C., Wise, H.M., Kudryavtseva, K., Curran, M.D., and Digard, P. (2009). Characterisation of influenza A viruses with mutations in segment 5 packaging signals. Vaccine *27*, 6270–6275.

Jennings, P.A., Finch, J.T., Winter, G., and Robertson, J.S. (1983). Does the higher order structure of the influenza virus ribonucleoprotein guide sequence rearrangements in influenza viral RNA? Cell *34*, 619–627.

Jo, S., Kawaguchi, A., Takizawa, N., Morikawa, Y., Momose, F., and Nagata, K. (2010). Involvement of vesicular trafficking system in membrane targeting of the progeny influenza virus genome. Microbes Infect. *12*, 1079–1084.

Jorba, N., Coloma, R., and Ortin, J. (2009). Genetic trans-complementation establishes a new model for influenza virus RNA transcription and replication. PLoS Pathog. *5*, e1000462.

Kakisaka, M., Sasaki, Y., Yamada, K., Kondoh, Y., Hikono, H., Osada, H., Tomii, K., Saito, T., and Aida, Y. (2015). A novel antiviral target structure involved in the RNA binding, dimerization, and nuclear export functions of the influenza A virus nucleoprotein. PLoS Pathog. *11*, e1005062.

Kao, R.Y., Yang, D., Lau, L.S., Tsui, W.H., Hu, L., Dai, J., Chan, M.P., Chan, C.M., Wang, P., Zheng, B.J., *et al.* (2010). Identification of influenza A nucleoprotein as an antiviral target. Nat. Biotechnol. *28*, 600–605.

Karlas, A., Machuy, N., Shin, Y., Pleissner, K.P., Artarini, A., Heuer, D., Becker, D., Khalil, H., Ogilvie, L.A., Hess, S., *et al.* (2010). Genome-wide RNAi screen identifies human host factors crucial for influenza virus replication. Nature *463*, 818–822.

Kashiwagi, T., Hara, K., Nakazono, Y., Uemura, Y., Imamura, Y., Hamada, N., and Watanabe, H. (2014). The N-terminal fragment of a PB2 subunit from the influenza A virus (A/Hong Kong/156/1997 H5N1) effectively inhibits RNP activity and viral replication. PLoS One *9*, e114502.

Kawaguchi, A., Momose, F., and Nagata, K. (2011). Replication-coupled and host factor-mediated encapsidation of the influenza virus genome by viral nucleoprotein. J. Virol. *85*, 6197–6204.
Kingsbury, D.W., Jones, I.M., and Murti, K.G. (1987). Assembly of influenza ribonucleoprotein in vitro using recombinant nucleoprotein. Virology *156*, 396–403.
Kiso, M., Takahashi, K., Sakai-Tagawa, Y., Shinya, K., Sakabe, S., Le, Q.M., Ozawa, M., Furuta, Y., and Kawaoka, Y. (2010). T-705 (favipiravir) activity against lethal H5N1 influenza A viruses. Proc. Natl. Acad. Sci. U.S.A. *107*, 882–887.
Klumpp, K., Ruigrok, R.W., and Baudin, F. (1997). Roles of the influenza virus polymerase and nucleoprotein in forming a functional RNP structure. EMBO J. *16*, 1248–1257.
Kobayashi, M., Toyoda, T., Adyshev, D.M., Azuma, Y., and Ishihama, A. (1994). Molecular dissection of influenza virus nucleoprotein: deletion mapping of the RNA binding domain. J. Virol. *68*, 8433–8436.
Konig, R., Stertz, S., Zhou, Y., Inoue, A., Hoffmann, H.H., Bhattacharyya, S., Alamares, J.G., Tscherne, D.M., Ortigoza, M.B., Liang, Y., *et al.* (2010). Human host factors required for influenza virus replication. Nature *463*, 813–817.
Kowalinski, E., Zubieta, C., Wolkerstorfer, A., Szolar, O.H., Ruigrok, R.W., and Cusack, S. (2012). Structural analysis of specific metal chelating inhibitor binding to the endonuclease domain of influenza pH1N1 (2009) polymerase. PLoS Pathog. *8*, e1002831.
Kukol, A., and Hughes, D.J. (2014). Large-scale analysis of influenza A virus nucleoprotein sequence conservation reveals potential drug-target sites. Virology *454–455*, 40–47.
Lamb, R.A., and Krug, R.M. (2001). Orthomyxoviridae: the viruses and their replication. In Fields Virology, Knipe, D.M., and Howley, P.M. eds. (Lippincott-Raven), pp. 1487–1531.
Lejal, N., Tarus, B., Bouguyon, E., Chenavas, S., Bertho, N., Delmas, B., Ruigrok, R.W., Di Primo, C., and Slama-Schwok, A. (2013). Structure-based discovery of the novel antiviral properties of naproxen against the nucleoprotein of influenza A virus. Antimicrob. Agents Chemother. *57*, 2231–2242.
Liang, Y., Hong, Y., and Parslow, T.G. (2005). cis-Acting packaging signals in the influenza virus PB1, PB2, and PA genomic RNA segments. J. Virol. *79*, 10348–10355.
Liang, Y., Huang, T., Ly, H., and Parslow, T.G. (2008). Mutational analyses of packaging signals in influenza virus PA, PB1, and PB2 genomic RNA segments. J. Virol. *82*, 229–236.
Longhi, S. (2009). Nucleocapsid structure and function. Curr. Top. Microbiol. Immunol. *329*, 103–128.
Luytjes, W., Krystal, M., Enami, M., Parvin, J.D., and Palese, P. (1989). Amplification, expression, and packaging of foreign gene by influenza virus. Cell *59*, 1107–1113.
Marjuki, H., Yen, H.L., Franks, J., Webster, R.G., Pleschka, S., and Hoffmann, E. (2007). Higher polymerase activity of a human influenza virus enhances activation of the hemagglutinin-induced Raf/MEK/ERK signal cascade. Virol. J. *4*, 134.
Marklund, J.K., Ye, Q., Dong, J., Tao, Y.J., and Krug, R.M. (2012). Sequence in the influenza A virus nucleoprotein required for viral polymerase binding and RNA synthesis. J. Virol. *86*, 7292–7297.
Marsh, G.A., Hatami, R., and Palese, P. (2007). Specific residues of the influenza A virus hemagglutinin viral RNA are important for efficient packaging into budding virions. J. Virol. *81*, 9727–9736.
Marsh, G.A., Rabadan, R., Levine, A.J., and Palese, P. (2008). Highly conserved regions of influenza a virus polymerase gene segments are critical for efficient viral RNA packaging. J. Virol. *82*, 2295–2304.
Martin-Benito, J., Area, E., Ortega, J., Llorca, O., Valpuesta, J.M., Carrascosa, J.L., and Ortin, J. (2001). Three-dimensional reconstruction of a recombinant influenza virus ribonucleoprotein particle. EMBO Rep. *2*, 313–317.
Mena, I., Jambrina, E., Albo, C., Perales, B., Ortin, J., Arrese, M., Vallejo, D., and Portela, A. (1999). Mutational analysis of influenza A virus nucleoprotein: identification of mutations that affect RNA replication. J. Virol. *73*, 1186–1194.
Moeller, A., Kirchdoerfer, R.N., Potter, C.S., Carragher, B., and Wilson, I.A. (2012). Organization of the influenza virus replication machinery. Science *338*, 1631–1634.
Momose, F., Basler, C.F., O'Neill, R.E., Iwamatsu, A., Palese, P., and Nagata, K. (2001). Cellular splicing factor RAF-2p48/NPI-5/BAT1/UAP56 interacts with the influenza virus nucleoprotein and enhances viral RNA synthesis. J. Virol. *75*, 1899–1908.
Momose, F., Handa, H., and Nagata, K. (1996). Identification of host factors that regulate the influenza virus RNA polymerase activity. Biochimie *78*, 1103–1108.
Momose, F., Kikuchi, Y., Komase, K., and Morikawa, Y. (2007). Visualization of microtubule-mediated transport of influenza viral progeny ribonucleoprotein. Microbes Infect. *9*, 1422–1433.
Momose, F., Naito, T., Yano, K., Sugimoto, S., Morikawa, Y., and Nagata, K. (2002). Identification of Hsp90 as a stimulatory host factor involved in influenza virus RNA synthesis. J. Biol. Chem. *277*, 45306–45314.

Mondal, A., Potts, G.K., Dawson, A.R., Coon, J.J., and Mehle, A. (2015). Phosphorylation at the homotypic interface regulates nucleoprotein oligomerization and assembly of the influenza virus replication machinery. PLoS Pathog. *11*, e1004826.

Monod, A., Swale, C., Tarus, B., Tissot, A., Delmas, B., Ruigrok, R.W., Crepin, T., and Slama-Schwok, A. (2015). Learning from structure-based drug design and new antivirals targeting the ribonucleoprotein complex for the treatment of influenza. Expert Opin. Drug Discov. *10*, 345–371.

Mukaigawa, J., and Nayak, D.P. (1991). Two signals mediate nuclear localization of influenza virus (A/WSN/33) polymerase basic protein 2. J. Virol. *65*, 245–253.

Muramoto, Y., Takada, A., Fujii, K., Noda, T., Iwatsuki-Horimoto, K., Watanabe, S., Horimoto, T., Kida, H., and Kawaoka, Y. (2006). Hierarchy among viral RNA (vRNA) segments in their role in vRNA incorporation into influenza A virions. J. Virol. *80*, 2318–2325.

Murti, K.G., Webster, R.G., and Jones, I.M. (1988). Localization of RNA polymerases on influenza viral ribonucleoproteins by immunogold labeling. Virology *164*, 562–566.

Naito, T., Kiyasu, Y., Sugiyama, K., Kimura, A., Nakano, R., Matsukage, A., and Nagata, K. (2007). An influenza virus replicon system in yeast identified Tat-SF1 as a stimulatory host factor for viral RNA synthesis. Proc. Natl. Acad. Sci. U.S.A. *104*, 18235–18240.

Nath, S.T., and Nayak, D.P. (1990). Function of two discrete regions is required for nuclear localization of polymerase basic protein 1 of A/WSN/33 influenza virus (H1 N1). Mol. Cell. Biol. *10*, 4139–4145.

Nayak, D.P., Sivasubramanian, N., Davis, A.R., Cortini, R., and Sung, J. (1982). Complete sequence analyses show that two defective interfering influenza viral RNAs contain a single internal deletion of a polymerase gene. Proc. Natl. Acad. Sci. U.S.A. *79*, 2216–2220.

Neumann, G., and Hobom, G. (1995). Mutational analysis of influenza virus promoter elements in vivo. J. Gen. Virol. *76*, 1709–1717.

Neumann, G., Brownlee, G.G., Fodor, E., and Kawaoka, Y. (2004). Orthomyxovirus replication, transcription, and polyadenylation. Curr. Top. Microbiol. Immunol. *283*, 121–143.

Neumann, G., Castrucci, M.R., and Kawaoka, Y. (1997). Nuclear import and export of influenza virus nucleoprotein. J. Virol. *71*, 9690–9700.

Neumann, G., Hughes, M.T., and Kawaoka, Y. (2000). Influenza A virus NS2 protein mediates vRNP nuclear export through NES-independent interaction with hCRM1. EMBO J. *19*, 6751–6758.

Newcomb, L.L., Kuo, R.L., Ye, Q., Jiang, Y., Tao, Y.J., and Krug, R.M. (2009). Interaction of the influenza a virus nucleocapsid protein with the viral RNA polymerase potentiates unprimed viral RNA replication. J. Virol. *83*, 29–36.

Ng, A.K., Lam, M.K., Zhang, H., Liu, J., Au, S.W., Chan, P.K., Wang, J., and Shaw, P.C. (2012). Structural basis for RNA binding and homo-oligomer formation by influenza B virus nucleoprotein. J. Virol. *86*, 6758–6767.

Ng, A.K., Zhang, H., Tan, K., Li, Z., Liu, J.H., Chan, P.K., Li, S.M., Chan, W.Y., Au, S.W., Joachimiak, A., *et al.* (2008). Structure of the influenza virus A H5N1 nucleoprotein: implications for RNA binding, oligomerization, and vaccine design. FASEB J. *22*, 3638–3647.

Nieto, A., de la Luna, S., Barcena, J., Portela, A., and Ortin, J. (1994). Complex structure of the nuclear translocation signal of influenza virus polymerase PA subunit. J. Gen. Virol. *75*, 29–36.

Noble, S., and Dimmock, N.J. (1995). Characterization of putative defective interfering (DI) A/WSN RNAs isolated from the lungs of mice protected from an otherwise lethal respiratory infection with influenza virus A/WSN (H1N1): a subset of the inoculum DI RNAs. Virology *210*, 9–19.

Noda, T., Sagara, H., Yen, A., Takada, A., Kida, H., Cheng, R.H., and Kawaoka, Y. (2006). Architecture of ribonucleoprotein complexes in influenza A virus particles. Nature *439*, 490–492.

Noda, T., Sugita, Y., Aoyama, K., Hirase, A., Kawakami, E., Miyazawa, A., Sagara, H., and Kawaoka, Y. (2012). Three-dimensional analysis of ribonucleoprotein complexes in influenza A virus. Nat. Commun. *3*, 639.

O'Neill, R.E., Jaskunas, R., Blobel, G., Palese, P., and Moroianu, J. (1995). Nuclear import of influenza virus RNA can be mediated by viral nucleoprotein and transport factors required for protein import. J. Biol. Chem. *270*, 22701–22704.

O'Neill, R.E., Talon, J., and Palese, P. (1998). The influenza virus NEP (NS2 protein) mediates the nuclear export of viral ribonucleoproteins. EMBO J. *17*, 288–296.

Obayashi, E., Yoshida, H., Kawai, F., Shibayama, N., Kawaguchi, A., Nagata, K., Tame, J.R., and Park, S.Y. (2008). The structural basis for an essential subunit interaction in influenza virus RNA polymerase. Nature *454*, 1127–1131.

Odagiri, T., and Tashiro, M. (1997). Segment-specific noncoding sequences of the influenza virus genome RNA are involved in the specific competition between defective interfering RNA and its progenitor RNA segment at the virion assembly step. J. Virol. *71*, 2138–2145.

Ortega, J., Martin-Benito, J., Zurcher, T., Valpuesta, J.M., Carrascosa, J.L., and Ortin, J. (2000). Ultrastructural and functional analyses of recombinant influenza virus ribonucleoproteins suggest dimerization of nucleoprotein during virus amplification. J. Virol. *74*, 156–163.

Ozawa, M., Fujii, K., Muramoto, Y., Yamada, S., Yamayoshi, S., Takada, A., Goto, H., Horimoto, T., and Kawaoka, Y. (2007). Contributions of two nuclear localization signals of influenza A virus nucleoprotein to viral replication. J. Virol. *81*, 30–41.

Ozawa, M., Maeda, J., Iwatsuki-Horimoto, K., Watanabe, S., Goto, H., Horimoto, T., and Kawaoka, Y. (2009). Nucleotide sequence requirements at the 5′ end of the influenza A virus M RNA segment for efficient virus replication. J. Virol. *83*, 3384–3388.

Parvin, J.D., Palese, P., Honda, A., Ishihama, A., and Krystal, M. (1989). Promoter analysis of influenza virus RNA polymerase. J. Virol. *63*, 5142–5152.

Pautus, S., Sehr, P., Lewis, J., Fortune, A., Wolkerstorfer, A., Szolar, O., Guilligay, D., Lunardi, T., Decout, J.L., and Cusack, S. (2013). New 7-methylguanine derivatives targeting the influenza polymerase PB2 cap-binding domain. J. Med. Chem. *56*, 8915–8930.

Pflug, A., Guilligay, D., Reich, S., and Cusack, S. (2014). Structure of influenza A polymerase bound to the viral RNA promoter. Nature *516*, 355–360.

Pleschka, S., Wolff, T., Ehrhardt, C., Hobom, G., Planz, O., Rapp, U.R., and Ludwig, S. (2001). Influenza virus propagation is impaired by inhibition of the Raf/MEK/ERK signalling cascade. Nat. Cell. Biol. *3*, 301–305.

Poch, O., Sauvaget, I., Delarue, M., and Tordo, N. (1989). Identification of four conserved motifs among the RNA-dependent polymerase encoding elements. EMBO J. *8*, 3867–3874.

Pons, M.W., Schulze, I.T., Hirst, G.K., and Hauser, R. (1969). Isolation and characterization of the ribonucleoprotein of influenza virus. Virology *39*, 250–259.

Portela, A., and Digard, P. (2002). The influenza virus nucleoprotein: a multifunctional RNA-binding protein pivotal to virus replication. J. Gen. Virol. *83*, 723–734.

Reich, S., Guilligay, D., Pflug, A., Malet, H., Berger, I., Crepin, T., Hart, D., Lunardi, T., Nanao, M., Ruigrok, R.W., *et al.* (2014). Structural insight into cap-snatching and RNA synthesis by influenza polymerase. Nature *516*, 361–366.

Resa-Infante, P., Jorba, N., Coloma, R., and Ortin, J. (2011). The influenza virus RNA synthesis machine: advances in its structure and function. RNA Biol. *8*, 207–215.

Reuther, P., Manz, B., Brunotte, L., Schwemmle, M., and Wunderlich, K. (2011). Targeting of the influenza A virus polymerase PB1-PB2 interface indicates strain-specific assembly differences. J. Virol. *85*, 13298–13309.

Robertson, J.S. (1979). 5′ and 3′ terminal nucleotide sequences of the RNA genome segments of influenza virus. Nucleic Acids Res. *6*, 3745–3757.

Ruigrok, R.W., and Baudin, F. (1995). Structure of influenza virus ribonucleoprotein particles. II. Purified RNA-free influenza virus ribonucleoprotein forms structures that are indistinguishable from the intact influenza virus ribonucleoprotein particles. J. Gen. Virol. *76*, 1009–1014.

Ruigrok, R.W., Crepin, T., Hart, D.J., and Cusack, S. (2010). Towards an atomic resolution understanding of the influenza virus replication machinery. Curr. Opin. Struct. Biol. *20*, 104–113.

Sagong, H.Y., Bauman, J.D., Patel, D., Das, K., Arnold, E., and LaVoie, E.J. (2014). Phenyl substituted 4-hydroxypyridazin-3(2H)-ones and 5-hydroxypyrimidin-4(3H)-ones: inhibitors of influenza A endonuclease. J. Med. Chem. *57*, 8086–8098.

Shapira, S.D., Gat-Viks, I., Shum, B.O., Dricot, A., de Grace, M.M., Wu, L., Gupta, P.B., Hao, T., Silver, S.J., Root, D.E., *et al.* (2009). A physical and regulatory map of host-influenza interactions reveals pathways in H1N1 infection. Cell *139*, 1255–1267.

Shen, Y.F., Chen, Y.H., Chu, S.Y., Lin, M.I., Hsu, H.T., Wu, P.Y., Wu, C.J., Liu, H.W., Lin, F.Y., Lin, G., *et al.* (2011). E339...R416 salt bridge of nucleoprotein as a feasible target for influenza virus inhibitors. Proc. Natl. Acad. Sci. U.S.A. *108*, 16515–16520.

Skehel, J.J., and Hay, A.J. (1978). Nucleotide sequences at the 5′ termini of influenza virus RNAs and their transcripts. Nucleic Acids Res. *5*, 1207–1219.

Sugita, Y., Sagara, H., Noda, T., and Kawaoka, Y. (2013). Configuration of viral ribonucleoprotein complexes within the influenza A virion. J. Virol. *87*, 12879–12884.

Sugiyama, K., Obayashi, E., Kawaguchi, A., Suzuki, Y., Tame, J.R., Nagata, K., and Park, S.Y. (2009). Structural insight into the essential PB1-PB2 subunit contact of the influenza virus RNA polymerase. EMBO J. *28*, 1803–1811.

Tao, Y., Farsetta, D.L., Nibert, M.L., and Harrison, S.C. (2002). RNA synthesis in a cage—structural studies of reovirus polymerase lambda3. Cell *111*, 733–745.

Tarendeau, F., Boudet, J., Guilligay, D., Mas, P.J., Bougault, C.M., Boulo, S., Baudin, F., Ruigrok, R.W., Daigle, N., Ellenberg, J., *et al.* (2007). Structure and nuclear import function of the C-terminal domain of influenza virus polymerase PB2 subunit. Nat. Struct. Mol. Biol. *14*, 229–233.

Tarendeau, F., Crepin, T., Guilligay, D., Ruigrok, R.W., Cusack, S., and Hart, D.J. (2008). Host determinant residue lysine 627 lies on the surface of a discrete, folded domain of influenza virus polymerase PB2 subunit. PLoS Pathog. *4*, e1000136.

Tarus, B., Bakowiez, O., Chenavas, S., Duchemin, L., Estrozi, L.F., Bourdieu, C., Lejal, N., Bernard, J., Moudjou, M., Chevalier, C., *et al.* (2012). Oligomerization paths of the nucleoprotein of influenza A virus. Biochimie *94*, 776–785.

Tarus, B., Bertrand, H., Zedda, G., Di Primo, C., Quideau, S., and Slama-Schwok, A. (2015). Structure-based design of novel naproxen derivatives targeting monomeric nucleoprotein of Influenza A virus. J. Biomol. Struct. Dyn. *33*, 1899–1912.

Torreira, E., Schoehn, G., Fernandez, Y., Jorba, N., Ruigrok, R.W., Cusack, S., Ortin, J., and Llorca, O. (2007). Three-dimensional model for the isolated recombinant influenza virus polymerase heterotrimer. Nucleic Acids Res. *35*, 3774–3783.

Tsurumura, T., Qiu, H., Yoshida, T., Tsumori, Y., Hatakeyama, D., Kuzuhara, T., and Tsuge, H. (2013). Conformational polymorphism of m7GTP in crystal structure of the PB2 middle domain from human influenza A virus. PLoS One *8*, e82020.

Turrell, L., Hutchinson, E.C., Vreede, F.T., and Fodor, E. (2015). Regulation of influenza A virus nucleoprotein oligomerization by phosphorylation. J. Virol. *89*, 1452–1455.

Verhelst, J., Parthoens, E., Schepens, B., Fiers, W., and Saelens, X. (2012). Interferon-inducible protein Mx1 inhibits influenza virus by interfering with functional viral ribonucleoprotein complex assembly. J. Virol. *86*, 13445–13455.

Wang, P., Palese, P., and O'Neill, R.E. (1997). The NPI-1/NPI-3 (karyopherin alpha) binding site on the influenza a virus nucleoprotein NP is a nonconventional nuclear localization signal. J. Virol. *71*, 1850–1856.

Wang, Z., Liu, X., Zhao, Z., Xu, C., Zhang, K., Chen, C., Sun, L., Gao, G.F., Ye, X., and Liu, W. (2011). Cyclophilin E functions as a negative regulator to influenza virus replication by impairing the formation of the viral ribonucleoprotein complex. PLoS One *6*, e22625.

Watanabe, T., Watanabe, S., and Kawaoka, Y. (2010). Cellular networks involved in the influenza virus life cycle. Cell Host Microbe *7*, 427–439.

Watanabe, T., Watanabe, S., Noda, T., Fujii, Y., and Kawaoka, Y. (2003). Exploitation of nucleic acid packaging signals to generate a novel influenza virus-based vector stably expressing two foreign genes. J. Virol. *77*, 10575–10583.

Weber, F., Kochs, G., Gruber, S., and Haller, O. (1998). A classical bipartite nuclear localization signal on Thogoto and influenza A virus nucleoproteins. Virology *250*, 9–18.

Wu, C.Y., Jeng, K.S., and Lai, M.M. (2011). The SUMOylation of matrix protein M1 modulates the assembly and morphogenesis of influenza A virus. J. Virol. *85*, 6618–6628.

Wu, W.W., Sun, Y.H., and Pante, N. (2007a). Nuclear import of influenza A viral ribonucleoprotein complexes is mediated by two nuclear localization sequences on viral nucleoprotein. Virol. J. *4*, 49.

Wu, W.W., Weaver, L.L., and Pante, N. (2007b). Ultrastructural analysis of the nuclear localization sequences on influenza A ribonucleoprotein complexes. J. Mol. Biol. *374*, 910–916.

Wunderlich, K., Mayer, D., Ranadheera, C., Holler, A.S., Manz, B., Martin, A., Chase, G., Tegge, W., Frank, R., Kessler, U., *et al.* (2009). Identification of a PA-binding peptide with inhibitory activity against influenza A and B virus replication. PLoS One *4*, e7517.

Yamanaka, K., Ishihama, A., and Nagata, K. (1990). Reconstitution of influenza virus RNA-nucleoprotein complexes structurally resembling native viral ribonucleoprotein cores. J. Biol. Chem. *265*, 11151–11155.

Ye, Q., Guu, T.S., Mata, D.A., Kuo, R.L., Smith, B., Krug, R.M., and Tao, Y.J. (2012). Biochemical and structural evidence in support of a coherent model for the formation of the double-helical influenza A virus ribonucleoprotein. MBio *4*, e00467–00412.

Ye, Q., Krug, R.M., and Tao, Y.J. (2006). The mechanism by which influenza A virus nucleoprotein forms oligomers and binds RNA. Nature *444*, 1078–1082.

York, A., Hengrung, N., Vreede, F.T., Huiskonen, J.T., and Fodor, E. (2013). Isolation and characterization of the positive-sense replicative intermediate of a negative-strand RNA virus. Proc. Natl. Acad. Sci. U.S.A. *110*, E4238–4245.

Yuan, P., Bartlam, M., Lou, Z., Chen, S., Zhou, J., He, X., Lv, Z., Ge, R., Li, X., Deng, T., *et al.* (2009). Crystal structure of an avian influenza polymerase PA(N) reveals an endonuclease active site. Nature *458*, 909–913.

Zheng, W., Olson, J., Vakharia, V., and Tao, Y.J. (2013). The crystal structure and RNA-binding of an orthomyxovirus nucleoprotein. PLoS Pathog. *9*, e1003624.

Zhou, Z., Cao, M., Guo, Y., Zhao, L., Wang, J., Jia, X., Li, J., Wang, C., Gabriel, G., Xue, Q., *et al.* (2014). Fragile X mental retardation protein stimulates ribonucleoprotein assembly of influenza A virus. Nat. Commun. *5*, 3259.

Host Factors Regulating the Influenza Virus Replication Machinery

5

James Kirui*, Vy Tran* and Andrew Mehle

Abstract

The influenza replication machinery drives gene expression and genome replication. Whereas the viral polymerase contains all of the intrinsic enzymatic activity required for these processes, it is dependent upon interactions with host cell factors for a successful infection. Here we describe the host factors that have been shown to interact with and modulate the viral polymerase. These include host factors repurposed by the virus, factors whose normal activities have been disrupted, viral and host proteins that regulate polymerase function, and host mechanisms that antagonize the viral replication machinery in an unsuccessful attempt to stop replication.

Introduction

Influenza A virus is a negative-stranded RNA viruses whose genome contains eight separate genome segments. Infection initiates via receptor-mediated endocytosis (Fig. 5.1). Maturation of the endosome results in a decrease in endosomal pH with two major consequences for the incoming virion: pH-dependent fusion of viral and host membranes performed by the viral haemagglutinin; and the acidification and disassembly of the viral core due to an influx of protons via the viral M2 ion channel. Both of these events are required for the release of the viral genome into the cytoplasm of the infected cell.

The viral genome is packaged as a large ribonucleoprotein (RNP) complex composed of the negative-sense vRNA, the viral nucleoprotein (NP), and the viral polymerase (Fig. 5.2). The polymerase is a ~250 kDa heterotrimer composed of the polypeptides PB1, PB2, and PA. The polymerase associates with the termini of the genomic RNA and NP in the RNP where it mediates transcription and replication. These components and processes are described in detail in Chapters 2 and 4. Briefly, PB1 is catalytic subunit of the polymerase and binds to PB2 and PA to form the trimeric holoenzyme (Digard *et al.*, 1989; Hao *et al.*, 2008; Obayashi *et al.*, 2008; Sugiyama *et al.*, 2009). PB1 also binds NP and genomic RNAs in the course of vRNPs assembly (Biswas *et al.*, 1998; Li *et al.*, 1998; Medcalf *et al.*, 1999). PB2 binds directly to PB1 and NP in the RNP. PB2 also binds to host mRNAs via the m^7G cap appended to their 5′ end during transcription of viral mRNAs (Biswas *et al.*, 1998; Poole *et al.*, 2004; Ulmanen *et al.*, 1981). PA binds to PB1 as well, and is an essential part of the polymerase, possessing the endonuclease activity required for transcription (Dias *et al.*, 2009; Yuan *et al.*, 2009). PA and PB2 do not form a stable interaction, but bimolecular fluorescence complementation assays show that they are in close proximity (Hemerka *et al.*, 2009). The multiple

*These authors contributed equally.

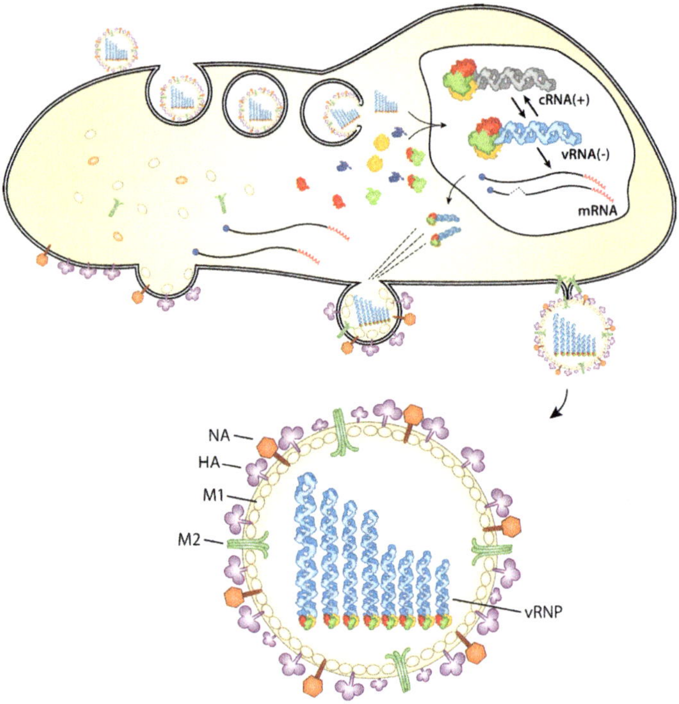

Figure 5.1 Overview of the influenza virus replication cycle.

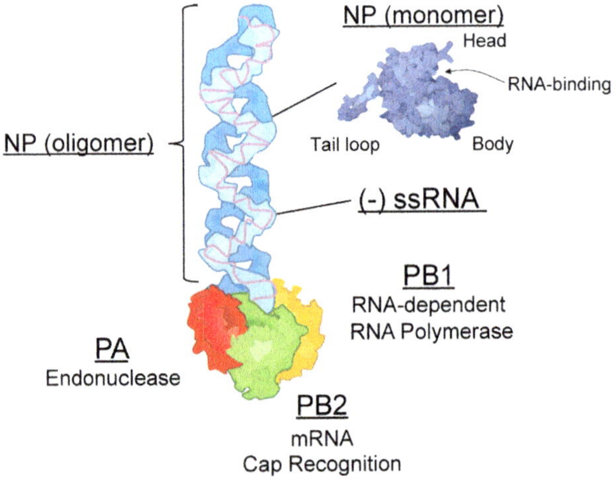

Figure 5.2 The influenza virus ribonucleoprotein complex.

interactions between the polymerase subunits have been confirmed in three-dimensional reconstructions from electron microscopy that reveal the polymerase as a compact globular structure (Area *et al.*, 2004; Arranz *et al.*, 2012; Coloma *et al.*, 2009; Moeller *et al.*, 2012). Indeed, the recently solved atomic-resolution structures of the polymerases from influenza A and B viruses show a U-shaped complex with all three subunits located close together in a compact core at the base of the U (Pflug *et al.*, 2014; Reich *et al.*, 2014).

Upon release into the cytoplasm, vRNPs are transported to the nucleus and undergo an initial round of transcription (Herz *et al.*, 1981). Influenza virus transcripts are produced by 'cap-snatching' wherein a short host-derived m^7G-capped RNA primes synthesis of viral mRNAs (Fig. 5.1) (Plotch *et al.*, 1981). The 5′ end of the minus-sense genomic RNA (vRNA) is bound by PB1 and activates cap binding by the PB2 subunit (Cianci *et al.*, 1995; Hagen *et al.*, 1994; Li *et al.*, 1998). PB2 uses a non-canonical cap binding pocket to bind the m^7G cap on host mRNAs (Fechter *et al.*, 2003; Guilligay *et al.*, 2008; Ulmanen *et al.*, 1981). PB1 also binds the 3′ end of vRNA (Li *et al.*, 2001). Host mRNA and snRNA transcripts are then cleaved 10–12 nucleotides downstream from the m^7G cap by the N-terminal endonuclease domain in PA (Dias *et al.*, 2009; Koppstein *et al.*, 2015; Yuan *et al.*, 2009). These short, capped RNAs are used to prime synthesis of viral mRNA. The terminal nucleotide of the capped primer base-pairs with the template vRNA and nascent chain synthesis is performed by PB1 (Romanos and Hay, 1984). Transcription continues to a conserved poly(U) stretch of 5–7 nucleotides at the 5′ end of all vRNAs. Repeated copying and slippage on the poly(U) tract produces a non-templated poly(A) tail of ~20 nucleotides on the 3′ end of viral messages (Li and Palese, 1994; Poon *et al.*, 1999; Robertson *et al.*, 1981). In this way, the completed viral transcript contains the 5′ cap and 3′ poly(A) tail characteristic of efficiently translated mRNAs.

The viral genome is replicated by the same machinery used for transcription. vRNA templates in the incoming vRNPs are copied to plus-sense complementary RNA (cRNA) intermediates that are packaged into cRNPs (Fig. 5.1). PB1 again binds both of the genome termini and catalyses extension (Li *et al.*, 1998). Unlike transcription, cRNA synthesis is primer-independent and by-passes the polyadenylation signal to produce full-length copies (Hay *et al.*, 1982). Full-length cRNA synthesis also requires free NP that oligomerizes along the length of the nascent RNA to form cRNPs (Honda *et al.*, 1988; Shapiro and Krug, 1988; Vreede *et al.*, 2011). cRNPs then use an analogous process to copy new genomic vRNAs and produce vRNPs. Finally, the newly made vRNPs can initiation another round of replication, template more mRNA synthesis, or be packaged into newly budding virions.

Whereas all of the enzymatic activity required for replication and transcription are contained solely in the viral polymerase, the viral replication cycle is dependent upon the host cell and interaction with host factors. This chapter summarizes our current knowledge of the host factors that are exploited by the viral replication machinery, and in some cases factors that attempt to regulate or restrict its activity (Table 5.1). By no means is this an exhaustive description, and the reader is referred to FluMap for a more comprehensive list of host proteins that impact replication (http://www.influenza-x.org/flumap/ (Matsuoka *et al.*, 2013)). And while this chapter focuses on those interactions with proposed functional consequences, the viral replication machinery has an even larger 'interactome' that almost certainly plays a role in viral replication, host range and pathogenicity (Bortz *et al.*, 2011; Bradel-Tretheway *et al.*, 2011; Jorba *et al.*, 2008; Mayer *et al.*, 2007; Munier *et al.*, 2013; Shapira *et al.*, 2009; Tafforeau *et al.*, 2011; Watanabe *et al.*, 2014; York *et al.*, 2014).

Table 5.1 An abbreviated list of host factors regulating the influenza virus replication machinery

Influenza protein	Host interactor	Identified activity	Reference
vRNP			
	Importin α1 and α2	Nuclear import	Cros *et al.* (2005), Wang *et al.* (1997)
	Chromatin	Replication, nuclear export	Chase *et al.* (2011)
	YB-1	Nuclear export, cytoplasmic trafficking	Kawaguchi *et al.* (2012)
	HRB	Nuclear export	Eisfeld *et al.* (2011b)
	Rab11-positive endosomes	Cytoplasmic trafficking	Amorim *et al.* (2011), Eisfeld *et al.* (2011a)
	Microtubules/MTOC	Cytoplasmic trafficking	Amorim *et al.* (2011), Momose *et al.* (2007)
	RNA pol II	Cap-snatching	Engelhardt *et al.* (2005)
	Cyclin T1/Cdk9	Cap-snatching	Zhang *et al.* (2010)
	SFPQ/PSF	Polyadenylation	Landeras-Bueno *et al.* (2011)
	NPM1	Replication/ transcription	Mayer *et al.* (2007)
	PP6	Replication/ transcription	York, *et al.* (2014)
	RBL2	Antagonism of vRNP	Kakugawa *et al.* (2009)
	RIG-I	Antagonism of vRNP	Kakugawa *et al.* (2009), Weber *et al.* (2013)
	RIG-I	Species-specific inhibitor	Weber *et al.* (2015)
Polymerase			
	Crm1 (via NEP)	Nuclear export	Manz *et al.* (2012)
	Crm1 (via M1 and NEP)	Nuclear export	Paterson and Fodor, (2012)
	Hsp90	Chaperone	Momose *et al.* (2002).
	p23	Chaperone	Ge *et al.* (2011)
	ANP32A/ANP32B (pp32/APRIL)	Replication	Sugiyama *et al.* (2016)
	ANP32A	Species-specific enhancer	Long *et al.* (2016)
PB1			
	RanBP5	Nuclear import	Deng *et al.* (2006), Hutchinson *et al.* (2011)
	Ebp1	Antagonism of vRNP	Honda *et al.* (2007)
	RED/SMU1	NS splicing	Fournier, *et al.* (2014)
	TRIM32	Ubiquitination of PB1	Fu, *et al.* (2015)
	DDX21	Antagonize polymerase assembly	Chen, *et al.* (2014)

Influenza protein	Host interactor	Identified activity	Reference
PB1-F2			
	MAVS	Disruption of antiviral response	Dudek *et al.* (2011), Varga *et al.* (2011)
PB2			
	Importin α1, α3, α5, α7	Nuclear import	Gabriel *et al.* (2008, 2011), Resa-Infante *et al.* (2008), Tarendeau *et al.* (2007)
	m^7G cap on mRNA	Cap-snatching	Guilligay *et al.* (2008)
	Hsp90	Chaperone, replication	Momose *et al.* (2002)
	CCT	Chaperone	Fislova *et al.* (2010)
	Rab11	Cytoplasmic trafficking	Avilov *et al.* (2012)
	MAVS	Disruption of antiviral response	Graef *et al.* (2010), Iwai *et al.* (2010)
	RED/SMU1	NS splicing	Fournier, *et al.* (2014)
PA			
	hCLE	Transcription/ replication	Huarte *et al.* (2001)
	MCM2–7	Replication	Kawaguchi and Nagata (2007)
NP			
	Importin α1 and α2	Nuclear import	Cros *et al.* (2005), Wang *et al.* (1997)
	Crm1	Nuclear export	Elton *et al.* (2001)
	HMGB1 and 2	Chromatin association	Moisy *et al.* (2012)
	RAF-2p48 (DDX39B/ UAP59/Bat1)	Replication	Kawaguchi *et al.* (2011), Momose *et al.* (2001)
	Tat-SF1	Replication	Naito *et al.* (2007a)
	FMRP	RNP assembly	Naito *et al.* (2007a)
	MxA/Mx1	Antagonism of vRNP	Dittmann *et al.* (2008)
	RBL2	Antagonism of vRNP	Kakugawa *et al.* (2009)
	NF90	Antagonism of vRNP	Wang *et al.* (2009)
	CypE	Antagonism of vRNP	Wang *et al.* (2011)

Assembling the replication machinery in the nucleus

Unlike many other RNA viruses whose replication occurs in the cytoplasm, influenza virus replication and transcription occurs exclusively inside the nucleus of the host cell (Herz *et al.*, 1981; Jackson *et al.*, 1982; Shapiro *et al.*, 1987). This therefore requires that following release from the viral core the vRNPs transit to the nucleus. As vRNPs are massive molecular complexes from ~2.5 to 6 MDa, they are incapable of passive diffusion across the nuclear envelope and are imported by an active, energy-dependent process. Incoming vRNPs exploit the classical import pathway to enter the nucleus via the nuclear pore complex (NPC) within 20 minutes pos infection (Chou *et al.*, 2013; Martin and Helenius, 1991b; O'Neill *et al.*, 1995). In the classical import pathway, a nuclear localization signal (NLS) on the cargo is bound by importin α, which is in turn bound by importin β (also known as karyopherin α and β1, respectively). Importin β then engages the NPC to allow import. Once inside the nucleus, importin β is bound by RanGTP and the import complex dissociates releasing the cargo into the nucleoplasm. The newly formed importin β:RanGTP complex shuttles back to the cytoplasm where GTP is hydrolysed, importin β dissociates and the cycle begins again. An unconventional NLS at the N-terminus of NP interacts with importin α1 or α2 to drive the import of incoming vRNPs; this is the same NLS that mediates import of NP alone (Cros *et al.*, 2005; Wang *et al.*, 1997). Biochemical evidence localized the NLS to amino acids 3–13 of NP and showed that this region interacts with the importin α proteins (Wang *et al.*, 1997). Supporting these findings, the crystal structure of the NP trimer revealed that the proposed NLS is solvent exposed and disordered, and thus accessible for binding by import factors in the context of the NP oligomers present in the vRNP (Ng *et al.*, 2008; Ye *et al.*, 2006). The eight incoming vRNPs appear to remain associated throughout the transit process and only dissociate after nuclear import (Chou *et al.*, 2013; Nevalainen *et al.*, 2010). By 60 minutes post infection, the viral genome has already gained access to nucleus, dispersed throughout the nucleoplasm and undergone initial rounds of replication and mRNA synthesis (Chou *et al.*, 2013; Smith and Hay, 1982).

The viral mRNAs are exported to the cytoplasm for translation. All of the newly made RNP components are then imported back into the nucleus for assembly of polymerase trimers, RNPs and further rounds of genome replication and transcription. As mentioned, NP is imported by interacting with importin α1 or α2. PB2 also utilizes the classical import pathway via an NLS identified at the extreme C-terminus of PB2 (Gabriel *et al.*, 2008; Mukaigawa and Nayak, 1991; Tarendeau *et al.*, 2007). Structural analysis of the C-terminus of PB2 revealed a compact a-b structure that undergoes a large rearrangement into an elongated conformation with a bipartite NLS bound by importin α5 (Tarendeau *et al.*, 2007). PB2 has also been shown to interact with importin α1, α3 and α7 (Boivin and Hart, 2011; Gabriel *et al.*, 2008, 2011; Resa-Infante *et al.*, 2008). Which of these importins is preferentially used during infection or whether they function redundantly for PB2 is unclear. However, which importin α proteins are present in the infected cell impacts viral pathogenicity and host range as they have been proposed as species-specific regulators of viral infection (Gabriel *et al.*, 2008). As viruses move from birds to people, adaptive mutations in both NP and PB2 increase their usage of human importin as versus their avian homologues, enhancing nuclear import, virus replication and pathogenicity (Gabriel *et al.*, 2005, 2008; Resa-Infante *et al.*, 2008).

PA and PB1 both contain sequences that mediate nuclear import when the proteins are expressed alone; classical bipartite NLSs are located in residues 124–139 for PA and 187–211 for PB1 (Nath and Nayak, 1990; Nieto *et al.*, 1994). However, import is inefficient for individually expressed subunits. Current data best support a model where PB1 and PA form a complex in the cytoplasm and are then imported into the nucleus as a dimer by the cellular import factor RanBP5 (Deng *et al.*, 2006; Fodor and Smith, 2004). RanBP5, also known as importin β3 or importin 5, is a non-classical nuclear import factor that binds cargo directly, precluding the requirement for an importin α adaptor and facilitating entry through the NPC. RanBP5 binds to PB1 in the presence or absence of PA, but not in the context of the polymerase trimer, and may prevent premature association of PB2 with the PB1–PA complex (Deng *et al.*, 2006). The NLS in PB1 mediates interaction with RanBP5 and enhances, but is not required for nuclear localization of the PB1-PA dimer (Hutchinson *et al.*, 2011). The largest stimulator of PB1 nuclear import is binding to PA, although it is not known how this alters localization (Fodor and Smith, 2004; Hutchinson *et al.*, 2011). Once inside the nucleus, RanBP5 is bound by RanGTP and releases its cargo allowing polymerase assembly to continue.

Atomic structures show that the polymerase trimer is assembled through direct interactions at defined interfaces between domains in PB1 and PA and between domains in PB1 and PB2, along with a number of more dispersed interactions between PB1 and interdomain linker regions from PB2 and PA that are crucial for assembly (Hengrung *et al.*, 2015; Pflug *et al.*, 2014; Reich *et al.*, 2014; Thierry *et al.*, 2016). The PB1–PA interface involves the insertion of the extreme N-terminus of PB1 into the 'jaws' of the C-terminal domain of PA (He *et al.*, 2008; Obayashi *et al.*, 2008). PA almost encircles the PB1 peptide. The PB1–PB2 interfaces includes the extreme C-terminus of PB1 and the N-terminus of PB2. Helices from both proteins interleave to form the binding site (Sugiyama *et al.*, 2009). These complex interfaces are possibly assembled through co-folding of the two separate polypeptides, and evidence suggests an important role for cellular chaperones during this process. Chaperones are involved in various protein related functions including *de novo* protein folding, refolding of stress-denatured proteins, assembling oligomers, protein trafficking and assistance in proteolytic degradation (Hartl *et al.*, 2011). A number of chaperones interact with the influenza replication proteins. Hsp90 was identified by biochemical fractionation as a PB2-interacting factor with a stimulatory effect on *in vitro* viral polymerase activity (Momose *et al.*, 2002). It was subsequently shown that PB2 re-localizes Hsp90 to the nucleus of infected cells (Naito *et al.*, 2007b). Hsp90 dissociates from PB2 upon polymerase formation, consistent with a role in aiding assembly of PB2 onto the pre-formed PB1-PA dimer. This is supported by experiments showing that chemical inhibitors of Hsp90 reduce polymerase activity and virus replication (Chase *et al.*, 2008). Another chaperone identified to interact with PB2 is the eight-membered cytosolic chaperonin containing TCP-1 (CCT) complex (Fislova *et al.*, 2010). CCT binds PB2, but not the polymerase trimer, and is thought to be involved in the correct folding of the PB2 subunit. Silencing of CCT reduced PB2 levels, polymerase activity and virus replication. Other chaperones that associate with the polymerase include the Hsp90 co-chaperone p23, Hsp60 and Hsp70, but their functions during infection are less defined (Ge *et al.*, 2011; Fislova *et al.*, 2010; Hirayama *et al.*, 2004). Finally, in addition to their role in nuclear import, is has been suggested that importins may also help chaperone protein folding. In the case of influenza, importins may stabilize assembly intermediates as the polymerase subunits and NP move to the nucleus where the final supermolecular complexes are formed (Hutchinson and Fodor, 2012). A key observation of the recent atomic structures is that the C-terminus of PB2 undergoes large-scale conformational rearrangements within the trimer (Hengrung *et al.*, 2015; Thierry *et al.*, 2016). It will be important to determine whether chaperones play a role in this remodelling and how the different states of PB2 impact polymerase function.

Replication and transcription in the nucleus

Both transcription and replication of the influenza viral genome occurs in the nucleus. Thus, for both the virus and the host cell, the nuclear compartment serves as the site for initiating gene expression. The nuclear landscape in the host is densely packed with chromatin, subnuclear domains (the nucleolus, PML bodies, nuclear matrix, etc.), and a diversity of host proteins, enzymes and nucleic acids. Influenza viruses have evolved an important replication strategy to take advantage of these factors present in the host nucleus making its viral life cycle unique among other RNA viruses. By hijacking cellular factors, influenza viral proteins and complexes are able to navigate through the nucleus facilitating gene expression, traffic throughout the cell, modulate their catalytic activities, and counteract antiviral host factors.

Host factors required for transcription and processing of viral messages

Upon import into the nucleus, influenza RNPs associate with nuclear host factors to immediately begin viral gene expression. Incoming vRNA genomes have negative polarity and thus cannot be immediately translated into protein upon entry. Because all viral RNA synthesis is performed by the viral polymerase, cellular factors and entire cellular pathways are required to process these transcripts and express them as proteins. Transcription occurs by cap-snatching, thus an essential host factor is the m^7G cap located at the 5′ end of cellular mRNAs that is bound by the PB2 subunit (Guilligay *et al.*, 2008). The m^7G cap and a short stretch of heterogeneous cellular RNA fragments are appended to all influenza viral messages. As a consequence, influenza transcription is functionally dependent on host transcription and blocking host transcription with a-amanitin prevents viral mRNA synthesis (Lamb and Choppin, 1977).

In host cells, transcription, capping, splicing, and assembly of nuclear-export competent RNAs is performed by the DNA-dependent RNA polymerase II (Pol II) and Pol II-associated factors. The influenza polymerase localizes to sites of active transcription initiation and physically interacts with Pol II (Chan *et al.*, 2006; Engelhardt *et al.*, 2005). Pol II associated with the influenza polymerase is specifically enriched for phosphorylation at serine 5 in the C-terminal domain (CTD). This differentially phosphorylated form of Pol II is present early in the cellular transcription cycle when capping of nascent transcripts occurs. Additionally, the CTD also serves as an important docking site for accessory factors necessary for capping and splicing pre-mRNAs. Interaction between the viral polymerase and Pol II presumably enables the viral machinery to preferentially access newly capped pre-mRNAs and a high concentration of host factors that regulate mRNA processing. Caps are stolen from a diverse array of host mRNAs, and in an unexpected finding, the most abundant class of host RNAs used by influenza virus for cap-snatching are snRNA (Koppstein *et al.*, 2015). In addition to its role in cap-snatching, the cleavage of nascent transcripts likely reduces the number of host mRNAs and contributes to the shut off of host protein synthesis characteristic of influenza virus infection. Binding between the influenza polymerase of the Pol II CTD also results in inhibition of Pol II elongation and ubiquitination and degradation of Pol II late in infection, further reducing the synthesis of host mRNA and possibly providing temporal regulation of viral polymerase activity during infection (Chan *et al.*, 2006; Vreede *et al.*, 2010). Cap-snatching and virally induced premature transcriptional termination thus results in a reduction of complete cellular mRNAs, and the recycling of Pol II and further generation of short, capped transcripts that can then be co-opted by the viral replication machinery.

Pol II accessory factors have further elucidated the coupling between the cellular transcription and influenza replication machineries. The vRNP has been shown to interact with cyclin T1/cyclin-dependent kinase 9, a dimer of Pol II-associated transcription elongation regulators involved in the phosphorylation of the Pol II CTD (Zhang *et al.*, 2010). Cyclin

T1/CDK9 is proposed to recruit the vRNP to hyperphosphorylated forms of the CTD, although in this case phosphorylation was enriched at serine 2, a modification associated with transcriptional elongation. Similarly, human CLE/C14orf166 (*hCLE*) has been shown to interact with PA (Huarte *et al.*, 2001). hCLE/C14orf166 localizes to sites of active transcription and co-precipitates with different phosphorylated states of Pol II, potentially functioning as a modulator of mRNA transcription and a positive regulator of influenza infection (Pérez-González *et al.*, 2006; Rodriguez *et al.*, 2011). Whereas silencing of both hCLE and cyclin T1 results in decreased viral mRNA, cRNA and mRNA, further experiments are needed to determine if this is a direct effect on interactions between the influenza polymerase and Pol II, the consequence of global changes in Pol II activity, or a combination of pleotropic effects.

Interaction between the viral polymerase and the cellular Pol II occurs at fixed locations within the nucleus in tight association with chromatin and the nuclear matrix (Chan *et al.*, 2006; Chase *et al.*, 2011; Jackson *et al.*, 1982; Takizawa *et al.*, 2006). *In vitro* analyses demonstrated that viral RNPs associate with histone tails and nucleosomes through interactions with NP (Garcia-Robles *et al.*, 2005). NP also interacts with high-mobility group box proteins (HMGB) 1 and 2, well-described DNA-binding chromatin remodellers (Moisy *et al.*, 2012). Experiments in cells suggest that binding to HMGB1 may help recruit vRNPs to chromatin and facilitate efficient transcription and replication, although neither HMGB1 nor HMGB2 is essential for infection. Interestingly, the influenza structural protein M1 also binds nucleosomes *in vitro* and is associated with chromatin in cells (Chase *et al.*, 2011; Garcia-Robles *et al.*, 2005; Zhirnov and Klenk, 1997). These disparate findings were brought together in recent work that suggests that chromatin targeting by vRNPs and M1 may be important not only for cap-snatching, but also for recruitment and preferential export of vRNPs complexes (see below) (Chase *et al.*, 2011).

Transcriptional termination, polyadenylation and mRNA splicing

A five- to seven-nucleotide stretch of uracil nucleotides is conserved at the 5′ end of each viral RNA segment approximately 17 nucleotides from the terminus (Robertson *et al.*, 1981). Upon reaching this stretch of U's, the transcribing polymerase stutters over this sequence generating a polyadenosine tail resulting in premature termination (Poon *et al.*, 1999; Zheng *et al.*, 1999). This differs from cellular mRNA polyadenylation where cellular mRNAs are cleaved downstream of a defined poly(A) signal sequence and a tail is later added by a poly(A) polymerase. Regardless, in both cases the presence of a poly(A) tail allows for efficient recognition by the host splicing, export and translational machinery. During this polyadenylation step, the host cellular splicing factor SFPQ/PSF enhances polyadenylation of viral messages and is necessary for optimal gene expression (Landeras-Bueno *et al.*, 2011). SFPQ/PSF co-precipitates with the vRNPs and its silencing in host cells selectively reduces replication of influenza virus, but not adenovirus or vesicular stomatitis virus. Another host factor involved in 3′ end processing, CPSF30 (the 30-kDa subunit of the cellular cleavage and polyadenylation specificity factor) also interacts with the polymerase complex in the presence of the viral NS1 (Kuo and Krug, 2009). In this case, binding appears to block normal processing and maturation of host messages and prevent antiviral responses (Noah *et al.*, 2003).

Within the influenza A genome, only segments 7 and 8 undergo splicing. The primary, unspliced transcripts from these segments correspond to genes M1 and NS1 whereas spliced transcripts code for M2 and NEP. Because the virus does not encode splicing factors, the series of splicing reactions are performed by the host. The human spliceosomal factors RED and SMU1 associate with PB1 and P and influence splicing of the NS gene to produce transcripts for NEP, but not splicing of the M gene (Fournier *et al.*, 2014). Given that NEP is essential for nuclear export of the replicated vRNP, knock-down of RED/SMU1 decreased levels of NS splicing and reduced viral replication. Little is known about the regulation and stoichiometric control for influenza spliced transcripts. NS splicing efficiency may in large part be programmed by the virus itself. NEP transcripts are inefficiently spliced from NS due to a weak splice donor site in the gene (Chua *et al.*, 2013). On the other hand, two host proteins, NS1-BP and hnRNP K, have been identified as important regulators of splicing for the M mRNA segment (Tsai *et al.*, 2013). NS1-BP and hnRNP K do not affect splicing of the NS mRNA, indicating that differential splicing factors and mechanisms occur between the two influenza segments.

Host factors implicated in viral RNA replication

After an initial period of protein synthesis, viral genomic RNA accumulates as the infection proceeds. For the virus, this accumulation of RNA genomes marks a critical switch in the viral life cycle from gene expression to the assembly of progeny virus. The switch is not necessarily binary, but rather a gradient from primarily gene expression early in infection to genome replication at later stages. The regulated switch from transcription, to cRNA synthesis, to vRNA synthesis is a complicated and incompletely understood process. A speculative model supported by current findings suggests that the viral nuclear export protein (NEP), whose synthesis is intentionally delayed by suboptimal splicing, biases the polymerase late in infection to produce cRNA (Chua *et al.*, 2013; Robb *et al.*, 2009). Subsequent replication using the cRNA template initially produces abortive replication products, termed small viral RNAs (svRNAs). svRNAs are thought to trigger vRNA synthesis by eventually accumulating to high enough levels to bind PA and stimulate creation of full-length products (Perez *et al.*, 2010, 2012). Increased concentrations of the polymerase proteins and NP may also stimulate the transition between transcription and replication by supply the raw material to create new RNPs (Honda *et al.*, 1988; Olson *et al.*, 2010; Shapiro and Krug, 1988; Vreede *et al.*, 2011). Additionally, recent work has shown that phosphorylation of NP negatively regulates its oligomerization and RNP assembly, suggesting that host kinase activity may also impact the transition towards replication (Chenavas *et al.*, 2013; Mondal *et al.*, 2015; Turrell *et al.*, 2015). The structures of the viral polymerase also suggest large-scale conformational rearrangements that regulate the enzymatic activity of the polymerase, and possibly influence whether the polymerase initiates mRNA, cRNA or vRNA synthesis (Hengrung *et al.*, 2015; Reich *et al.*, 2014; Thierry *et al.*, 2016).

In contrast to transcription, the viral genome is replicated *de novo* in a primer-independent fashion. Both cRNA and vRNA are rapidly encapsidated by NP, possibly concomitant with their synthesis, to ensure that naked viral RNAs are never present in the infected cell (Kawaguchi *et al.*, 2011; Vreede *et al.*, 2004). Complementing the viral factors that regulate replication, host proteins also contribute. MCM2–7, replicative DNA helicase minichromosome maintenance complex (MCM) subunits 2 through 7, have been shown to act as processivity factors to stimulate full-length cRNA synthesis (Kawaguchi and Nagata, 2007). MCM2–7 interacts with PA and is proposed to stabilize the nascent chain complex through the process of promoter escape as the polymerase transitions from initiation to elongation.

Promoter escape and early elongation is enhanced by NP and the cellular splicing factor RAF-2p48 (also designated as DDX39B, UAP59, NPI-5 and BAT1) (Kawaguchi *et al.*, 2011; Momose *et al.*, 2001). RAF-2p48 binds free NP and facilitates cRNA encapsidation to further stabilize newly made cRNA.

Several stimulatory factors that enhance vRNA synthesis have been identified. Biochemical fractionation identified ANP32A [acidic (leucine-rich) nuclear phosphoprotein 32 family, member A, also called pp32] and ANP32B (APRIL) as nuclear factors that stimulate the primer-independent replication of vRNA from a cRNA template (Sugiyama *et al.*, 2016). ANP32A and B interact with the trimeric polymerase, but not NP or individual sub-complexes of the polymerase. How these proteins modulate polymerase function, and how the regulate species-specific polymerase activity (see below), remains to be determined. Host factors also associate with many individual subunits of the RNP to drive vRNA synthesis. Tat-SF1, an elongation factor of DNA transcription, was identified in a yeast single-gene deletion library (Naito *et al.*, 2007a). Through interactions with NP, Tat-SF1 is proposed to act as a chaperone for the formation of RNA–NP complexes stabilizing replication intermediates during vRNA synthesis. NP also associates with fragile X mental retardation protein (FMRP) via RNA-mediated interactions and this also stimulates RNP assembly (Zhou *et al.*, 2014). Hsp90, likely independent of its chaperone activity, partially relocalizes to the nucleus shortly after infection to stimulate vRNA synthesis. Through interactions with PB2, Hsp90 is able to modulate the activity of the replicating polymerase, enhancing RNA synthesis and elongation (Momose *et al.*, 2002). Protein phosphatase 6 (PP6), a multisubunit serine/threonine protein phosphatase, co-purified with RNPs during infection and was shown to be important for both c- and vRNA synthesis (York *et al.*, 2014). Whether the phosphatase activity of PP6 is essential, and, if so, whether it targets viral or cellular proteins, remains unknown. Lastly, nucleophosmin 1 (NPM1) interacts with RNP complexes, co-localizes to sites of transcription and replication in cells, and functions through unknown means as a positive regulator of polymerase activity (Mayer *et al.*, 2007). These factors, along with others, support the replication and synthesis of viral genomes for downstream export and release. Recent advances have allowed the selective isolation of vRNP and cRNP (York *et al.*, 2013), offering the potential to identify more host factors that selectively associate with minus- and plus-sense genomes and possibly regulate activity of the associated polymerase.

Antagonists of the influenza replication machinery

In addition to requisite host factors or host factors that ensure optimal gene expression and replication, several cellular proteins specifically inhibit influenza multiplication at the nuclear level. Negative regulators of influenza replication represent an important facet of molecular virus–host interplay and evolution. All viruses co-opt host cellular machinery and processes for efficient replication and spread. In response, cells have co-evolved to express a number of diverse proteins that subvert the viral life cycle.

Murine Mx1, and the human homologue MxA, are well-known IFN-inducible proteins with antiviral activity against a broad range of RNA viruses. For influenza virus, Mx1 accumulates in the nucleus of infected murine cells and inhibits viral mRNA synthesis (Krug *et al.*, 1985). MxA, on the other hand, is thought to recognize vRNPs in the cytoplasm of infected human cells and prevent their nuclear import (Kochs and Haller, 1999). Genetic analysis revealed that NP is the main target of both Mx proteins, and that adaptive mutations in the virus located within NP permit escape from Mx-mediated restriction (Dittmann *et al.*, 2008; Manz *et al.*, 2013). vRNPs appear to be targeted in the cytoplasm by RIG-I as well. RIG-I is a well-known sensor of viral RNAs and stimulates innate immune responses. RIG-I co-precipitates with the individual polymerase subunits PB1, PB2 and PA (Li *et al.*, 2014) and it has been proposed that RIG-I detects incoming vRNPs shortly after infection to initiate antiviral signalling (Weber *et al.*, 2013). When avian-origin viruses infect mammalian cells, it was further suggested that RIG-I destablizes the vRNP and dissociates the polymerase (Weber *et al.*, 2015). The RuvB-Like Protein 2 (RBL2, also termed Rvb2) was identified as another inhibitor of vRNA synthesis (Kakugawa *et al.*, 2009). RBL2 is a AAA+ protein with homology to a bacterial ATP-dependent DNA helicase important for branch migration and resolution of holiday junctions during homologous recombination and repair of DNA damage. RBL2, in association with RBL1, also performs chaperone activities for a number of different cellular protein and nucleic acid:protein complexes (Nano and Houry, 2013). In human cells, RBL2 interacts with the RNP and with NP alone. Overexpression of RBL2 disrupts NP oligomerization and ultimately inhibits viral polymerase activity (Kakugawa *et al.*, 2009). RBL2 has not been tested during a viral infection, but RBL1 was identified as a positive regulator of IFN signalling during infection in a genome-wide analysis, suggesting a possible activity during replication (Shapira *et al.*, 2009). Nuclear factor 90 (NF90/interleukin enhancer binding factor 3) and the peptidyl-prolyl isomerase cyclophilin E (CypE) were identified as other negative regulators of influenza polymerase activity and replication that interact with NP (Wang *et al.*, 2009, 2011). In the cell, NF90 functions as a double-stranded RNA binding protein that complexes with proteins and non-coding RNAs to regulate and stabilize mRNAs. In contrast to its role in the cell, down-regulation of NF90 results in enhanced accumulation of viral mRNAs and vRNAs. NF90 was later validated by yeast two hybrid experiments to interact with and negatively regulate PB2 (Bortz *et al.*, 2011; Shapira *et al.*, 2009). CypE appears to function by directly interacting with NP and preventing self-assembly into the oligomers that form RNPs and by preventing NP-PB1 and NP-PB2 binding. The mechanism of action is unclear, and whether is involves conformational rearrangement of proteins through proline isomerization is an open question.

Most of the identified antagonists of the replication machinery target NP. This may result from technical limitations of the experiments; NP is one of the most abundantly expressed viral proteins and is readily purified from infected cells, increasing the likelihood of identifying co-factors. Alternatively, and perhaps more intriguing, NP may be targeted due to its essential role in replication and its presence as a regularly repeating structural subunit in a complex whose global architecture is largely independent of the minor polymorphism present in NP of different strains. This would be analogous to how Trim5a recognizes retroviral capsids – by using the repeated structure in the capsid to scaffold assembly of an active Trim5a (Ganser-Pornillos *et al.*, 2011; Pertel *et al.*, 2011). This would also partially explain how Mx proteins effectively control a diverse collection of negative-stranded RNA virus families.

Individual subunits of the polymerase do not escape targeting by host factors. The E3 ubiquitin ligase TRIM32 is an antiviral factor that binds to PB1 (Fu *et al.*, 2015). The coiled-coil of TRIM32 interacts with the C-terminus of PB1, causing its ubiquitination and degradation. Depletion or knock-out of TRIM32 restores PB1 levels, enhancing polymerase activity and increasing viral titres during replication about 10-fold. PB2 and PA are similarly targeted for proteasomal degradation. An unknown E3 ubiquitin ligase targets PB2 and PA prior to trimer assembly, possibly mediated by the protein ZAPL, a well-characterized antiviral protein first shown to inhibit retroviral RNA production (Gao *et al.*, 2002; Liu *et al.*, 2015). PB1 is also the target of the cellular RNA helicase DDX21 (Chen *et al.*, 2014). It has been proposed that DDX21 binding to PB1 inhibits assembly of the polymerase trimer, thus reducing polymerase function and virus replication. The viral protein NS1 is thought to compete for binding with DDX21, displacing it from PB1 and permitting polymerase formation. Finally, Ebp1 (ErbB3-binding protein also designated proliferation-associated protein 2G4, PA2G4), a nucleolar growth regulating protein, interacts specifically with the PB1 subunit of the polymerase, interfering with mRNA synthesis both in cells and *in vitro* (Honda *et al.*, 2007). Ebp1 gene expression is induced following infection and is then thought to interact with PB1 in its primer binding domain to inhibit viral transcriptase activity (Ejima *et al.*, 2011; Honda *et al.*, 2007). Of course, in addition to these factors the replication machinery will be indirectly affected by the large number of antiviral countermeasures mounted by an infected host. Given that cellular regulators of the viral replication machinery highlight naturally occurring activities that may be targeted for therapeutic intervention, it is important to continue to identify host factors and the molecular mechanisms by which they antagonize the replication machinery

Nuclear host factors with an undefined mechanism

Although numerous studies have identified putative influenza host factors that target or are targeted by the influenza machinery in the nucleus, only a limited number of these proteins have a well-defined mechanism or functional significance in the nuclear phase of the viral replication cycle. Within 12–18 hours of infection, the nuclear proteome changes dramatically with over 600 proteins significantly over- or under-expressed across a diversity of functional groups including gene expression, metabolism, and signalling-related proteins (Lietzen *et al.*, 2011). Proteomics-based studies have identified nucleolar and ribosomal proteins as recurring binding partners in addition to proteins involved in mRNA processing, splicing, transport and translation (Jorba *et al.*, 2008; Mayer *et al.*, 2007). Several DNA damage or chromatin-associated factors involved in the modification, modulation or structural components of DNA packing have been identified through both proteomic and RNAi screens including: poly(ADP-ribose) polymerase 1 (PARP1), a nuclear protein that post-translationally modifies targets by ADP ribosylation; DNA damage binding protein 1 (DDB1), a protein involved in UV-mediated DNA damage responses (Mayer *et al.*, 2007), and chromodomain helicase *in vitro*-binding domain-containing protein 6 (CHD6), a member of a chromatin remodelling complex which was identified as a negative modulator of infection that interacts with RNPs at late times post infection (Alfonso *et al.*, 2011). Moreover, several factors have been identified that positively affect virus replication and transcription upon over-expression and knockdown causes the opposite effect: COPS5, a COP9 signalosome subunit; MNAT1, a component of the CDK-activating kinase enzymatic complex; NMI, an N-Myc and STAT transcription factor interactor; EIF3L, a translation initiation factor; NUP54, a component of the nuclear pore; FANCG, a Fanconi anaemia pathway member involved in DNA damage response; and PRKRA, an IFN-inducible protein kinase, although their mechanism of action has yet to be determined (Tafforeau *et al.*, 2011). Gene ontology analysis on the current nuclear influenza interactome is enriched in biological processes involved in post-translational modifications, kinase cascades, RNA localization, intracellular signalling cascades, positive regulation of DNA-dependent transcription and innate immune response. Further experimentation is required to determine how these proteins interact with the RNP and modulate its activity.

Cellular factors that control host range

The viral polymerase is a major determinant of host range. Avian influenza polymerases support high levels of activity and virus replication in avian cells, but function poorly in mammalian hosts (Subbarao *et al.*, 1993). Adaptive mutations within the polymerase restore polymerase activity as viruses move from birds to humans, most notably the charge change from the avian-style glutamic acid to a human-style lysine at position 627 in PB2 or the acquisition of a basic residue at position 591 in PB2 (Mehle and Doudna, 2009; Subbarao *et al.*, 1993; Yamada *et al.*, 2010). Heterokaryon analyses provided evidence for both an inhibitory factor in mammalian cells that impairs avian-origin polymerases as well as an enhancing factor in avian cells that supports high-level activity of the avian-origin polymerase (Mehle and Doudna, 2008; Moncorge *et al.*, 2010). Subsequent work has shown that RIG-I in mammalian cells preferentially targets avian-origin polymerase (Weber *et al.*, 2015). As RIG-I is not present in domestic chickens, this suggests that RIG-I may be the inhibitory factor alluded to by the heterokaryon analysis. More recent work provided compelling evidence that ANP32A functions as a species-specific enhancer of polymerase function (Long *et al.*, 2016). Avian-origin polymerases required avian ANP32A for high-level activity and expressing avian ANP32A in human cells alleviated the species-specific restriction on polymerase function and viral replication. As predicted, the impact of avian ANP32A was dependent on the presence of the avian-style glutamic acid at PB2 residue 627. Avian ANP32A did not enhance activity of polymerases containing the mammalian-style lysine at PB2 residue 627, nor did human ANP32A enhance avian polymerase. The species specificity for ANP32A mapped to a simple 33 amino insert that was acquired during avian evolution (except ratites) and is absent in mammals (Long *et al.*, 2016). Avian-origin polymerases are well tuned to use avian ANP32A containing this insert, but must adapt to use the mammalian version lacking the insert. How ANP32A functions remains unclear, nonetheless ANP32A is likely the major regulator of influenza polymerase host range. It will be important to determine if the role of ANP32A in restricting host range is related to the recent identification of ANP32A and ANP32B as co-factors that stimulate vRNA synthesis (Sugiyama *et al.*, 2016).

Minor polymerase products

In addition to the full-length PB1, PB2 and PA proteins, the polymerase genes also code for multiple other minor protein products via an internal open reading frame (PB1-F2) (Chen *et al.*, 2001), frame shifting (PA-X) (Jagger *et al.*, 2012) and leaking scanning (PB1 N40, PA-N155 and –N182) (Muramoto *et al.*, 2013; Wise *et al.*, 2009). PB1-F2 is produced by leaky scanning and initiation at the fourth start codon in the +1 reading frame. PB1-F2 is a short polypeptide up to 90 amino acids in length whose presence and length varies from strain to strain (Chen *et al.*, 2001). Although PB1-F2 is not essential for virus replication, polymorphism present in the protein can significantly alter the pathogenesis of influenza infection and secondary pneumonia (Conenello *et al.*, 2007; McAuley *et al.*, 2007). PB1-F2 localizes to the mitochondria where it binds the cellular protein MAVS (Dudek *et al.*, 2011; Varga *et al.*, 2011). MAVS is an adaptor protein for signalling via RIG-I and RIG-I-like receptors (RLR) that induces type I IFN production. RLRs signalling is critical for controlling viral infection. PB1-F2 disrupts signalling through MAVS, potentially explaining its effect on the pathogenesis of infection. A small population of PB2 also localizes to the mitochondria where it too disrupts signalling via MAVS (Carr *et al.*, 2006; Graef *et al.*, 2010; Iwai *et al.*, 2010). Polymorphisms in the mitochondrial targeting signal of PB2 alter localization and antagonism of IFN expression, influencing the pathogenesis of infection in mice (Carr *et al.*, 2006; Graef *et al.*, 2010). In addition to polymerase proteins targeting MAVS, the viral protein NS1 also binds to and disrupts the activity of TRIM25, an upstream regulator of RLRs (Gack *et al.*, 2007, 2009). Thus, multiple viral proteins target the RLR signalling pathway to suppress antiviral responses.

The recently discovered PA-X protein contains the N-terminal 191 amino acids of PA fused to a C-terminal extension accessed by +1 frameshifting (Jagger *et al.*, 2012). In the original case, frameshifting translates an additional 61 amino acids, although the length and sequence of the extension is variable (Shi *et al.*, 2012). PA-X is present at low levels during infection and contains the N-terminal nuclease domain of PA. Its expression non-specifically degrades mRNAs and suppresses the expression of host proteins, including proinflammatory cytokines (Desmet *et al.*, 2013; Jagger *et al.*, 2012). Eliminating PA-X in the 1918 strain of influenza virus increases the pathogenicity of infection, possibly due to immunopathology caused by higher levels of cytokines. Defining the complete repertoire of PA-X function and the role of the C-terminal extension and host factors that recognize it is an area of active investigation.

PB1 N40 is produced by leaking scanning and subsequent initiation at a conserved methionine located 40 amino acids downstream from the N-terminus of PB1 (Wise *et al.*, 2009). PA-N155 and -N183 are similarly produced by leaking scanning and initiation at the 11th and 13th start codons in the PA gene, truncating 155 and 183 amino acids, respectively (Muramoto *et al.*, 2013). The function of these N-terminally truncated variants is less well known. None of them is required for virus replication. The PA-binding site, located at the N-terminus of PB1 (Perez and Donis, 2001), is absent from PB1 N40. As PB1 is thought to be imported into the nucleus only when complexed with PA (see above), PB1 N40 remains in the cytoplasm. Viruses lacking PB1 N40 display slightly delayed replication kinetics and a minor increase in PB1 levels early in infection (Wise *et al.*, 2009). PA-N155 and -N183 cannot reconstitute polymerase activity and replication of viruses lacking these products is only modestly reduced (Muramoto *et al.*, 2013). Whether these truncations function in a dominant-negative fashion by binding other viral proteins, saturate binding to host factors, potentially act as decoys for inhibitors, or have other essential functions remains to be determined.

vRNP export and cytoplasmic transport

Following successful replication of the viral genome, newly made vRNPs must be exported from the nucleus. This is an active process where vRNPs exit through the NPC directed by the host importin β Crm1, as treatment of infected cells with the Crm1 inhibitor leptomycin B blocks vRNP export (Elton *et al.*, 2001). Only the vRNP, but not the cRNP is exported, possibly due to different secondary structures present in the minus- versus plus-sense genomic RNA (Tchatalbachev *et al.*, 2001). Like other importin βs, Crm1 is activated by binding the cofactor RanGTP and recognizes hydrophobic nuclear export signals (NES) on cargo proteins. RanGDP is converted to the active RanGTP by the chromatin-bound Ran guanine exchange factor Rcc1. It has recently been shown that vRNPs are tethered to regions of host chromatin that are also enriched in Crm1 and Rcc1, suggesting a mechanism by which the vRNP preferentially engages active export complexes (Chase *et al.*, 2011). Because a portion of cellular Crm1-Ran-Rcc1 is sequestered on chromatin, this interaction may further contribute to virus-mediated host shut-off.

In addition to the vRNP, the viral proteins M1 and NEP are also important players during export. M1 coats vRNPs and a fraction is bound by NEP. NESs have be characterized in NEP (Huang *et al.*, 2013; Neumann *et al.*, 2000; O'Neill *et al.*, 1998), M1 (Cao *et al.*, 2012) and NP (Yu *et al.*, 2012). There are at least three non-exclusive models proposed for how vRNPs interact with the host export machinery: the 'daisy chain' model where vRNPs bind to M1, M1 binds to NEP and NEP binds to Crm1 (Paterson and Fodor, 2012); the viral polymerase interacts directly with NEP and NEP binds Crm1 (Manz *et al.*, 2012); or the NESs present in NP and M1 interact directly with Crm1 to export RNPs (Bui *et al.*, 2000; Elton *et al.*, 2001). A Crm1-independent pathway driven by NP has also been suggested (Elton *et al.*, 2001). Once in the cytoplasm, RanGTP is hydrolysed to RanGDP, causing a conformational rearrangement and disassembly of the export complexes. During the export process, the vRNPs are also known to interact with the host proteins HIV Rev-binding protein (HRB) and Y-box binding protein 1 (YB-1), which may aid dissociation of the export complex and interaction with microtubules for cytoplasmic trafficking, respectively (Eisfeld *et al.*, 2011b; Kawaguchi *et al.*, 2012).

Exported vRNPs are initially dispersed throughout the cytoplasm but ultimately accumulate in the perinuclear region containing the microtubule-organizing centre (MTOC) (Amorim *et al.*, 2011; Momose *et al.*, 2007). As the released vRNPs are coated by M1, which occludes the NLSs present on the vRNP, they do not undergo re-importation (Martin and Helenius, 1991a). vRNPs are then localized to Rab11-positive vesicles on recycling endosome, possibly through interactions between PB2 and Rab11 (Amorim *et al.*, 2011; Avilov *et al.*, 2012; Eisfeld *et al.*, 2011a). Rab11 is a small GTPase that regulates recycling of endocytic vesicles from the plasma membrane to distinct cytoplasmic compartments and back to the plasma membrane. It is required for the production of influenza virions (Bruce *et al.*, 2010). It is here that the eight different vRNPs co-localize again and begin to assemble into the higher-order genome complex that is presumptively packaged into virions (Chou *et al.*, 2013). vRNPs travel with Rab11-positive vesicles to the apical surface of the cell primarily in a microtubule-dependent fashion (Amorim *et al.*, 2011; Momose *et al.*, 2007). Finally, in a process that is poorly understood, vRNPs migrate from the vesicle to the plasma membrane and sites of assembly. Virions bud from the plasma membrane and are ready to initiate the next round of infection.

Perspective

Between proteomic and genomic approaches, over 2000 genes have been implicated as host factors impacting influenza virus replication, of which 400 have been suggested to physically interact with the RNP or its components. Only a small number of these have been validated to modulated influenza infection, and even a smaller number with a proposed mechanism of action are described here. As advances in screening and proteomic technologies reveal new essential host factors, the list of these and other unidentified pro- and antiviral host proteins will certainly grow revealing more about the molecular mechanisms that underlie influenza polymerase function, adaptation and virus–host co-evolution.

Acknowledgements

It was not possible to make this a comprehensive analysis and we apologize to our colleagues whose exciting results may not have been included or discussed in depth. Work in our laboratory is supported in part by the National Institute of General Medical Sciences (R00GM088484), the American Lung Association (RG-310016), a Shaw Scientist Award, and a Wisconsin Partnership Education and Research Committee New Investigator Program grant (#2563) to A.M. and an NIH National Research Service Award (T32 GM07215) to V.T.

References

Alfonso, R., Lutz, T., Rodriguez, A., Chavez, J.P., Rodriguez, P., Gutierrez, S., and Nieto, A. (2011). CHD6 chromatin remodeler is a negative modulator of influenza virus replication that relocates to inactive chromatin upon infection. Cell. Microbiol. *13*, 1894–1906.

Amorim, M.J., Bruce, E.A., Read, E.K., Foeglein, A., Mahen, R., Stuart, A.D., and Digard, P. (2011). A Rab11- and microtubule-dependent mechanism for cytoplasmic transport of influenza A virus viral RNA. J. Virol. *85*, 4143–4156.

Area, E., Martin-Benito, J., Gastaminza, P., Torreira, E., Valpuesta, J.M., Carrascosa, J.L., and Ortin, J. (2004). 3D structure of the influenza virus polymerase complex: localization of subunit domains. Proc. Natl. Acad. Sci. U.S.A. *101*, 308–313.

Arranz, R., Coloma, R., Chichon, F.J., Conesa, J.J., Carrascosa, J.L., Valpuesta, J.M., Ortin, J., and Martin-Benito, J. (2012). The structure of native influenza virion ribonucleoproteins. Science *338*, 1634–1637.

Avilov, S.V., Moisy, D., Naffakh, N., and Cusack, S. (2012). Influenza A virus progeny vRNP trafficking in live infected cells studied with the virus-encoded fluorescently tagged PB2 protein. Vaccine *30*, 7411–7417.

Biswas, S.K., Boutz, P.L., and Nayak, D.P. (1998). Influenza virus nucleoprotein interacts with influenza virus polymerase proteins. J. Virol. *72*, 5493–5501.

Boivin, S., and Hart, D.J. (2011). Interaction of the influenza A virus polymerase PB2 C-terminal region with importin alpha isoforms provides insights into host adaptation and polymerase assembly. J. Biol. Chem. *286*, 10439–10448.

Bortz, E., Westera, L., Maamary, J., Steel, J., Albrecht, R.A., Manicassamy, B., Chase, G., Martinez-Sobrido, L., Schwemmle, M., and Garcia-Sastre, A. (2011). Host- and strain-specific regulation of influenza virus polymerase activity by interacting cellular proteins. MBio 2.

Bradel-Tretheway, B.G., Mattiacio, J.L., Krasnoselsky, A., Stevenson, C., Purdy, D., Dewhurst, S., and Katze, M.G. (2011). Comprehensive proteomic analysis of influenza virus polymerase complex reveals a novel association with mitochondrial proteins and RNA polymerase accessory factors. J. Virol. *85*, 8569–8581.

Bruce, E.A., Digard, P., and Stuart, A.D. (2010). The Rab11 pathway is required for influenza A virus budding and filament formation. J. Virol. *84*, 5848–5859.

Bui, M., Wills, E.G., Helenius, A., and Whittaker, G.R. (2000). Role of the influenza virus M1 protein in nuclear export of viral ribonucleoproteins. J. Virol. *74*, 1781–1786.

Cao, S., Liu, X., Yu, M., Li, J., Jia, X., Bi, Y., Sun, L., Gao, G.F., and Liu, W. (2012). A nuclear export signal in the matrix protein of Influenza A virus is required for efficient virus replication. J. Virol. *86*, 4883–4891.

Carr, S.M., Carnero, E., Garcia-Sastre, A., Brownlee, G.G., and Fodor, E. (2006). Characterization of a mitochondrial-targeting signal in the PB2 protein of influenza viruses. Virology *344*, 492–508.

Chan, A.Y., Vreede, F.T., Smith, M., Engelhardt, O.G., and Fodor, E. (2006). Influenza virus inhibits RNA polymerase II elongation. Virology *351*, 210–217.

Chase, G., Deng, T., Fodor, E., Leung, B.W., Mayer, D., Schwemmle, M., and Brownlee, G. (2008). Hsp90 inhibitors reduce influenza virus replication in cell culture. Virology 377, 431–439.

Chase, G.P., Rameix-Welti, M.-A., Zvirbliene, A., Zvirblis, G., Götz, V., Wolff, T., Naffakh, N., and Schwemmle, M. (2011). Influenza virus ribonucleoprotein complexes gain preferential access to cellular export machinery through chromatin targeting. PLoS Pathog. *7*, e1002187.
Chen, G., Liu, C.H., Zhou, L., and Krug, R.M. (2014). Cellular DDX21 RNA helicase inhibits influenza A virus replication but is counteracted by the viral NS1 protein. Cell Host Microbe *15*, 484–493.
Chen, W., Calvo, P.A., Malide, D., Gibbs, J., Schubert, U., Bacik, I., Basta, S., O'Neill, R., Schickli, J., Palese, P., *et al.* (2001). A novel influenza A virus mitochondrial protein that induces cell death. Nat. Med. *7*, 1306–1312.
Chenavas, S., Estrozi, L.F., Slama-Schwok, A., Delmas, B., Di Primo, C., Baudin, F., Li, X., Crepin, T., and Ruigrok, R.W. (2013). Monomeric nucleoprotein of influenza A virus. PLoS Pathog. *9*, e1003275.
Chou, Y.Y., Heaton, N.S., Gao, Q., Palese, P., Singer, R.H., and Lionnet, T. (2013). Colocalization of different influenza viral RNA segments in the cytoplasm before viral budding as shown by single-molecule sensitivity FISH analysis. PLoS Pathog. *9*, e1003358.
Chua, M.A., Schmid, S., Perez, J.T., Langlois, R.A., and Tenoever, B.R. (2013). Influenza A virus utilizes suboptimal splicing to coordinate the timing of infection. Cell Rep. *3*, 23–29.
Cianci, C., Tiley, L., and Krystal, M. (1995). Differential activation of the influenza virus polymerase via template RNA binding. J. Virol. *69*, 3995–3999.
Coloma, R., Valpuesta, J.M., Arranz, R., Carrascosa, J.L., Ortin, J., and Martin-Benito, J. (2009). The structure of a biologically active influenza virus ribonucleoprotein complex. PLoS Pathog. *5*, e1000491.
Conenello, G.M., Zamarin, D., Perrone, L.A., Tumpey, T., and Palese, P. (2007). A single mutation in the PB1-F2 of H5N1 (HK/97) and 1918 influenza A viruses contributes to increased virulence. PLoS Pathog. *3*, 1414–1421.
Cros, J.F., Garcia-Sastre, A., and Palese, P. (2005). An unconventional NLS is critical for the nuclear import of the influenza A virus nucleoprotein and ribonucleoprotein. Traffic *6*, 205–213.
Deng, T., Engelhardt, O.G., Thomas, B., Akoulitchev, A.V., Brownlee, G.G., and Fodor, E. (2006). Role of ran binding protein 5 in nuclear import and assembly of the influenza virus RNA polymerase complex. J. Virol. *80*, 11911–11919.
Desmet, E.A., Bussey, K.A., Stone, R., and Takimoto, T. (2013). Identification of the N-terminal domain of the influenza virus PA responsible for the suppression of host protein synthesis. J. Virol. *87*, 3108–3118.
Dias, A., Bouvier, D., Crepin, T., McCarthy, A.A., Hart, D.J., Baudin, F., Cusack, S., and Ruigrok, R.W. (2009). The cap-snatching endonuclease of influenza virus polymerase resides in the PA subunit. Nature *458*, 914–918.
Digard, P., Blok, V.C., and Inglis, S.C. (1989). Complex formation between influenza virus polymerase proteins expressed in Xenopus oocytes. Virology *171*, 162–169.
Dittmann, J., Stertz, S., Grimm, D., Steel, J., García-Sastre, A., Haller, O., and Kochs, G. (2008). Influenza A virus strains differ in sensitivity to the antiviral action of Mx-GTPase. J. Virol. *82*, 3624–3631.
Dudek, S.E., Wixler, L., Nordhoff, C., Nordmann, A., Anhlan, D., Wixler, V., and Ludwig, S. (2011). The influenza virus PB1-F2 protein has interferon antagonistic activity. Biol. Chem. *392*, 1135–1144.
Eisfeld, A.J., Kawakami, E., Watanabe, T., Neumann, G., and Kawaoka, Y. (2011a). RAB11A is essential for transport of the influenza virus genome to the plasma membrane. J. Virol. *85*, 6117–6126.
Eisfeld, A.J., Neumann, G., and Kawaoka, Y. (2011b). Human immunodeficiency virus rev-binding protein is essential for influenza A virus replication and promotes genome trafficking in late-stage infection. J. Virol. *85*, 9588–9598.
Ejima, M., Kadoi, K., and Honda, A. (2011). Influenza virus infection induces cellular Ebp1 gene expression. Genes Cells *16*, 927–937.
Elton, D., Simpson-Holley, M., Archer, K., Medcalf, L., Hallam, R., McCauley, J., and Digard, P. (2001). Interaction of the influenza virus nucleoprotein with the cellular CRM1-mediated nuclear export pathway. J. Virol. *75*, 408–419.
Engelhardt, O.G., Smith, M., and Fodor, E. (2005). Association of the influenza A virus RNA-dependent RNA polymerase with cellular RNA polymerase II. J. Virol. *79*, 5812–5818.
Fechter, P., Mingay, L., Sharps, J., Chambers, A., Fodor, E., and Brownlee, G.G. (2003). Two aromatic residues in the PB2 subunit of influenza A RNA polymerase are crucial for cap binding. J. Biol. Chem. *278*, 20381–20388.
Fislova, T., Thomas, B., Graef, K.M., and Fodor, E. (2010). Association of the influenza virus RNA polymerase subunit PB2 with the host chaperonin CCT. J. Virol. *84*, 8691–8699.
Fodor, E., and Smith, M. (2004). The PA subunit is required for efficient nuclear accumulation of the PB1 subunit of the influenza A virus RNA polymerase complex. J. Virol. *78*, 9144–9153.

Fournier, G., Chiang, C., Munier, S., Tomoiu, A., Demeret, C., Vidalain, P.O., Jacob, Y., and Naffakh, N. (2014). Recruitment of RED-SMU1 complex by Influenza A Virus RNA polymerase to control Ciral mRNA splicing. PLoS Pathog. *10*, e1004164.

Fu, B., Wang, L., Ding, H., Schwamborn, J.C., Li, S., and Dorf, M.E. (2015). TRIM32 senses and restricts influenza a virus by ubiquitination of PB1 Polymerase. PLoS Pathog. *11*, e1004960.

Gabriel, G., Dauber, B., Wolff, T., Planz, O., Klenk, H.D., and Stech, J. (2005). The viral polymerase mediates adaptation of an avian influenza virus to a mammalian host. Proc. Natl. Acad. Sci. U.S.A. *102*, 18590–18595.

Gabriel, G., Herwig, A., and Klenk, H.D. (2008). Interaction of polymerase subunit PB2 and NP with importin alpha1 is a determinant of host range of influenza A virus. PLoS Pathog. *4*, e11.

Gabriel, G., Klingel, K., Otte, A., Thiele, S., Hudjetz, B., Arman-Kalcek, G., Sauter, M., Shmidt, T., Rother, F., Baumgarte, S., *et al.* (2011). Differential use of importin-alpha isoforms governs cell tropism and host adaptation of influenza virus. Nat. Commun. *2*, 156.

Gack, M.U., Albrecht, R.A., Urano, T., Inn, K.S., Huang, I.C., Carnero, E., Farzan, M., Inoue, S., Jung, J.U., and Garcia-Sastre, A. (2009). Influenza A virus NS1 targets the ubiquitin ligase TRIM25 to evade recognition by the host viral RNA sensor RIG-I. Cell Host Microbe *5*, 439–449.

Gack, M.U., Shin, Y.C., Joo, C.H., Urano, T., Liang, C., Sun, L., Takeuchi, O., Akira, S., Chen, Z., Inoue, S., *et al.* (2007). TRIM25 RING-finger E3 ubiquitin ligase is essential for RIG-I-mediated antiviral activity. Nature *446*, 916–920.

Ganser-Pornillos, B.K., Chandrasekaran, V., Pornillos, O., Sodroski, J.G., Sundquist, W.I., and Yeager, M. (2011). Hexagonal assembly of a restricting TRIM5alpha protein. Proc. Natl. Acad. Sci. U.S.A. *108*, 534–539.

Gao, G., Guo, X., and Goff, S.P. (2002). Inhibition of retroviral RNA production by ZAP, a CCCH-type zinc finger protein. Science *297*, 1703–1706.

Garcia-Robles, I., Akarsu, H., Muller, C.W., Ruigrok, R.W., and Baudin, F. (2005). Interaction of influenza virus proteins with nucleosomes. Virology *332*, 329–336.

Ge, X., Rameix-Welti, M.-A., Gault, E., Chase, G., dos Santos Afonso, E., Picard, D., Schwemmle, M., and Naffakh, N. (2011). Influenza virus infection induces the nuclear relocalization of the Hsp90 co-chaperone p23 and inhibits the glucocorticoid receptor response. PLoS One *6*, e23368.

Graef, K.M., Vreede, F.T., Lau, Y.F., McCall, A.W., Carr, S.M., Subbarao, K., and Fodor, E. (2010). The PB2 subunit of the influenza virus RNA polymerase affects virulence by interacting with the mitochondrial antiviral signaling protein and inhibiting expression of beta interferon. J. Virol. *84*, 8433–8445.

Guilligay, D., Tarendeau, F., Resa-Infante, P., Coloma, R., Crepin, T., Sehr, P., Lewis, J., Ruigrok, R.W., Ortin, J., Hart, D.J., *et al.* (2008). The structural basis for cap binding by influenza virus polymerase subunit PB2. Nat. Struct. Mol. Biol. *15*, 500–506.

Hagen, M., Chung, T.D., Butcher, J.A., and Krystal, M. (1994). Recombinant influenza virus polymerase: requirement of both 5′ and 3′ viral ends for endonuclease activity. J. Virol. *68*, 1509–1515.

Hao, L., Sakurai, A., Watanabe, T., Sorensen, E., Nidom, C.A., Newton, M.A., Ahlquist, P., and Kawaoka, Y. (2008). Drosophila RNAi screen identifies host genes important for influenza virus replication. Nature *454*, 890–893.

Hartl, F.U., Bracher, A., and Hayer-Hartl, M. (2011). Molecular chaperones in protein folding and proteostasis. Nature *475*, 324–332.

Hay, A.J., Skehel, J.J., and McCauley, J. (1982). Characterization of influenza virus RNA complete transcripts. Virology *116*, 517–522.

He, X., Zhou, J., Bartlam, M., Zhang, R., Ma, J., Lou, Z., Li, X., Li, J., Joachimiak, A., Zeng, Z., *et al.* (2008). Crystal structure of the polymerase PA(C)-PB1(N) complex from an avian influenza H5N1 virus. Nature *454*, 1123–1126.

Hemerka, J.N., Wang, D., Weng, Y., Lu, W., Kaushik, R.S., Jin, J., Harmon, A.F., and Li, F. (2009). Detection and characterization of influenza A virus PA-PB2 interaction through a bimolecular fluorescence complementation assay. J. Virol. *83*, 3944–3955.

Hengrung, N., El Omari, K., Serna Martin, I., Vreede, F.T., Cusack, S., Rambo, R.P., Vonrhein, C., Bricogne, G., Stuart, D.I., Grimes, J.M., *et al.* (2015). Crystal structure of the RNA-dependent RNA polymerase from influenza C virus. Nature *527*, 114–117.

Herz, C., Stavnezer, E., Krug, R., and Gurney, T., Jr. (1981). Influenza virus, an RNA virus, synthesizes its messenger RNA in the nucleus of infected cells. Cell *26*, 391–400.

Hirayama, E., Atagi, H., Hiraki, A., and Kim, J. (2004). Heat shock protein 70 is related to thermal inhibition of nuclear export of the influenza virus ribonucleoprotein complex. J. Virol. *78*, 1263–1270.

Honda, A., Okamoto, T., and Ishihama, A. (2007). Host factor Ebp1: selective inhibitor of influenza virus transcriptase. Genes Cells *12*, 133–142.

Honda, A., Ueda, K., Nagata, K., and Ishihama, A. (1988). RNA polymerase of influenza virus: role of NP in RNA chain elongation. J. Biochem. *104*, 1021–1026.

Huang, S., Chen, J., Chen, Q., Wang, H., Yao, Y., Chen, J., and Chen, Z. (2013). A second CRM1-dependent nuclear export signal in the influenza A virus NS2 protein contributes to the nuclear export of viral ribonucleoproteins. J. Virol. *87*, 767–778.

Huarte, M., Sanz-Ezquerro, J.J., Roncal, F., Ortin, J., and Nieto, A. (2001). PA subunit from influenza virus polymerase complex interacts with a cellular protein with homology to a family of transcriptional activators. J. Virol. *75*, 8597–8604.

Hutchinson, E.C., and Fodor, E. (2012). Nuclear import of the influenza A virus transcriptional machinery. Vaccine *30*, 7353–7358.

Hutchinson, E.C., Orr, O.E., Man Liu, S., Engelhardt, O.G., and Fodor, E. (2011). Characterization of the interaction between the influenza A virus polymerase subunit PB1 and the host nuclear import factor Ran-binding protein 5. J. Gen. Virol. *92*, 1859–1869.

Iwai, A., Shiozaki, T., Kawai, T., Akira, S., Kawaoka, Y., Takada, A., Kida, H., and Miyazaki, T. (2010). Influenza A virus polymerase inhibits type I interferon induction by binding to interferon beta promoter stimulator 1. J. Biol. Chem. *285*, 32064–32074.

Jackson, D.A., Caton, A.J., McCready, S.J., and Cook, P.R. (1982). Influenza virus RNA is synthesized at fixed sites in the nucleus. Nature *296*, 366–368.

Jagger, B.W., Wise, H.M., Kash, J.C., Walters, K.A., Wills, N.M., Xiao, Y.L., Dunfee, R.L., Schwartzman, L.M., Ozinsky, A., Bell, G.L., *et al.* (2012). An overlapping protein-coding region in influenza A virus segment 3 modulates the host response. Science *337*, 199–204.

Jorba, N., Juarez, S., Torreira, E., Gastaminza, P., Zamarreno, N., Albar, J.P., and Ortin, J. (2008). Analysis of the interaction of influenza virus polymerase complex with human cell factors. Proteomics *8*, 2077–2088.

Kakugawa, S., Shimojima, M., Neumann, G., Goto, H., and Kawaoka, Y. (2009). RuvB-like protein 2 Is a Suppressor of influenza A virus polymerases. J. Virol. *83*, 6429–6434.

Kawaguchi, A., Matsumoto, K., and Nagata, K. (2012). YB-1 functions as a porter to lead influenza virus ribonucleoprotein complexes to microtubules. J. Virol. *86*, 11086–11095.

Kawaguchi, A., Momose, F., and Nagata, K. (2011). Replication-coupled and host factor-mediated encapsidation of the influenza virus genome by viral nucleoprotein. J. Virol. *85*, 6197–6204.

Kawaguchi, A., and Nagata, K. (2007). De novo replication of the influenza virus RNA genome is regulated by DNA replicative helicase, MCM. EMBO J. *26*, 4566–4575.

Kochs, G., and Haller, O. (1999). Interferon-induced human MxA GTPase blocks nuclear import of Thogoto virus nucleocapsids. Proc. Natl. Acad. Sci. U.S.A. *96*, 2082–2086.

Koppstein, D., Ashour, J., and Bartel, D.P. (2015). Sequencing the cap-snatching repertoire of H1N1 influenza provides insight into the mechanism of viral transcription initiation. Nucleic Acids Res. *43*, 5052–5064.

Krug, R.M., Shaw, M., Broni, B., Shapiro, G., and Haller, O. (1985). Inhibition of influenza viral mRNA synthesis in cells expressing the interferon-induced Mx gene product. J. Virol. *56*, 201–206.

Kuo, R.L., and Krug, R.M. (2009). Influenza a virus polymerase is an integral component of the CPSF30-NS1A protein complex in infected cells. J. Virol. *83*, 1611–1616.

Lamb, R.A., and Choppin, P.W. (1977). Synthesis of influenza virus polypeptides in cells resistant to alpha-amanitin: evidence for the involvement of cellular RNA polymerase II in virus replication. J. Virol. *23*, 816–819.

Landeras-Bueno, S., Jorba, N., Perez-Cidoncha, M., and Ortin, J. (2011). The splicing factor proline-glutamine rich (SFPQ/PSF) is involved in influenza virus transcription. PLoS Pathog. *7*, e1002397.

Li, M.L., Ramirez, B.C., and Krug, R.M. (1998). RNA-dependent activation of primer RNA production by influenza virus polymerase: different regions of the same protein subunit constitute the two required RNA-binding sites. EMBO J. *17*, 5844–5852.

Li, M.L., Rao, P., and Krug, R.M. (2001). The active sites of the influenza cap-dependent endonuclease are on different polymerase subunits. EMBO J. *20*, 2078–2086.

Li, W., Chen, H., Sutton, T., Obadan, A., and Perez, D.R. (2014). Interactions between the influenza A virus RNA polymerase components and retinoic acid-inducible gene I. J. Virol. *88*, 10432–10447.

Li, X., and Palese, P. (1994). Characterization of the polyadenylation signal of influenza virus RNA. J. Virol. *68*, 1245–1249.

Lietzen, N., Ohman, T., Rintahaka, J., Julkunen, I., Aittokallio, T., Matikainen, S., and Nyman, T.A. (2011). Quantitative subcellular proteome and secretome profiling of influenza A virus-infected human primary macrophages. PLoS Pathog. *7*, e1001340.

Liu, C.H., Zhou, L., Chen, G., and Krug, R.M. (2015). Battle between influenza A virus and a newly identified antiviral activity of the PARP-containing ZAPL protein. Proc. Natl. Acad. Sci. U.S.A. *112*, 14048–14053.

Long, J.S., Giotis, E.S., Moncorgé, O., Frise, R., Mistry, B., James, J., Morisson, M., Iqbal, M., Vignal, A., Skinner, M.A., *et al.* (2016). Species difference in ANP32A underlies influenza A virus polymerase host restriction. Nature *529*, 101–104.

Manz, B., Brunotte, L., Reuther, P., and Schwemmle, M. (2012). Adaptive mutations in NEP compensate for defective H5N1 RNA replication in cultured human cells. Nat. Commun. *3*, 802.

Manz, B., Dornfeld, D., Gotz, V., Zell, R., Zimmermann, P., Haller, O., Kochs, G., and Schwemmle, M. (2013). Pandemic influenza A viruses escape from restriction by human MxA through adaptive mutations in the nucleoprotein. PLoS Pathog. *9*, e1003279.

Martin, K., and Helenius, A. (1991a). Nuclear transport of influenza virus ribonucleoproteins: the viral matrix protein (M1) promotes export and inhibits import. Cell *67*, 117–130.

Martin, K., and Helenius, A. (1991b). Transport of incoming influenza virus nucleocapsids into the nucleus. J. Virol. *65*, 232–244.

Matsuoka, Y., Matsumae, H., Katoh, M., Eisfeld, A., Neumann, G., Hase, T., Ghosh, S., Shoemaker, J., Lopes, T., Watanabe, T., *et al.* (2013). A comprehensive map of the influenza A virus replication cycle. BMC Syst. Biol. *7*, 97.

Mayer, D., Molawi, K., Martinez-Sobrido, L., Ghanem, A., Thomas, S., Baginsky, S., Grossmann, J., Garcia-Sastre, A., and Schwemmle, M. (2007). Identification of cellular interaction partners of the influenza virus ribonucleoprotein complex and polymerase complex using proteomic-based approaches. J. Proteome Res. *6*, 672–682.

McAuley, J.L., Hornung, F., Boyd, K.L., Smith, A.M., McKeon, R., Bennink, J., Yewdell, J.W., and McCullers, J.A. (2007). Expression of the 1918 influenza A virus PB1-F2 enhances the pathogenesis of viral and secondary bacterial pneumonia. Cell Host Microbe *2*, 240–249.

Medcalf, L., Poole, E., Elton, D., and Digard, P. (1999). Temperature-sensitive lesions in two influenza A viruses defective for replicative transcription disrupt RNA binding by the nucleoprotein. J. Virol. *73*, 7349–7356.

Mehle, A., and Doudna, J.A. (2008). An inhibitory activity in human cells restricts the function of an avian-like influenza virus polymerase. Cell Host Microbe *4*, 111–122.

Mehle, A., and Doudna, J.A. (2009). Adaptive strategies of the influenza virus polymerase for replication in humans. Proc. Natl. Acad. Sci. U.S.A. *106*, 21312–21316.

Moeller, A., Kirchdoerfer, R.N., Potter, C.S., Carragher, B., and Wilson, I.A. (2012). Organization of the influenza virus replication machinery. Science *338*, 1631–1634.

Moisy, D., Avilov, S.V., Jacob, Y., Laoide, B.M., Ge, X., Baudin, F., Naffakh, N., and Jestin, J.L. (2012). HMGB1 protein binds to influenza virus nucleoprotein and promotes viral replication. J. Virol. *86*, 9122–9133.

Momose, F., Basler, C.F., O'Neill, R.E., Iwamatsu, A., Palese, P., and Nagata, K. (2001). Cellular splicing factor RAF-2p48/NPI-5/BAT1/UAP56 interacts with the influenza virus nucleoprotein and enhances viral RNA synthesis. J. Virol. *75*, 1899–1908.

Momose, F., Kikuchi, Y., Komase, K., and Morikawa, Y. (2007). Visualization of microtubule-mediated transport of influenza viral progeny ribonucleoprotein. Microbes Infect. *9*, 1422–1433.

Momose, F., Naito, T., Yano, K., Sugimoto, S., Morikawa, Y., and Nagata, K. (2002). Identification of Hsp90 as a stimulatory host factor involved in influenza virus RNA synthesis. J. Biol. Chem. *277*, 45306–45314.

Moncorge, O., Mura, M., and Barclay, W.S. (2010). Evidence for avian and human host cell factors that affect the activity of influenza virus polymerase. J. Virol. *84*, 9978–9986.

Mondal, A., Potts, G.K., Dawson, A.R., Coon, J.J., and Mehle, A. (2015). Phosphorylation at the homotypic interface regulates nucleoprotein oligomerization and assembly of the influenza virus replication machinery. PLoS Pathog. *11*, e1004826.

Mukaigawa, J., and Nayak, D.P. (1991). Two signals mediate nuclear localization of influenza virus (A/WSN/33) polymerase basic protein 2. J. Virol. *65*, 245–253.

Munier, S., Rolland, T., Diot, C., Jacob, Y., and Naffakh, N. (2013). Exploration of binary virus-host interactions using an infectious protein complementation assay. Mol. Cell. Proteomics *12*, 2845–2855.

Muramoto, Y., Noda, T., Kawakami, E., Akkina, R., and Kawaoka, Y. (2013). Identification of novel influenza A virus proteins translated from PA mRNA. J. Virol. *87*, 2455–2462.

Naito, T., Kiyasu, Y., Sugiyama, K., Kimura, A., Nakano, R., Matsukage, A., and Nagata, K. (2007a). An influenza virus replicon system in yeast identified Tat-SF1 as a stimulatory host factor for viral RNA synthesis. Proc. Natl. Acad. Sci. U.S.A. *104*, 18235–18240.

Naito, T., Momose, F., Kawaguchi, A., and Nagata, K. (2007b). Involvement of Hsp90 in assembly and nuclear import of influenza virus RNA polymerase subunits. J. Virol. *81*, 1339–1349.

Nano, N., and Houry, W.A. (2013). Chaperone-like activity of the AAA+ proteins Rvb1 and Rvb2 in the assembly of various complexes. Philos. Trans. R. Soc. Lond. B Biol. Sci. *368*.

Nath, S.T., and Nayak, D.P. (1990). Function of two discrete regions is required for nuclear localization of polymerase basic protein 1 of A/WSN/33 influenza virus (H1 N1). Mol. Cell. Biol. *10*, 4139–4145.

Neumann, G., Hughes, M.T., and Kawaoka, Y. (2000). Influenza A virus NS2 protein mediates vRNP nuclear export through NES-independent interaction with hCRM1. EMBO J. *19*, 6751–6758.

Nevalainen, M., Nissinen, M., Kaakinen, M., and Metsikko, K. (2010). Influenza virus infection in multinucleated skeletal myofibers. Exp. Cell Res. *316*, 1784–1794.

Ng, A.K., Zhang, H., Tan, K., Li, Z., Liu, J.H., Chan, P.K., Li, S.M., Chan, W.Y., Au, S.W., Joachimiak, A., *et al.* (2008). Structure of the influenza virus A H5N1 nucleoprotein: implications for RNA binding, oligomerization, and vaccine design. FASEB J. *22*, 3638–3647.

Nieto, A., de la Luna, S., Barcena, J., Portela, A., and Ortin, J. (1994). Complex structure of the nuclear translocation signal of influenza virus polymerase PA subunit. J. Gen. Virol. *75*, 29–36.

Noah, D.L., Twu, K.Y., and Krug, R.M. (2003). Cellular antiviral responses against influenza A virus are countered at the posttranscriptional level by the viral NS1A protein via its binding to a cellular protein required for the 3′ end processing of cellular pre-mRNAS. Virology *307*, 386–395.

O'Neill, R.E., Jaskunas, R., Blobel, G., Palese, P., and Moroianu, J. (1995). Nuclear import of influenza virus RNA can be mediated by viral nucleoprotein and transport factors required for protein import. J. Biol. Chem. *270*, 22701–22704.

O'Neill, R.E., Talon, J., and Palese, P. (1998). The influenza virus NEP (NS2 protein) mediates the nuclear export of viral ribonucleoproteins. EMBO J. *17*, 288–296.

Obayashi, E., Yoshida, H., Kawai, F., Shibayama, N., Kawaguchi, A., Nagata, K., Tame, J.R., and Park, S.Y. (2008). The structural basis for an essential subunit interaction in influenza virus RNA polymerase. Nature *454*, 1127–1131.

Olson, A.C., Rosenblum, E., and Kuchta, R.D. (2010). Regulation of influenza RNA polymerase activity and the switch between replication and transcription by the concentrations of the vRNA 5′ end, the cap source, and the polymerase. Biochemistry *49*, 10208–10215.

Paterson, D., and Fodor, E. (2012). Emerging roles for the influenza A virus nuclear export protein (NEP). PLoS Pathog. *8*, e1003019.

Perez, D.R., and Donis, R.O. (2001). Functional analysis of PA binding by influenza a virus PB1: effects on polymerase activity and viral infectivity. J. Virol. *75*, 8127–8136.

Perez, J.T., Varble, A., Sachidanandam, R., Zlatev, I., Manoharan, M., Garcia-Sastre, A., and tenOever, B.R. (2010). Influenza A virus-generated small RNAs regulate the switch from transcription to replication. Proc. Natl. Acad. Sci. U.S.A. *107*, 11525–11530.

Perez, J.T., Zlatev, I., Aggarwal, S., Subramanian, S., Sachidanandam, R., Kim, B., Manoharan, M., and tenOever, B.R. (2012). A small-RNA enhancer of viral polymerase activity. J. Virol. *86*, 13475–13485.

Pérez-González, A., Rodriguez, A., Huarte, M., Salanueva, I.J., and Nieto, A. (2006). hCLE/CGI-99, a human protein that interacts with the influenza virus polymerase, is a mRNA transcription modulator. J. Mol. Biol. *362*, 887–900.

Pertel, T., Hausmann, S., Morger, D., Zuger, S., Guerra, J., Lascano, J., Reinhard, C., Santoni, F.A., Uchil, P.D., Chatel, L., *et al.* (2011). TRIM5 is an innate immune sensor for the retrovirus capsid lattice. Nature *472*, 361–365.

Pflug, A., Guilligay, D., Reich, S., and Cusack, S. (2014). Structure of influenza A polymerase bound to the viral RNA promoter. Nature *516*, 355–360.

Plotch, S.J., Bouloy, M., Ulmanen, I., and Krug, R.M. (1981). A unique cap(m7GpppXm)-dependent influenza virion endonuclease cleaves capped RNAs to generate the primers that initiate viral RNA transcription. Cell *23*, 847–858.

Poole, E., Elton, D., Medcalf, L., and Digard, P. (2004). Functional domains of the influenza A virus PB2 protein: identification of NP- and PB1-binding sites. Virology *321*, 120–133.

Poon, L.L., Pritlove, D.C., Fodor, E., and Brownlee, G.G. (1999). Direct evidence that the poly(A) tail of influenza A virus mRNA is synthesized by reiterative copying of a U track in the virion RNA template. J. Virol. *73*, 3473–3476.

Reich, S., Guilligay, D., Pflug, A., Malet, H., Berger, I., Crepin, T., Hart, D., Lunardi, T., Nanao, M., Ruigrok, R.W., *et al.* (2014). Structural insight into cap-snatching and RNA synthesis by influenza polymerase. Nature *516*, 361–366.

Resa-Infante, P., Jorba, N., Zamarreno, N., Fernandez, Y., Juarez, S., and Ortin, J. (2008). The host-dependent interaction of alpha-importins with influenza PB2 polymerase subunit is required for virus RNA replication. PLoS One *3*, e3904.

Robb, N.C., Smith, M., Vreede, F.T., and Fodor, E. (2009). NS2/NEP protein regulates transcription and replication of the influenza virus RNA genome. J. Gen. Virol. *90*, 1398–1407.

Robertson, J.S., Schubert, M., and Lazzarini, R.A. (1981). Polyadenylation sites for influenza virus mRNA. J. Virol. *38*, 157–163.

Rodriguez, A., Pérez-González, A., and Nieto, A. (2011). Cellular human CLE/C14orf166 protein interacts with influenza virus polymerase and is required for viral replication. J. Virol. *85*, 12062–12066.

Romanos, M.A., and Hay, A.J. (1984). Identification of the influenza virus transcriptase by affinity-labeling with pyridoxal 5′-phosphate. Virology *132*, 110–117.

Shapira, S.D., Gat-Viks, I., Shum, B.O., Dricot, A., de Grace, M.M., Wu, L., Gupta, P.B., Hao, T., Silver, S.J., Root, D.E., *et al.* (2009). A physical and regulatory map of host–influenza interactions reveals pathways in H1N1 infection. Cell *139*, 1255–1267.

Shapiro, G.I., Gurney, T., Jr., and Krug, R.M. (1987). Influenza virus gene expression: control mechanisms at early and late times of infection and nuclear-cytoplasmic transport of virus-specific RNAs. J. Virol. *61*, 764–773.

Shapiro, G.I., and Krug, R.M. (1988). Influenza virus RNA replication in vitro: synthesis of viral template RNAs and virion RNAs in the absence of an added primer. J. Virol. *62*, 2285–2290.

Shi, M., Jagger, B.W., Wise, H.M., Digard, P., Holmes, E.C., and Taubenberger, J.K. (2012). Evolutionary conservation of the PA-X open reading frame in segment 3 of influenza A virus. J. Virol. *86*, 12411–12413.

Smith, G.L., and Hay, A.J. (1982). Replication of the influenza virus genome. Virology *118*, 96–108.

Subbarao, E.K., London, W., and Murphy, B.R. (1993). A single amino acid in the PB2 gene of influenza A virus is a determinant of host range. J. Virol. *67*, 1761–1764.

Sugiyama, K., Kawaguchi, A., Okuwaki, M., and Nagata, K. (2016). pp32 and APRIL are host cell-derived regulators of influenza virus RNA synthesis from cRNA. eLife *4*.

Sugiyama, K., Obayashi, E., Kawaguchi, A., Suzuki, Y., Tame, J.R.H., Nagata, K., and Park, S.Y. (2009). Structural insight into the essential PB1-PB2 subunit contact of the influenza virus RNA polymerase. EMBO J. *28*, 1803–1811.

Tafforeau, L., Chantier, T., Pradezynski, F., Pellet, J., Mangeot, P.E., Vidalain, P.-O., Andre, P., Rabourdin-Combe, C., and Lotteau, V. (2011). Generation and comprehensive analysis of an influenza virus polymerase cellular interaction network. J. Virol. *85*, 13010–13018.

Takizawa, N., Watanabe, K., Nouno, K., Kobayashi, N., and Nagata, K. (2006). Association of functional influenza viral proteins and RNAs with nuclear chromatin and sub-chromatin structure. Microbes Infect. *8*, 823–833.

Tarendeau, F., Boudet, J., Guilligay, D., Mas, P.J., Bougault, C.M., Boulo, S., Baudin, F., Ruigrok, R.W., Daigle, N., Ellenberg, J., *et al.* (2007). Structure and nuclear import function of the C-terminal domain of influenza virus polymerase PB2 subunit. Nat. Struct. Mol. Biol. *14*, 229–233.

Tchatalbachev, S., Flick, R., and Hobom, G. (2001). The packaging signal of influenza viral RNA molecules. RNA *7*, 979–989.

Thierry, E., Guilligay, D., Kosinski, J., Bock, T., Gaudon, S., Round, A., Pflug, A., Hengrung, N., El Omari, K., Baudin, F., *et al.* (2016). Influenza polymerase can adopt an alternative configuration involving a radical repacking of PB2 domains. Mol. Cell *61*, 125–137.

Tsai, P.-L., Chiou, N.-T., Kuss, S., García-Sastre, A., Lynch, K.W., and Fontoura, B.M.A. (2013). Cellular RNA binding proteins NS1-BP and hnRNP K regulate influenza A virus RNA splicing. PLoS Pathog. *9*, e1003460.

Turrell, L., Hutchinson, E.C., Vreede, F.T., and Fodor, E. (2015). Regulation of influenza a virus nucleoprotein oligomerization by phosphorylation. J. Virol. *89*, 1452–1455.

Ulmanen, I., Broni, B.A., and Krug, R.M. (1981). Role of two of the influenza virus core P proteins in recognizing cap 1 structures (m7GpppNm) on RNAs and in initiating viral RNA transcription. Proc. Natl. Acad. Sci. U.S.A. *78*, 7355–7359.

Varga, Z.T., Ramos, I., Hai, R., Schmolke, M., Garcia-Sastre, A., Fernandez-Sesma, A., and Palese, P. (2011). The influenza virus protein PB1-F2 inhibits the induction of type I interferon at the level of the MAVS adaptor protein. PLoS Pathog. 7, e1002067.

Vreede, F.T., Chan, A.Y., Sharps, J., and Fodor, E. (2010). Mechanisms and functional implications of the degradation of host RNA polymerase II in influenza virus infected cells. Virology *396*, 125–134.

Vreede, F.T., Jung, T.E., and Brownlee, G.G. (2004). Model suggesting that replication of influenza virus is regulated by stabilization of replicative intermediates. J. Virol. *78*, 9568–9572.

Vreede, F.T., Ng, A.K., Shaw, P.C., and Fodor, E. (2011). Stabilization of influenza virus replication intermediates is dependent on the RNA-binding but not the homo-oligomerization activity of the viral nucleoprotein. J. Virol. *85*, 12073–12078.

Wang, P., Palese, P., and O'Neill, R.E. (1997). The NPI-1/NPI-3 (karyopherin alpha) binding site on the influenza a virus nucleoprotein NP is a nonconventional nuclear localization signal. J. Virol. *71*, 1850–1856.

Wang, P., Song, W., Mok, B.W.-Y., Zhao, P., Qin, K., Lai, A., Smith, G.J.D., Zhang, J., Lin, T., Guan, Y., *et al.* (2009). Nuclear factor 90 negatively regulates influenza virus replication by interacting with viral nucleoprotein. J. Virol. *83*, 7850–7861.

Wang, Z., Liu, X., Zhao, Z., Xu, C., Zhang, K., Chen, C., Sun, L., Gao, G.F., Ye, X., and Liu, W. (2011). Cyclophilin E functions as a negative regulator to influenza virus replication by impairing the formation of the viral ribonucleoprotein complex. PLoS One *6*, e22625.

Watanabe, T., Kawakami, E., Shoemaker, J.E., Lopes, T.J., Matsuoka, Y., Tomita, Y., Kozuka-Hata, H., Gorai, T., Kuwahara, T., Takeda, E., *et al.* (2014). Influenza virus-host interactome screen as a platform for antiviral drug development. Cell Host Microbe *16*, 795–805.

Weber, M., Gawanbacht, A., Habjan, M., Rang, A., Borner, C., Schmidt, A.M., Veitinger, S., Jacob, R., Devignot, S., Kochs, G., *et al.* (2013). Incoming RNA virus nucleocapsids containing a 5′-triphosphorylated genome activate RIG-I and antiviral signaling. Cell Host Microbe *13*, 336–346.

Weber, M., Sediri, H., Felgenhauer, U., Binzen, I., Banfer, S., Jacob, R., Brunotte, L., Garcia-Sastre, A., Schmid-Burgk, J.L., Schmidt, T., *et al.* (2015). Influenza virus adaptation PB2-627K modulates nucleocapsid inhibition by the pathogen sensor RIG-I. Cell Host Microbe *17*, 309–319.

Wise, H.M., Foeglein, A., Sun, J., Dalton, R.M., Patel, S., Howard, W., Anderson, E.C., Barclay, W.S., and Digard, P. (2009). A complicated message: identification of a novel PB1-related protein translated from influenza A virus segment 2 mRNA. J. Virol. *83*, 8021–8031.

Yamada, S., Hatta, M., Staker, B.L., Watanabe, S., Imai, M., Shinya, K., Sakai-Tagawa, Y., Ito, M., Ozawa, M., Watanabe, T., *et al.* (2010). Biological and structural characterization of a host-adapting amino acid in influenza virus. PLoS Pathog. *6*, e1001034.

Ye, Q., Krug, R.M., and Tao, Y.J. (2006). The mechanism by which influenza A virus nucleoprotein forms oligomers and binds RNA. Nature *444*, 1078–1082.

York, A., Hengrung, N., Vreede, F.T., Huiskonen, J.T., and Fodor, E. (2013). Isolation and characterization of the positive-sense replicative intermediate of a negative-strand RNA virus. Proc. Natl. Acad. Sci. U.S.A. *110*, E4238–4245.

York, A., Hutchinson, E.C., and Fodor, E. (2014). Interactome analysis of the influenza A virus transcription/ replication machinery identifies protein phosphatase 6 as a cellular factor required for efficient virus replication. J. Virol. *88*, 13284–13299.

Yu, M., Liu, X., Cao, S., Zhao, Z., Zhang, K., Xie, Q., Chen, C., Gao, S., Bi, Y., Sun, L., *et al.* (2012). Identification and characterization of three novel nuclear export signals in the influenza A virus nucleoprotein. J. Virol. *86*, 4970–4980.

Yuan, P., Bartlam, M., Lou, Z., Chen, S., Zhou, J., He, X., Lv, Z., Ge, R., Li, X., Deng, T., *et al.* (2009). Crystal structure of an avian influenza polymerase PA(N) reveals an endonuclease active site. Nature *458*, 909–913.

Zhang, J., Li, G., and Ye, X. (2010). Cyclin T1/CDK9 interacts with influenza A virus polymerase and facilitates its association with cellular RNA polymerase II. J. Virol. *84*, 12619–12627.

Zheng, H., Lee, H.A., Palese, P., and Garcia-Sastre, A. (1999). Influenza A virus RNA polymerase has the ability to stutter at the polyadenylation site of a viral RNA template during RNA replication. J. Virol. *73*, 5240–5243.

Zhirnov, O.P., and Klenk, H.D. (1997). Histones as a target for influenza virus matrix protein M1. Virology *235*, 302–310.

Zhou, Z., Cao, M., Guo, Y., Zhao, L., Wang, J., Jia, X., Li, J., Wang, C., Gabriel, G., Xue, Q., *et al.* (2014). Fragile X mental retardation protein stimulates ribonucleoprotein assembly of influenza A virus. Nat. Commun. *5*, 3259.

Receptor Specificity in Surveillance of Natural Sequence Evolution of Influenza A Virus Haemagglutinin

6

Rahul Raman, Kannan Tharakaraman, Zachary Shriver, Akila Jayaraman, V. Sasisekharan and Ram Sasisekharan

Abstract

Influenza A viruses are rapidly evolving pathogens with potential for novel strains to emerge and cause human pandemics. H1N1, H2N2 and H3N2 influenza A virus (known as human viruses) haemagglutinin (HA) binds to glycan receptors in the human upper respiratory epithelia that are terminated by α2→6-linked sialic acid (also known as human receptors), a critical feature that permits the virus to efficiently infect and transmit via aerosol in humans. The avian-adapted H5N1, H9N1, H7N7, H7N2 and H7N9 have shown binding to human receptors, cause severe infections in humans and are rapidly evolving in various species but are yet to adapt to the human host to establish sustained circulation. There is a need to better understand and differentiate glycan receptor binding properties between these avian-adapted and human viruses. This chapter offers perspectives on structural and biochemical analyses of HA–glycan receptor interactions from standpoint of distinguishing receptor specificity of human and avian viruses and also in the context of their natural evolution. The perspectives offered in this chapter are intended to expand the current thinking and hence understanding of HA–glycan specificity to facilitate improved surveillance and preparedness in the event of an emergence of a novel strain with pandemic potential.

Introduction and significance

Influenza A, a zoonotic disease, represents a substantial public health burden, especially in the case of epidemic or pandemic outbreaks (Ahmed *et al.*, 2007; Perez Velasco *et al.*, 2012). Influenza A virus subtypes, found naturally in aquatic birds, are identified according to their surface antigens: haemagglutinin (HA) and neuraminidase (NA). Influenza A viruses are known to rapidly evolve resulting in novel strains arising due to mutations (antigenic drift) and reassortment among subtypes (antigenic shift). Additionally, individuals with compromised immune systems are more susceptible to infection with this virus, which can spread from person-to-person through respiratory droplets On what appears to be a semi-periodic basis, predominantly through the process of antigenic shift, altered influenza viruses can emerge that efficiently infect humans, are highly transmissible via aerosol between humans and potentially pathogenic, resulting in a pandemic outbreak (Layne *et al.*, 2009; Neumann *et al.*, 2009; Russell and Webster, 2005; Taubenberger and Morens, 2008). Such pandemics have occurred several times in the 20th century, including in 1918 (H1N1), 1958 (H2N2) and 1967 (H3N2). Among these subtypes, H1N1 and H3N2 have established sustained circulation in the human population by underdoing antigenic drift, which results in seasonal flu outbreaks each year. More recently even among these human virus subtypes, novel strains including 2009 H1N1 and 2010 H3N2 have emerged from reassortment of viral gene segments among avian, swine, and human viral strains and were able to successfully establish circulation via efficient human-to-human transmission (Fraser *et al.*, 2009; Itoh *et al.*, 2009; Pearce *et al.*, 2012).

The previous rapid introduction and spread of novel influenza strains/subtypes in the population has increased the surveillance and study of avian-adapted strains that have been documented to infect (but not spread in) humans. Of particular interest are the H5 (N1), H7 (N2, N7 and N9) and H9 (N1 and N2) subtypes. Quite recently in fact, a novel avian-adapted H7N9 strain emerged in China that caused severe infection and was ultimately fatal in some instances. Although this subtype has not completely adapted yet to humans, it already possesses partial phenotypic features characteristic of human adapted-viruses (Belser *et al.*, 2013; Chen *et al.*, 2013; Gao *et al.*, 2013; Kageyama *et al.*, 2013; Tharakaraman *et al.*, 2013a; Watanabe *et al.*, 2013). Therefore, the adaptation of avian-adapted subtypes to the human host poses a constant threat of pandemic outbreak (due to the poor pre-sexisting immunity for novel subtypes). Significant effort has been focused on determining the genetic determinants for human host adaptation, virulence, and aerosol transmissibility (Palese, 2004; Pappas *et al.*, 2008; Van Hoeven *et al.*, 2009) (summarized in Table 6.1).

The binding specificity of the viral surface HA to sialylated glycan receptors (glycans terminated by α-D-N-acetyl neuraminic acid; Neu5Ac) on the host cell surface is one of many factors that critically govern adaptation of influenza to the human host. Avian virus HA binds with high specificity and affinity to glycans terminated by α2→3-linked sialic acid which are found in abundance in avian gut and deep lung of humans (these glycans will henceforth be referred to as α2→3 glycans or *avian receptors*) (Gambaryan *et al.*, 1997; Russell *et al.*, 2006; Shinya *et al.*, 2006; van Riel *et al.*, 2006). Human virus HA possess characteristic glycan receptor binding properties; their HA predominantly binds with high affinity (or avidity) to glycan receptors terminated by α2→6-linked sialic acid, which are predominantly expressed in the upper respiratory epithelia of humans (these glycans will henceforth be referred to as α2→6 glycans or human receptors) (Chandrasekaran *et al.*, 2008; Shinya *et al.*, 2006; Stevens *et al.*, 2006a). The human upper respiratory epithelium is the primary target site for infection of human-adapted viruses and is thought to be a prerequisite for efficient human-to-human transmission via respiratory droplets. Thus, it appears that human adaptation of

Table 6.1 Mutations in gene segments/protein products

Protein	Mutation	Effect
Polymerase (PB2)	E627K	Increased replication
Polymerase (PA)	F666L	Increased replication
Non-structural protein (NS1)	V137F	Evasion of immune response
Nucleoprotein (NP)	E136K	Increased replication
Neuraminidase (NA)	Several	Efficient particle release
Haemagglutinin	?	Receptor binding and virus uptake

an HA is associated with a switch in its binding preference from avian to human receptors. Notably, this switch is a necessary but not sufficient change required for human adaptation, which ultimately involves other genetic modifications within the viral genome (Table 6.1) and emergence of phenotypic characteristics such as efficient respiratory droplet transmission in ferret animal models (Van Hoeven *et al.*, 2009).

To address in greater detail the binding of HA to its glycan receptors, advances in the synthesis of complex glycan structures have been coupled with technologies to display these structures on various glycan array platforms and interrogate HA receptor specificity (Liang *et al.*, 2008; Song *et al.*, 2011; Stevens *et al.*, 2006b). Using such technologies, the glycan receptor binding properties has been defined in many ways in different studies. For example, some studies using glycan arrays describe the ratio of the number of $\alpha2\rightarrow6$ to $\alpha2\rightarrow3$ sialylated glycans that show binding to a specific HA or virus analysed at a high titre or concentration (Stevens *et al.*, 2006a,c). Other studies describe the ratio of binding affinity (or avidity) of HA (or virus) to $\alpha2\rightarrow6$ versus $\alpha2\rightarrow3$ glycans (Imai *et al.*, 2012; Xiong *et al.*, 2013).

In parallel with these advances, efforts have been ongoing to routinely solve co-crystal structures of HA–glycan complexes for a variety of HA subtypes, including H1, H2, H3, H5, H7, and H9 (Gamblin *et al.*, 2004; Ha *et al.*, 2001, 2003; Lin *et al.*, 2009, 2012; Stevens *et al.*, 2006c; Xu *et al.*, 2010; Yang *et al.*, 2010b, 2012; Zhang *et al.*, 2013). Detailed structural information has provided a wealth of information on key interactions within the glycan-receptor binding site (RBS) of HA with surrogates of either avian or human receptors or both, leading to the identification of hallmark residues that distinguish binding of HAs to both avian and human receptors.

The gaps that remain to be addressed in the context of what is known about HA–glycan interactions based on the aforementioned studies are the following. First, how do changes in the RBS in the context of natural sequence evolution impact glycan receptor-binding properties of HA, and more importantly from the standpoint of avian virus HAs acquiring human receptor specificity? As an example, introducing amino acid changes in different natural strains of avian-adapted H5 HA based on prototypic amino acids that contribute to human receptor-binding in human-adapted H1, H2 or H3 HAs results in drastically different glycan binding properties unrelated to the human receptor binding preference (Stevens *et al.*, 2008; Tharakaraman *et al.*, 2013b). Second, how does binding of viral HA to defined glycans on glycan array platforms relate to its binding to physiological glycan receptors in the human respiratory tract? For example, the glycan-array binding properties of the recently emerged H7N9 HA do not correlate with its tissue tropism in the human upper and lower respiratory tract (Tharakaraman *et al.*, 2013a). Third, the varying definitions of glycan receptor binding have complicated the distinction between binding of human and avian virus HA to human receptors and thus made it difficult to assess the path towards acquisition of human receptor binding properties by avian virus HAs in the context of their natural sequence evolution.

In the context of the above questions, this chapter reviews the different measurements of HA–glycan interactions. This chapter also offers perspectives on addressing the aforementioned gaps by describing an integrated framework. This framework incorporates structural and biochemical analyses and data. The structural analyses take into account glycan conformation and the network of inter-residue interactions in the RBS responsible for interactions with human (and avian) receptors. The biochemical analyses involve measuring both quantitative binding affinity to representative glycan receptors and the physiological tropism of

HA within the human respiratory tract. The perspectives offered in this chapter are broadly aimed at augmenting current understanding of HA–glycan interactions with the eventual goal of improving surveillance methods to advance preparedness in the event of emergence of novel influenza strains.

HA–glycan receptor interactions: structural and biochemical aspects of receptor specificity

This section of the chapter covers analyses of X-ray co-crystal structures of HA–glycan complexes to understand role and relevance of glycan conformation, topology, hallmark RBS residues in distinguishing avian and human receptor binding of HA. The experimental tools to measure HA–glycan interactions (to link back to the structural observations) along with their caveats, strengths and limitations are also discussed. The summary of this section highlights the need to take an integrated approach that incorporates all the measurements described below to robustly distinguish avian and human receptor-binding of HA

Glycan conformation and concept of hallmark residues defined based on HA–glycan co-crystal structures

Several X-ray crystallographic structures of HA–glycan receptor complexes have been solved (Gamblin *et al.*, 2004; Ha *et al.*, 2001, 2003; Lin *et al.*, 2012; Liu *et al.*, 2009; Stevens *et al.*, 2006c; Xu *et al.*, 2010; Yang *et al.*, 2010b, 2012; Zhang *et al.*, 2013). Notably, the most commonly used glycans to represent avian and human receptors, respectively are LS-tetrasaccharide a (or LSTa; Neu5Acα2–3Galβ1–3GlcNAcβ1–3Galβ1–4Glc) and LS-tetrasaccharide c (or LSTc; Neu5Acα2–6Galβ1–4GlcNAcβ1–3Galβ1–4Glc). In the co-crystal structures of avian-adapted HAs (such as H5N1, H7N2, H7N7) with LSTa, the coordinates are typically available only for the non-reducing end trisaccharide (Neu5Acα2–3Galβ1–3GlcNAc). On the other hand, in the case of co-crystal structures of human-adapted HAs with LSTc, depending on the structure, the coordinates are available for either the entire pentasaccharide or the non-reducing end tetra- or trisaccharide. Based on some of the earliest X-ray co-crystal structures, the conformations of LSTa and LSTc have been characterized primarily by the glycosidic torsion angles of the terminal sialic acid linkage (Fig. 6.1A) (Russell *et al.*, 2006). In the case of the Neu5Acα2–3Gal- linkage in LSTa complexed with avian-adapted HA, the torsion angle j (C-1–C-2–O-C-3) is ~180° and is described as the *trans* conformation. In the *trans* conformation the glycosidic oxygen is pointed towards the base of the RBS. In contrast, the Neu5Acα2–6Gal linkage in LSTc complexed with human-adapted HA, j (C-1–C-2–O-C-3), is ~ –60°, or a *cis* conformation. In this conformation the glycosidic oxygen points away from the base of the RBS and the C-6 atom of the penultimate Gal sugar points towards the base of the RBS.

The *cis* and *trans* definition of glycan receptor conformation enabled distinguishing key contacts of residues within the RBS of to either LSTa or LSTc, leading to the concept of 'hallmark' residues within the RBS of avian- and human-adapted HAs. In the case of avian-adapted HAs, residue Glu-190 and Gln-226 (residue numbering based on H3 HA throughout the text) are hallmark residues wherein Glu-190 is positioned to interact with sialic acid and Gln-226 in the base of the RBS is positioned to make ionic contacts with the glycosidic oxygen of Neu5Acα2–3Gal in the *trans* conformation (Russell *et al.*, 2006). In the case of human-adapted H2N2 and H3N2 HAs, the 226-position typically has a hydrophobic

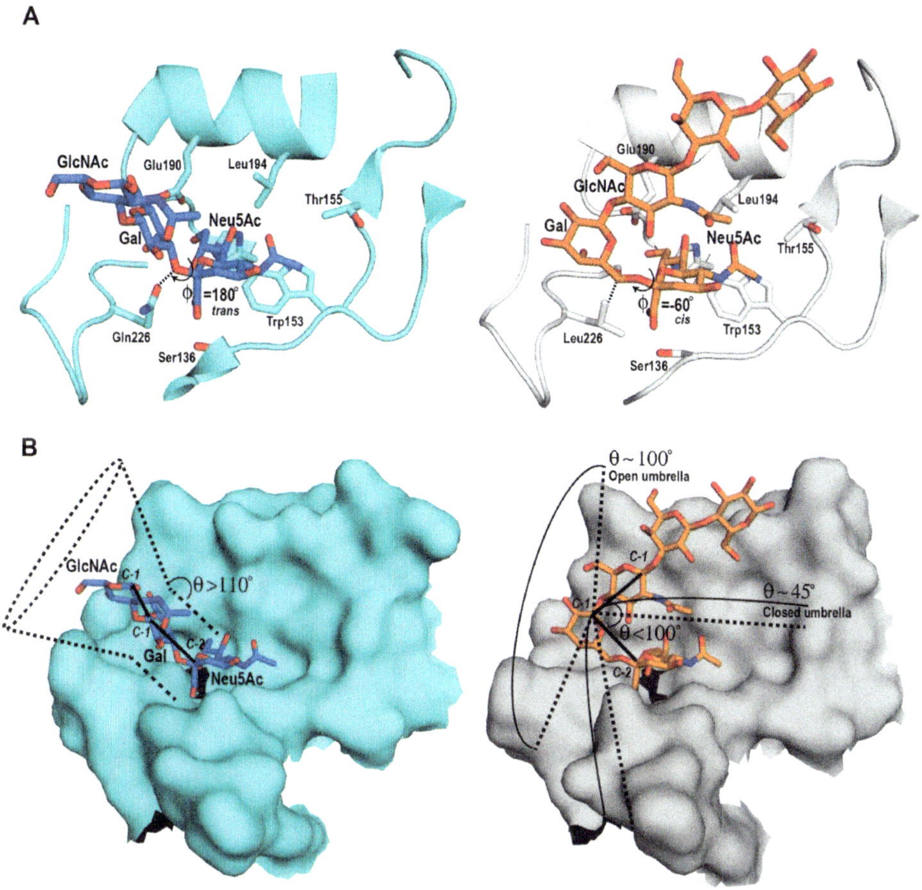

Figure 6.1 Glycan receptor conformation and topology in HA RBS. (A) Shown on the left is the *trans* conformation adopted by LSTa in receptor binding site of avian-adapted H3 HA (A/duck/Ukraine/63; PDB ID: 1MQM). The LSTa glycan is shown in stick representation coloured by atom (C, blue; O, red; N, dark blue) and HA RBS is shown in cartoon representation coloured cyan with key side-chains of key RBS residues interacting with the Neu5Acα2→3Gal motif labelled and shown in stick representation. The interaction between characteristic Gln-226 and glycosidic oxygen atom is shown in dotted line. Shown on the right is the *cis* conformation adopted by LSTc in receptor binding site of pandemic H3 HA (PDB ID:2YPG). The LSTc glycan is shown in stick representation coloured by atom (C, orange; O, red; N, dark blue) and HA RBS is shown in cartoon representation coloured grey with key side-chains of key RBS residues interacting with the Neu5Acα2→6Gal motif labelled and shown in stick representation. The interaction between characteristic Leu-226 and C-6 atom of Gal is shown in dotted line. (B) Shown on the left is the topological description of the same avian HA-LSTa–glycan complex shown in A (RBS is shown as a surface) with the description of the θ angle as angle between C-2 atom of Neu5Ac, C-1 atom of Gal and *C*-1 atom of GlcNAc. For θ >110°, the possible conformations sampled by the avian receptor spans a surface on the RBS that resembles a cone (shown in dotted lines). Shown on the right is the topological description of the same human HA-LSTc–glycan complex shown in A (RBS is shown as a surface) where for θ <100°, the possible conformations sampled by the human receptor spans a much larger surface on the RBS that resembles an umbrella in an open state (at the boundary of θ ~100°) to a closed state (θ ~45°) which is shown as a dotted line and the curvature of the umbrella in the open and closed form is shown as a solid line arc.

residue such as Leu, Ile or Val, which facilitates hydrophobic interactions with the *C6* atom of Neu5Acα2–6Gal in the *cis* conformation (Russell *et al.*, 2006). Additionally, the presence of a hydrophobic residue in the 226-position does not enable favorable contacts with the glycosidic oxygen of Neu5Acα2–3Gal and hence is detrimental for avian-receptor binding. Therefore, the Gln226→Leu amino acid change has been considered a hallmark mutation for switching the receptor preference (leading to human adaptation) for H2 and H3 HAs.

On the other hand, considering H1, both avian- and human-adapted HAs have Gln-226, which based on the RBS structure of this subtype is less favoured for making hydrophobic interactions with the C-6 atom of Neu5Acα2–6Gal in the *cis* conformation. Instead, an Asp in the 225 position (which is typically a Gly in avian-adapted H1 HAs) in human-adapted H1 HA provides additional contacts with the penultimate Gal sugar in the *trans* conformation (Gamblin *et al.*, 2004; Russell *et al.*, 2006; Zhang *et al.*, 2013). In H1 HA, the differences in contacts between avian and human receptors go beyond the distinct contacts with Neu5Acα2–6Gal and Neu5Acα2–3Gal in the base of the RBS. Another amino acid typically observed in human-adapted H1 HA is Asp-190, which favors specific contacts with the third GlcNAc sugar (from the non-reducing end) which is not the case with Glu-190, which is typically present within avian-adapted HAs (Gamblin *et al.*, 2004; Russell *et al.*, 2006). Therefore the Glu versus Asp in the 190-position in H1 HA likely plays a key role in distinguishing avian and human receptor specificity (Glaser *et al.*, 2005). Consequently, in H1 HA, Glu190→Asp and Gly225→Asp have been considered as hallmark amino acid changes to switch receptor specificity leading to human adaptation (Glaser *et al.*, 2005; Tumpey *et al.*, 2007).

While, the *cis* and *trans* definition of glycan conformation has been useful to characterize the distinct interactions with terminal Neu5Ac α2→3Gal or Neu5Ac α2→6Gal motif, this definition does not fully describe HA binding to a range of structurally diverse glycans, either present on glycan array platforms or present in glycomic analysis of human respiratory cells and tissues (Chandrasekaran *et al.*, 2008). This limitation motivated studies that revisited the definition of glycan conformation, extending the conformational analysis beyond the terminal sialic acid linkage to describe overall topology and dynamics of the glycan receptor upon binding to the RBS of avian and human-adapted HAs (Chandrasekaran *et al.*, 2008; Xu *et al.*, 2009). To capture this topology, a parameter, θ, has been defined to measure the angle between the Neu5Ac, the penultimate Gal and the third GlcNAc sugar (measured using anomeric carbon atoms as shown in Fig. 6.1B). The θ parameter permits classification of the ensemble of conformations sampled by the avian and human receptors within the HA binding site.

In the case of avian receptors, the conformations sampled by the Neu5Acα2→3Gal linkage (keeping the Neu5Ac anchored) and the sugars beyond this linkage (at the reducing end) span a region on the binding surface of HA that resemble a 'cone'. Therefore the term *cone*-like topology has been used to capture the ensemble of these conformations – characterized by a θ angle > 110°. The different conformations sampled by Neu5Aca2→6Gal linkage (keeping the Neu5Ac anchored) and the sugars beyond this linkage (at the reducing end) span a wider area on the HA binding surface. A portion of these RBS-receptor contacts can be described by a cone-like surface, whereas the other portion is more correctly described as *umbrella*-like, and is characterized by θ angle < 100°. Given the conformationally more flexible form, depending on the attributes of the HA RBS and the receptor sequence, the umbrella-like conformation ensemble can be fully folded (θ–45°) to fully open (θ–90°).

Regardless, the stem of the umbrella is defined by the Neu5Aca2–6Gal-motif and the spokes of the umbrella are occupied by monosaccharides at the reducing end of Gal.

Examination of a range of avian-adapted HAs indicate that the defining characteristic of a *cone*-like topology is that the majority of contacts with the HA RBS are through a three-sugar (or trisaccharide) (Neu5Aca2→3/6Galb1→3/4GlcNAc-) motif as well as monosaccharide substitutions such as O-sulfation (of Gal or GlcNAc) or fucosylation (at GlcNAc). On the other hand, the *umbrella*-like topology was such that monosaccharides beyond a trisaccharide make substantial contacts with the HA RBS. Using these shape-based definitions of the flexible glycan conformation, it was shown that the *umbrella*-like topology is predominantly adopted by human receptors which possessed at least four sugars including the Neu5Ac, for example poly-lactosamine branches terminated by a2→6-linked Neu5Ac (referred to has long a2→6). The *cone*-like topology was shown to be adopted by both avian and human receptors.

Taken together, the shape- or topology-based definitions of glycan receptor conformation have been able to provide additional structural perspectives on HA–glycan interactions in the context of glycan diversity going beyond terminal sialic acid linkage. Furthermore, this framework has identification of additional key residue positions within the RBS of different HA subtypes that are involved in binding to avian and human receptors (Chandrasekaran *et al.*, 2008; Xu *et al.*, 2009). Finally, in conjunction with experimental information (detailed below), this structural framework has enabled robust classification of avian and human receptors.

Tools to measure and characterize HA–glycan interactions

As is the case with many virus–receptor interactions, binding between HA receptor is multivalent. A variety of biochemical methods have been used to characterize the specificity in the context of multivalent HA–glycan interactions [see review by Shriver *et al.*, (2009) for an overview of these methods]. Among the various tools, glycan array platforms are rapidly emerging as a popular tool to probe finer nuances of glycan structures that are recognized by various HAs (Liang *et al.*, 2008; Song *et al.*, 2011; Stevens *et al.*, 2006b).

Glycan platforms consist of hundreds of synthetic glycan motifs (typically present on N- and O-linked glycoproteins and glycolipids) displayed on the surface of the array. Multiple types of arrays have been developed that utilize different strategies including the formation of neoglycolipids (Fukui *et al.*, 2002), neoglycoproteins (Oyelaran and Gildersleeve, 2009), or the direct application of glycans to various surfaces (Blixt *et al.*, 2004; Grun *et al.*, 2006; Karamanska *et al.*, 2008; Liang *et al.*, 2008; Mercey *et al.*, 2008; Xia *et al.*, 2005). Studies have also begun to adapt these technologies towards the presentation of *natural* glycans by harvesting glycans from the surface of cells and imprinting these on a glycan array format (Song *et al.*, 2009), thus allowing one to probe the glycan repertoire of a biological system.

Both whole viruses and recombinantly expressed trimeric HA units have been analysed on glycan array platforms. While analysis of viruses on glycan arrays permits obtaining qualitative binding characteristics, it is exigent, for two major reasons, to quantify these interactions so as to compare binding properties across different viruses. *First*, unless directly labeled, virus concentration is commonly expressed as haemagglutination units (HAU) based on the virus's ability to agglutinate red blood cells. This is not a true measure of concentration; depending on agglutination potential of a virus, an HAU value could correspond to a very different concentration of HA. Emphasizing this fact, glycomic analysis of red blood cells has shown that the glycans on red blood cells do not necessarily recapitulate those observed in human respiratory cells (Aich *et al.*, 2011). Thus, viruses that bind well to human respiratory tissue may nonetheless fail to agglutinate red blood cells (Aich *et al.*, 2011). Second, depending on the morphology of the virus, the distribution of the trimeric HAs vary between different viruses. In turn, the differences in distribution of the trimeric HA units impinge on the avidity of glycan binding.

In contrast, analysing recombinantly expressed turmeric HA units offers a means to circumvent these challenges. First, HA concentration can be precisely measured. Also, an approach to precomplex the trimeric HA unit with primary and secondary antibodies (in HA primary–secondary ratio of 4:2:1) prior to analysis on glycan array enables one to address issues associated with multivalency (Srinivasan *et al.*, 2008; Stevens *et al.*, 2006b). Due to the stoichiometry of the precomplex, this approach ensures that the predominant species in the analyte correspond to four HA trimeric units that are spatially constrained relative to each other (due to the antibody interactions). The apparent affinity constant defined by such an assay can be used to compare quantitative binding of different HAs analysed. Notably, this parameter does not have any independent significance from the standpoint of physical chemistry.

A survey of studies completed to date indicates that the scope of array-binding assays varies across different studies. In many studies, glycan arrays are used as a primary screen for qualitatively analysing the frequency and type of α2→3 and α2→6 glycans that demonstrate binding to recombinant HA (or whole virus). In these studies, glycan-binding specificity is defined on the basis of the ratio of α2→6 to α2→3 glycans that show binding signals. This type of a screening approach, while informative, does not offer quantitative information, particularly relating to the relative human and avian receptor-binding affinity of an HA. Quantitative studies focus on selection of a small sampling of glycans representative of avian and human receptor and performing a dose response curve by varying either HA (virus) concentration or glycan concentration (Childs *et al.*, 2009; Liao *et al.*, 2010; Srinivasan *et al.*, 2008; Xiong *et al.*, 2013). The trade-off of using this approach is, of course, the loss of information regarding the diversity of glycan structures that are recognized by a given HA.

Although glycan array platforms display hundreds of diverse glycan structures, they still likely do not capture the physiological context or diversity of glycan receptors encountered by influenza A viruses in human or animal models. This issue has been addressed in part by examining binding of HA or whole virus to tissue sections of the respiratory tract of humans (upper respiratory tract: pharynx, trachea; middle respiratory tract: bronchus and deep lung/alveolar) and/or animal models, such as mice, ferrets, or pigs (Chandrasekaran *et al.*, 2008; Jayaraman *et al.*, 2012a; Nicholls *et al.*, 2007; Shinya *et al.*, 2006; van Riel *et al.*, 2006). Plant lectins such as SNA-I (specifically binds to α2→6 glycans), MAL-II (shows binding to α2→3 glycans), Jacalin (marker for O-linked mucin glycans), Con A (marked for N-linked glycans), etc. can be used to characterize the glycans present in these sections and hence provide structural information on HA recognition. Additionally, analytical tools such as mass spectrometry have been used to perform detailed structural characterization of sialylated glycans isolated from the respiratory tissues and cell lines (Bateman *et al.*, 2010; Chandrasekaran *et al.*, 2008; Walther *et al.*, 2013).

Avian-adapted viruses and HA extensively stain the alveolar sections in human deep lung which predominantly express avian receptors (van Riel *et al.*, 2006). On the other hand human-adapted viruses and HA show characteristic binding to apical surface of human tracheal sections that predominantly express human receptors (Chandrasekaran *et al.*, 2008; Jayaraman *et al.*, 2012a; Shinya *et al.*, 2006). Also within the human respiratory epithelium, avian-adapted viruses have been shown to primarily infect ciliated cells while human-adapted viruses have been shown to infect non-ciliated cells (Matrosovich *et al.*, 2004). This cell tropism may be important to the physiology of influenza transmission, especially for human-adapted viruses. Binding to non-ciliated, goblet cells, especially heavily glycosylated mucins on their surface, may play a role in droplet formation and transmission.

It is clear that these tools provide diverse yet related information on HA–glycan interactions. Therefore, integration of information from analysis of HA or virus binding to glycan arrays and physiological tissues can provide additional information beyond that available in arrays, including tropism of HA. In our view, integrated information from both tissue staining and array analysis provides the most detailed biochemical information on HA–glycan interactions that is best suited to phenotypic characterization of HA. To ensure accurate assessment of results, an important step is to benchmark the measurements made to prototypic human-adapted viruses such as the pandemic strains.

Benchmarking measurements of HA–glycan interactions and their relationship to aerosol transmissibility of pandemic viruses

Given that pandemic viruses have been extensively studied in terms of glycan receptor binding and their relationship to other phenotypic properties such as aerosol transmission in ferrets, this section of the chapter discusses how these properties can be benchmarked from the standpoint of analysing how avian virus HAs acquire human receptor binding specificity.

1918 H1N1 pandemic

The 1918 H1N1 subtype is among the most studied viruses. The ability to reconstruct the pandemic 1918 H1N1 virus through reverse genetics and test its virulence in ferrets permitted a systematic exploration of the roles for various viral genes in its virulence and transmissibility (Palese, 2004; Pappas *et al.*, 2008; Tumpey *et al.*, 2005; Van Hoeven *et al.*, 2009). Based on notion of hallmark Asp-190 and Asp-225 residues playing a key role in human-receptor binding of H1N1, single amino acid changes at these positions were made on a prototypic pandemic HA (A/South Carolina/1/1918). This resulted in two variants, NY18 (Asp225→Gly mutant of SC18) and AV18 (Asp-190→Glu mutant of NY18). Analysis of the aerosol transmissibility of these viruses in ferrets demonstrated that SC18 transmitted efficiently via respiratory droplet, NY18 showed transmission but was inefficient and AV18 did not transmit at all (Tumpey *et al.*, 2007). Given that all the other genes were identical between SC18, NY18 and AV18, these results showed a clear and direct link between altering the RBS of HA and transmissibility of the virus.

The glycan receptor-binding properties of SC18, NY18 and AV18 HA have been subsequently characterized in several other studies (Srinivasan *et al.*, 2008; Stevens *et al.*, 2006a) including recent crystallographic analysis of SC18 and NY18 HA binding to LSTa and LSTc (Zhang *et al.*, 2013). Dose-dependent direct binding of SC18, NY18 and AV18 analysed by precomplexing the HA on glycan array with representative avian and human receptors showed distinct quantitative binding properties (Srinivasan *et al.*, 2008). While SC18 showed exclusive binding to human receptors with an apparent affinity (K_d') in the picomolar range and minimal binding to avian receptors (Fig. 6.2), AV18 showed exclusive binding to avian receptors. NY18 demonstrated intermediate binding, with two orders of magnitude lower apparent affinity to human receptors and binding to avian receptors in the sub-nanomolar range. That NY18, having Asp-190, demonstrated similar binding affinity to both avian and human receptors was surprising given that Asp-190 should have enabled NY18 to distinguish between LSTa and LSTc (Glaser *et al.*, 2005; Zhang *et al.*, 2013).

SC18, NY18 and AV18 were also analysed on human tracheal and alveolar sections. Both SC18 and NY18 showed apical surface staining of tracheal section in a manner that was characteristic of human-adapted HAs. However, SC18 showed a characteristic predominant staining of non-ciliated goblet cells when compared with NY18, which stained ciliated cells to a greater extent than goblet cells (Srinivasan *et al.*, 2008). SC18 showed minimal to no staining of alveolar tissue section, while, consistent with their avian receptor-binding properties, NY18 and AV18 showed detectable staining of alveolar tissue.

1957–58 H2N2 pandemic

Similar to 1918 H1N1, ferret transmission and glycan-binding studies have been completed for the a prototypic strain (A/Albany/6/58 or Alb58) of the 1958 H2N2 pandemic. This virus transmitted efficiently via respiratory droplets in ferrets (Pappas *et al.*, 2010). Dose-dependent glycan array binding of Alb58 HA on the glycan array showed high affinity binding to human receptors (K_d' ~picomolar) (Viswanathan *et al.*, 2010). Interestingly, unlike SC18, Alb58 also showed observable binding to avian receptors, albeit at a binding affinity that was orders of magnitude lower than that to human receptors (K_d' ~nanomolar) (Fig. 6.2). Consistent with what was observed for SC18, Alb58 HA extensively stained the goblet cells. Additionally, Alb58 stained ciliated cells on the apical surface of human tracheal tissue sections as well as alveolar sections (Viswanathan *et al.*, 2010). Although cross-comparison of ferret transmission and glycan-binding properties have not been performed on the 1967–68 pandemic H3N2 strain, the glycan binding properties of a prototypic strain (A/Aichi/1/68 or Aichi68) have been analysed. Aichi68 shows comparable binding to both avian and human receptors with high-binding affinity (Lin *et al.*, 2012).

2009 swine-origin H1N1 pandemic

More recently, the aerosol transmission in ferrets and glycan-binding properties of the 2009 H1N1 pandemic strain (A/California/04/09 or Ca0409) were studied (Bradley *et al.*, 2011; Childs *et al.*, 2009; Maines *et al.*, 2009; Yang *et al.*, 2010a; Yen *et al.*, 2011). The dose-dependent glycan binding property of Ca0409 was very similar to that of SC18 wherein binding was observed exclusively to human receptors. Human tissue of Ca0409, confirmed this analysis, like SC18, binding of Ca0409 HA was restricted to the goblet cell region on the apical surface of the tracheal section (Maines *et al.*, 2009). Notably, however, the binding affinity of Ca0409 to human receptors (K_d' in subnanomolar range) was substantially lower than that of SC18 (Jayaraman *et al.*, 2011). Consequently, while the Ca0409 virus showed respiratory droplet transmission in ferrets, the efficiency of transmission was lower than that of SC18 (Maines *et al.*, 2009).

Based on the studies summarized above, it is observed that the HA of pandemic viruses (those that able to achieve respiratory droplet transmissions) has distinct glycan binding properties, which include high affinity binding to human receptors and a characteristic extensive staining of the goblet cells in the apical surface of human tracheal section (Fig.

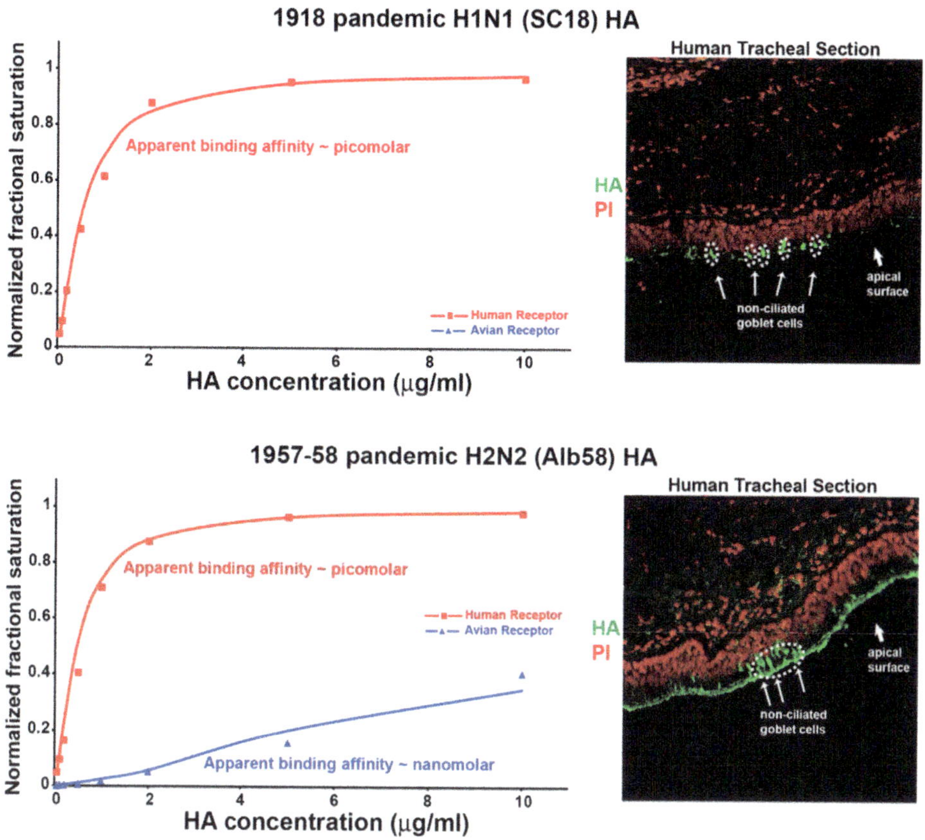

Figure 6.2 Glycan receptor binding properties of representative pandemic HAs. Shown in the figure are binding curves (on the left panels) for HA binding to representative human (Neu5Acα2–6Galβ1–4GlcNAcβ1–3Galβ1–4GlcNAcβ) and avian (Neu5Acα2–3Galβ1–4GlcNAcβ1–3Galβ1–4GlcNAcβ) receptors and representative binding of HA to human tracheal tissue sections (on right panels). The non-ciliated goblet cell regions on the apical surface of the human tracheal section are highlighted in dotted white circles.

6.2). On a comparative basis, the relative binding affinity of a given HA to human receptors correlates with the efficiency of transmission in the ferret model. Indeed, this analysis has demonstrated predictive power in the case of H1 (Srinivasan *et al.*, 2008), H2 (Pappas *et al.*, 2010; Viswanathan *et al.*, 2010), H5 (Maines *et al.*, 2011) and H7 (Fouchier *et al.*, 2004; Srinivasan *et al.*, 2013; Tharakaraman *et al.*, 2013a; Zhu *et al.*, 2013). Based on these observations, we postulate that the key HA determinant enabling human-to-human transmission via respiratory droplet, is the ability of the HA to bind distinct goblet cell-derived glycans in the upper airways. This is an attribute that is independently measurable (through experiments in the ferret) and is a necessary determinant of a virus capable of initiating an epidemic or pandemic. Conversely, infection can occur via multiple mechanisms, independent of HA glycan specificity or even that of HA itself, and is also a function of the immune status of the individual (Fukuyama and Kawaoka, 2011; Subbarao and Katz, 2000).

Residue interaction networks to analyse amino acid changes in the context of natural sequence evolution of HA

This section of the chapter mainly describes a framework that we had recently developed to define and analyse RBS in terms of molecular features that impact binding of avian versus human receptors and how amino acid changes in the context of natural HA sequence evolution impinge on these features.

The Ca0409 HA was shown to share high sequence identity, antigenic similarity and hallmark residues associated with human receptor binding with SC18 HA (Garten *et al.*, 2009; Soundararajan *et al.*, 2009). Despite these similarities, this HA showed substantially lower0affinity binding to human receptors relative to that of SC18 HA. A detailed structural analysis of the key residues in the RBS of CA0409 HA revealed a mismatch in the network of inter-residue interactions involving positions 219, 227, 222, 225 and 186 when compared to identical interactions in SC18 HA or seasonal H1N1 HAs (Jayaraman *et al.*, 2011). While this network was of a hydrophobic nature in SC18 HA, it is ionic in the case of seasonal HAs. In contrast to either case, in Ca0409, this network was neither hydrophobic nor ionic, affecting the positioning of the key Asp-190 residue. Introducing a single amino acid change Ile-219→ys in Ca0409, correcting this 'mismatch' made this interaction network ionic in character, which in turn substantially increased human receptor-binding affinity of Ca0409 (Jayaraman *et al.*, 2011).

Extending this analysis, others and we have examined the role of glycosylation on HA in mediating the receptor binding properties of HA (Kasson and Pande, 2008; Stevens *et al.*, 2008; Wang *et al.*, 2009; Wang *et al.*, 2010). Molecular dynamics simulation studies predicted that HA–glycans may form interactions near the binding pocket to influence receptor binding (Kasson and Pande, 2008). Site-directed mutagenesis to knock-out glycosylation sites on HA (Jayaraman *et al.*, 2012b; Stevens *et al.*, 2008) or modifying structure of N-linked glycans on the virus by enzymatic treatment or transgenic cell lines (Wang *et al.*, 2009) have shown distinct changes in glycan-receptor binding specificity. Our recent study showed that loss of glycosylation at a highly conserved sequon was detrimental to receptor binding by SC18 and NY18 HA, whereas it did not affect the binding of AV18 HA to avian receptors (Jayaraman *et al.*, 2012b). This observation was explained by analysing the network of inter-residue interactions in the RBS of SC18, NY18 and AV18 and describing the relationship of this network to the conserved glycosylation sequon. We found that removal of HA glycosylation at this sequon had minimal impact on the network involving the 220-loop in the RBS of AV18, whereas loss of glycosylation disrupted the network within NY18 and SC18 HA (Jayaraman *et al.*, 2012b) (Fig. 6.3).

Given these results, we believe that the presence of hallmark residues cannot be directly linked to conferring a specific glycan-binding property to any HA, particularly when extrapolating between subtypes. This is evidenced from attempts to introduce hallmark amino acids – observed in pandemic H1N1 or H2N2 or H3N2 HA – into H5 HA so as to confer so-called *gain of function* (i.e. aerosol transmissibility in ferrets). None of these H5 HA mutants showed comparable glycan receptor binding properties of pandemic HAs (Stevens *et al.*, 2008; Tharakaraman *et al.*, 2013b) or gain of function (Maines *et al.*, 2011). In addition to analysing HA–glycan contacts to identify key residues, it is important to consider interactions between key residues (and any proximal glycosylation) in the RBS, which can be mapped into a network of inter-residue interactions (Fig. 6.3).

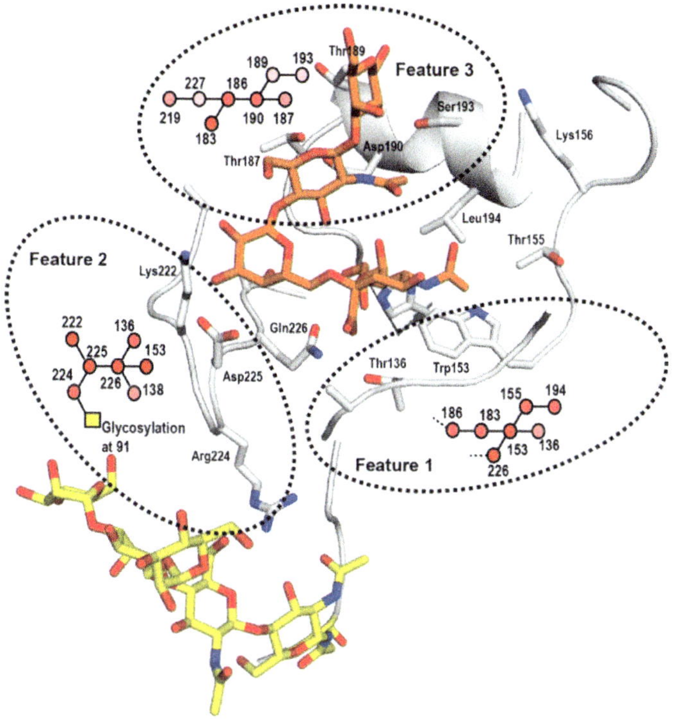

Figure 6.3 Residue interaction networks and molecular features of HA RBS. Shown in the figure is the RBS of SC18 complexed with LSTc. Also shown is an N-linked trimannosyl core glycan structure (shown in yellow) added at the Asn-91 position using the GlyProt tool (http://www.glycosciences.de/modeling/glyprot/php/main.php) where the SC18-LSTc cocrystal structure (PDB ID: 2WR7) was submitted for *in silico* glycosylation. The side chains of the key residues involved in contact with human receptor are shown and labeled. The residue interaction networks of representative residue positions are shown as interconnected circular nodes. The nodes are colored with varying shades of red where light pink corresponds to residues with lowest RBSN score and bright red corresponds to residues with highest RBSN score. The network of interactions involving the glycosylation is indicated as a yellow box in the RBSN diagram. The key residue positions along with their RBSN can be defined as molecular features characteristic of a given RBS and comparing these features with human-adapted HAs provides a more robust approach to investigate amino acid changes for human adaptation of HA.

These two key aspects are relevant to recent studies that have demonstrated mutations in 2004 (A/Vietnam/1203/04 or Viet04) and 2005 (A/Indonesia/5/05 or Ind05) strains of H5N1 HA that have conferred respiratory droplet transmission upon the virus strains (Herfst *et al.*, 2012; Imai *et al.*, 2012). Based on these results, several follow-on studies were inclined to fix these mutations as so-called hallmark changes for any H5 HA (Russell *et al.*, 2012). However, from surveillance data, we know that the sequences of HA from current circulating strains of H5 have diverged significantly from Viet04 and Indo05 HA. Given this divergence, introducing the same set of mutations that resulted in *gain of* function for Viet04 or Ind05 to currently circulating H5 HAs do result in a switch in receptor preference and a *gain of function* (Tharakaraman *et al.*, 2013b). Given the established framework, a detailed structural analysis of RBS of H5 HA was completed.

On the basis of phylogenetic 'closeness' of H5 to H2 HA, Alb58 HA was chosen as the reference human-adapted HA to identify key RBS properties within H5 HA. Four key differences were observed. First, the composition of the 130 loop of H2 HA is different from H5 HA in that the loop length is shorter by an amino acid. This deletion in the 130-loop in H5 HA relative to H2 HA was shown to critically govern the 130-loop. Second, amino acids in the 'base' of the RBS (such as those in 130-loop at positions 136–138, and 220-loop at positions 219–228) are different in H2 than in H5. Third, the 'top' of the RBS primarily comprising the '190-helix' (residues 188–196) that interacts with the sugars beyond terminal Neu5Acα2→6Gal motif in the human receptor are different in H2 than in H5 (specifically at positions 188, 189, 192 and 193). Fourth, position 158 is glycosylated in H5 HA but not in H2 HA. Glycosylation at this site has been shown to influence glycan receptor binding property of H5 HA (Stevens *et al.*, 2008).

Given these differences, and to understand amino acid changes that would enable the RBS of H5 HA match with that of H2, it was important to analyse the network of inter-residue interactions within the RBS. This analysis was performed by defining a map known as RBS network or RBSN, which showed interactions between RBS residues using a 2-D graph (Fig. 6.3). The extent of connectivity was quantified using a network score such that the higher the score of an amino acid within the RBS, the more structurally constrained it is to mutation. Finally, the differences between the RBS of H2 and H5 HA were captured using a new definition termed *molecular features* (one feature for each difference) which incorporated topological definition of glycan receptor in the RBS, RBS residues involved in the binding, and their RBSN maps. Four distinct features were identified that together constituted a complete description of the H5 RBS.

The molecular feature definition was then mapped onto the phylogenetic sequence analyses of H5 HA which showed that many of the clades, including currently circulating clade 1, clade 2.2, clade 2.2.1, and clade 7 had already acquired amino acid changes characteristic of one or two of Features 1, 3 and 4. However, only a subset of the rapidly evolving and currently circulating clades 2.2.1 and 7 had acquired amino acid changes to match Feature 1 and/or part of Feature 2, which are critical features of the RBS base. From this subset, it was demonstrated that select strains required as few as one or two amino acid changes to match the requisite features, switch in binding preference and demonstrate human receptor binding affinity in the same range as that of pandemic HAs (Tharakaraman *et al.*, 2013b).

Conclusions and significance

Influenza A viruses have always been viewed as 'unpredictable' pathogens based on their rapid evolution in response to immune selection pressure in different hosts and also past occurrences of novel subtype crossing species into humans leading to a widespread pandemic outbreaks. Given that glycan receptor specificity of HA is an important property in the host infection and adaptation by the virus, this property has to be carefully measured and interpreted to better understand its variations as a consequence of natural sequence evolution.

First, amino acid mutations that confer specific receptor binding properties to a particular strain and subtype of HA do not always (or even often) confer the same properties on an

HA of a different virus. For example, the extent of binding to different receptors appears to vary between different subtypes. While human-adapted viruses of group 1 viruses, such as H1N1 and H2N2, show minimal or low binding affinity to avian receptors, viruses within group 2, including H3N2, show comparable binding to both human and avian receptors. These studies question the simple definition of specificity as ratio of binding to $\alpha2\rightarrow6$ versus $\alpha2\rightarrow3$ glycan receptors and emphasize the importance of identifying and understanding the structural and biochemical aspects of HA–glycan receptor interactions. This is particularly relevant when looking at subtypes that are rapidly evolving, such as H5N1. We believe that the recently developed inter-residue interaction network can potentially be evolved into a metric that can assist such surveillance efforts and provide a method to identify strains of particular importance to monitor. Towards such a goal, additional studies need to be undertaken to systematically define network scores and network maps of RBS residues of avian-, swine- and human-adapted HAs and identifying a scoring system that discriminates the network properties of these HAs.

Second, the analyses of receptor binding properties of HA from multiple subtypes, including pandemic strains of H1 and H2, point to characteristic properties such as high-affinity binding to human receptors and also distinct goblet cell staining patterns, which are at least useful descriptors and may also provide insight into a mechanistic link between receptor binding preference and other phenotypic properties of the virus such as aerosol transmissibility. Goblet cells secrete mucins, which can potentially assist in the aerosolization of the virus, which in turn might facilitate efficient respiratory droplet transmission. Additionally, goblet cell tropism might also shed light on why many influenza strains, including H7N9, do not demonstrate efficient respiratory droplet transmission even though they have been shown to replicate efficiently in the human respiratory tract.

In summary, a better understanding of HA–glycan interactions can significantly improve surveillance methods to advance preparedness and potential countermeasures in the event of emergence of novel influenza strains.

Acknowledgements

This work was funded in part by National Institutes of Health (R37 GM057073-13) and the National Research Foundation supported Interdisciplinary Research group in Infectious Diseases of SMART (Singapore MIT alliance for Research and Technology).

References

Ahmed, R., Oldstone, M.B., and Palese, P. (2007). Protective immunity and susceptibility to infectious diseases: lessons from the 1918 influenza pandemic. Nat. Immunol. *8*, 1188–1193.

Aich, U., Beckley, N., Shriver, Z., Raman, R., Viswanathan, K., Hobbie, S., and Sasisekharan, R. (2011). Glycomics-based analysis of chicken red blood cells provides insight into the selectivity of the viral agglutination assay. FEBS J. *278*, 1699–1712.

Bateman, A.C., Karamanska, R., Busch, M.G., Dell, A., Olsen, C.W., and Haslam, S.M. (2010). Glycan analysis and influenza A virus infection of primary swine respiratory epithelial cells: the importance of NeuAc{alpha}2-6 glycans. J. Biol. Chem. *285*, 34016–34026.

Belser, J.A., Gustin, K.M., Pearce, M.B., Maines, T.R., Zeng, H., Pappas, C., Sun, X., Carney, P.J., Villanueva, J.M., Stevens, J., *et al.* (2013). Pathogenesis and transmission of avian influenza A (H7N9) virus in ferrets and mice. Nature *501*, 556–559.

Blixt, O., Head, S., Mondala, T., Scanlan, C., Huflejt, M.E., Alvarez, R., Bryan, M.C., Fazio, F., Calarese, D., Stevens, J., *et al.* (2004). Printed covalent glycan array for ligand profiling of diverse glycan binding proteins. Proc. Natl. Acad. Sci. U.S.A. *101*, 17033–17038.

Bradley, K.C., Jones, C.A., Tompkins, S.M., Tripp, R.A., Russell, R.J., Gramer, M.R., Heimburg-Molinaro, J., Smith, D.F., Cummings, R.D., and Steinhauer, D.A. (2011). Comparison of the receptor binding properties of contemporary swine isolates and early human pandemic H1N1 isolates (Novel 2009 H1N1). Virology *413*, 169–182.

Chandrasekaran, A., Srinivasan, A., Raman, R., Viswanathan, K., Raguram, S., Tumpey, T.M., Sasisekharan, V., and Sasisekharan, R. (2008). Glycan topology determines human adaptation of avian H5N1 virus hemagglutinin. Nat. Biotechnol. *26*, 107–113.

Chen, Y., Liang, W., Yang, S., Wu, N., Gao, H., Sheng, J., Yao, H., Wo, J., Fang, Q., Cui, D., *et al.* (2013). Human infections with the emerging avian influenza A H7N9 virus from wet market poultry: clinical analysis and characterisation of viral genome. Lancet *381*, 1916–1925.

Childs, R.A., Palma, A.S., Wharton, S., Matrosovich, T., Liu, Y., Chai, W., Campanero-Rhodes, M.A., Zhang, Y., Eickmann, M., Kiso, M., *et al.* (2009). Receptor-binding specificity of pandemic influenza A (H1N1) 2009 virus determined by carbohydrate microarray. Nat. Biotechnol. *27*, 797–799.

Fouchier, R.A., Schneeberger, P.M., Rozendaal, F.W., Broekman, J.M., Kemink, S.A., Munster, V., Kuiken, T., Rimmelzwaan, G.F., Schutten, M., Van Doornum, G.J., *et al.* (2004). Avian influenza A virus (H7N7) associated with human conjunctivitis and a fatal case of acute respiratory distress syndrome. Proc. Natl. Acad. Sci. U.S.A. *101*, 1356–1361.

Fraser, C., Donnelly, C.A., Cauchemez, S., Hanage, W.P., Van Kerkhove, M.D., Hollingsworth, T.D., Griffin, J., Baggaley, R.F., Jenkins, H.E., Lyons, E.J., *et al.* (2009). Pandemic potential of a strain of influenza A (H1N1): early findings. Science *324*, 1557–1561.

Fukui, S., Feizi, T., Galustian, C., Lawson, A.M., and Chai, W. (2002). Oligosaccharide microarrays for high-throughput detection and specificity assignments of carbohydrate-protein interactions. Nat. Biotechnol. *20*, 1011–1017.

Fukuyama, S., and Kawaoka, Y. (2011). The pathogenesis of influenza virus infections: the contributions of virus and host factors. Curr. Opin. Immunol. *23*, 481–486.

Gambaryan, A.S., Tuzikov, A.B., Piskarev, V.E., Yamnikova, S.S., Lvov, D.K., Robertson, J.S., Bovin, N.V., and Matrosovich, M.N. (1997). Specification of receptor-binding phenotypes of influenza virus isolates from different hosts using synthetic sialylglycopolymers: non-egg-adapted human H1 and H3 influenza A and influenza B viruses share a common high binding affinity for 6′-sialyl(N-acetyllactosamine). Virology *232*, 345–350.

Gamblin, S.J., Haire, L.F., Russell, R.J., Stevens, D.J., Xiao, B., Ha, Y., Vasisht, N., Steinhauer, D.A., Daniels, R.S., Elliot, A., *et al.* (2004). The structure and receptor binding properties of the 1918 influenza hemagglutinin. Science *303*, 1838–1842.

Gao, R., Cao, B., Hu, Y., Feng, Z., Wang, D., Hu, W., Chen, J., Jie, Z., Qiu, H., Xu, K., *et al.* (2013). Human infection with a novel avian-origin influenza A (H7N9) virus. N. Engl. J. Med. *368*, 1888–1897.

Garten, R.J., Davis, C.T., Russell, C.A., Shu, B., Lindstrom, S., Balish, A., Sessions, W.M., Xu, X., Skepner, E., Deyde, V., *et al.* (2009). Antigenic and genetic characteristics of swine-origin 2009 A(H1N1) influenza viruses circulating in humans. Science *325*, 197–201.

Glaser, L., Stevens, J., Zamarin, D., Wilson, I.A., Garcia-Sastre, A., Tumpey, T.M., Basler, C.F., Taubenberger, J.K., and Palese, P. (2005). A single amino acid substitution in 1918 influenza virus hemagglutinin changes receptor binding specificity. J. Virol. *79*, 11533–11536.

Grun, C.H., van Vliet, S.J., Schiphorst, W.E., Bank, C.M., Meyer, S., van Die, I., and van Kooyk, Y. (2006). One-step biotinylation procedure for carbohydrates to study carbohydrate-protein interactions. Anal. Biochem. *354*, 54–63.

Ha, Y., Stevens, D.J., Skehel, J.J., and Wiley, D.C. (2001). X-ray structures of H5 avian and H9 swine influenza virus hemagglutinins bound to avian and human receptor analogs. Proc. Natl. Acad. Sci. U.S.A. *98*, 11181–11186.

Ha, Y., Stevens, D.J., Skehel, J.J., and Wiley, D.C. (2003). X-ray structure of the hemagglutinin of a potential H3 avian progenitor of the 1968 Hong Kong pandemic influenza virus. Virology *309*, 209–218.

Herfst, S., Schrauwen, E.J.A., Linster, M., Chutinimitkul, S., de Wit, E., Munster, V.J., Sorrell, E.M., Bestebroer, T.M., Burke, D.F., Smith, D.J., *et al.* (2012). Airborne transmission of influenza A/H5N1 virus between ferrets. Science *336*, 1534–1541.

Imai, M., Watanabe, T., Hatta, M., Das, S.C., Ozawa, M., Shinya, K., Zhong, G., Hanson, A., Katsura, H., Watanabe, S., *et al.* (2012). Experimental adaptation of an influenza H5 HA confers respiratory droplet transmission to a reassortant H5 HA/H1N1 virus in ferrets. Nature *486*, 420–428.

Itoh, Y., Shinya, K., Kiso, M., Watanabe, T., Sakoda, Y., Hatta, M., Muramoto, Y., Tamura, D., Sakai-Tagawa, Y., Noda, T., *et al.* (2009). In vitro and in vivo characterization of new swine-origin H1N1 influenza viruses. Nature *460*, 1021–1025.

Jayaraman, A., Chandrasekharan, A., Viswanathan, K., Raman, R., Fox, J.G., and Sasisekharan, R. (2012a). Decoding the distribution of glycan receptors for human-adapted influenza A viruses in ferret respiratory tract. PLoS ONE *7*, e27517.

Jayaraman, A., Koh, X., Li, J., Raman, R., Viswanathan, K., Shriver, Z., and Sasisekharan, R. (2012b). Glycosylation at Asn91 of H1N1 haemagglutinin affects binding to glycan receptors. Biochem. J. *444*, 429–435.

Jayaraman, A., Pappas, C., Raman, R., Belser, J.A., Viswanathan, K., Shriver, Z., Tumpey, T.M., and Sasisekharan, R. (2011). A single base-pair change in 2009 H1N1 hemagglutinin increases human receptor affinity and leads to efficient airborne viral transmission in ferrets. PloS ONE *6*, e17616.

Kageyama, T., Fujisaki, S., Takashita, E., Xu, H., Yamada, S., Uchida, Y., Neumann, G., Saito, T., Kawaoka, Y., and Tashiro, M. (2013). Genetic analysis of novel avian A(H7N9) influenza viruses isolated from patients in China, February to April 2013. Euro Surveill. *18*, 20453.

Karamanska, R., Clarke, J., Blixt, O., Macrae, J.I., Zhang, J.Q., Crocker, P.R., Laurent, N., Wright, A., Flitsch, S.L., Russell, D.A., *et al.* (2008). Surface plasmon resonance imaging for real-time, label-free analysis of protein interactions with carbohydrate microarrays. Glycoconj. J. *25*, 69–74.

Kasson, P.M., and Pande, V.S. (2008). Structural basis for influence of viral glycans on ligand binding by influenza hemagglutinin. Biophys. J. *95*, L48–50.

Layne, S.P., Monto, A.S., and Taubenberger, J.K. (2009). Pandemic influenza: an inconvenient mutation. Science *323*, 1560–1561.

Liang, P.H., Wu, C.Y., Greenberg, W.A., and Wong, C.H. (2008). Glycan arrays: biological and medical applications. Curr. Opin. Chem. Biol. *12*, 86–92.

Liao, H.Y., Hsu, C.H., Wang, S.C., Liang, C.H., Yen, H.Y., Su, C.Y., Chen, C.H., Jan, J.T., Ren, C.T., Cheng, T.J., *et al.* (2010). Differential receptor binding affinities of influenza hemagglutinins on glycan arrays. J. Am. Chem. Soc. *132*, 14849–14856.

Lin, Y.P., Xiong, X., Wharton, S.A., Martin, S.R., Coombs, P.J., Vachieri, S.G., Christodoulou, E., Walker, P.A., Liu, J., Skehel, J.J., *et al.* (2012). Evolution of the receptor binding properties of the influenza A(H3N2) hemagglutinin. Proc. Natl. Acad. Sci. U.S.A. *109*, 21474–21479.

Liu, J., Stevens, D.J., Haire, L.F., Walker, P.A., Coombs, P.J., Russell, R.J., Gamblin, S.J., and Skehel, J.J. (2009). Structures of receptor complexes formed by hemagglutinins from the Asian Influenza pandemic of 1957. Proc. Natl. Acad. Sci. U.S.A. *106*, 17175–17180.

Maines, T.R., Chen, L.M., Van Hoeven, N., Tumpey, T.M., Blixt, O., Belser, J.A., Gustin, K.M., Pearce, M.B., Pappas, C., Stevens, J., *et al.* (2011). Effect of receptor binding domain mutations on receptor binding and transmissibility of avian influenza H5N1 viruses. Virology *413*, 139–147.

Maines, T.R., Jayaraman, A., Belser, J.A., Wadford, D.A., Pappas, C., Zeng, H., Gustin, K.M., Pearce, M.B., Viswanathan, K., Shriver, Z.H., *et al.* (2009). Transmission and pathogenesis of swine-origin 2009 A(H1N1) influenza viruses in ferrets and mice. Science *325*, 484–487.

Matrosovich, M.N., Matrosovich, T.Y., Gray, T., Roberts, N.A., and Klenk, H.D. (2004). Human and avian influenza viruses target different cell types in cultures of human airway epithelium. Proc. Natl. Acad. Sci. U.S.A. *101*, 4620–4624.

Mercey, E., Sadir, R., Maillart, E., Roget, A., Baleux, F., Lortat-Jacob, H., and Livache, T. (2008). Polypyrrole oligosaccharide array and surface plasmon resonance imaging for the measurement of glycosaminoglycan binding interactions. Anal. Chem. *80*, 3476–3482.

Neumann, G., Noda, T., and Kawaoka, Y. (2009). Emergence and pandemic potential of swine-origin H1N1 influenza virus. Nature *459*, 931–939.

Nicholls, J.M., Bourne, A.J., Chen, H., Guan, Y., and Peiris, J.S. (2007). Sialic acid receptor detection in the human respiratory tract: evidence for widespread distribution of potential binding sites for human and avian influenza viruses. Respir. Res. *8*, 73.

Oyelaran, O., and Gildersleeve, J.C. (2009). Glycan arrays: recent advances and future challenges. Curr. Opin. Chem. Biol. *13*, 406–413.

Palese, P. (2004). Influenza: old and new threats. Nat. Med. *10*, S82–87.

Pappas, C., Aguilar, P.V., Basler, C.F., Solorzano, A., Zeng, H., Perrone, L.A., Palese, P., Garcia-Sastre, A., Katz, J.M., and Tumpey, T.M. (2008). Single gene reassortants identify a critical role for PB1, HA, and NA in the high virulence of the 1918 pandemic influenza virus. Proc. Natl. Acad. Sci. U.S.A. *105*, 3064–3069.

Pappas, C., Viswanathan, K., Chandrasekaran, A., Raman, R., Katz, J.M., Sasisekharan, R., and Tumpey, T.M. (2010). Receptor specificity and transmission of H2N2 subtype viruses isolated from the pandemic of 1957. PLoS One. *5*, e11158.

Pearce, M.B., Jayaraman, A., Pappas, C., Belser, J.A., Zeng, H., Gustin, K.M., Maines, T.R., Sun, X., Raman, R., Cox, N.J., *et al.* (2012). Pathogenesis and transmission of swine origin A(H3N2)v influenza viruses in ferrets. Proc. Natl. Acad. Sci. U.S.A. *109*, 3944–3949.

Perez Velasco, R., Praditsitthikorn, N., Wichmann, K., Mohara, A., Kotirum, S., Tantivess, S., Vallenas, C., Harmanci, H., and Teerawattananon, Y. (2012). Systematic review of economic evaluations of preparedness strategies and interventions against influenza pandemics. PloS ONE *7*, e30333.

Russell, C.A., Fonville, J.M., Brown, A.E.X., Burke, D.F., Smith, D.L., James, S.L., Herfst, S., van Boheemen, S., Linster, M., Schrauwen, E.J., *et al.* (2012). The potential for respiratory droplet-transmissible A/H5N1 influenza virus to evolve in a mammalian host. Science *336*, 1541–1547.

Russell, C.J., and Webster, R.G. (2005). The genesis of a pandemic influenza virus. Cell *123*, 368–371.

Russell, R.J., Stevens, D.J., Haire, L.F., Gamblin, S.J., and Skehel, J.J. (2006). Avian and human receptor binding by hemagglutinins of influenza A viruses. Glycoconj. J. 23, 85–92.

Shinya, K., Ebina, M., Yamada, S., Ono, M., Kasai, N., and Kawaoka, Y. (2006). Avian flu: influenza virus receptors in the human airway. Nature *440*, 435–436.

Shriver, Z., Raman, R., Viswanathan, K., and Sasisekharan, R. (2009). Context-specific target definition in influenza a virus hemagglutinin-glycan receptor interactions. Chem. Biol. *16*, 803–814.

Song, X., Xia, B., Stowell, S.R., Lasanajak, Y., Smith, D.F., and Cummings, R.D. (2009). Novel fluorescent glycan microarray strategy reveals ligands for galectins. Chem. Biol. *16*, 36–47.

Song, X., Yu, H., Chen, X., Lasanajak, Y., Tappert, M.M., Air, G.M., Tiwari, V.K., Cao, H., Chokhawala, H.A., Zheng, H., *et al.* (2011). A sialylated glycan microarray reveals novel interactions of modified sialic acids with proteins and viruses. J. Biol. Chem. *286*, 31610–31622.

Soundararajan, V., Tharakaraman, K., Raman, R., Raguram, S., Shriver, Z., Sasisekharan, V., and Sasisekharan, R. (2009). Extrapolating from sequence—the 2009 H1N1 'swine' influenza virus. Nat. Biotechnol. *27*, 510–513.

Srinivasan, A., Viswanathan, K., Raman, R., Chandrasekaran, A., Raguram, S., Tumpey, T.M., Sasisekharan, V., and Sasisekharan, R. (2008). Quantitative biochemical rationale for differences in transmissibility of 1918 pandemic influenza A viruses. Proc. Natl. Acad. Sci. U.S.A. *105*, 2800–2805.

Srinivasan, K., Raman, R., Jayaraman, A., Viswanathan, K., and Sasisekharan, R. (2013). Quantitative description of glycan-receptor binding of influenza A virus H7 hemagglutinin. PLoS ONE *8*, e49597.

Stevens, J., Blixt, O., Chen, L.M., Donis, R.O., Paulson, J.C., and Wilson, I.A. (2008). Recent avian H5N1 viruses exhibit increased propensity for acquiring human receptor specificity. J. Mol. Biol. *381*, 1382–1394.

Stevens, J., Blixt, O., Glaser, L., Taubenberger, J.K., Palese, P., Paulson, J.C., and Wilson, I.A. (2006a). Glycan microarray analysis of the hemagglutinins from modern and pandemic influenza viruses reveals different receptor specificities. J. Mol. Biol. *355*, 1143–1155.

Stevens, J., Blixt, O., Paulson, J.C., and Wilson, I.A. (2006b). Glycan microarray technologies: tools to survey host specificity of influenza viruses. Nat. Rev. Microbiol. *4*, 857–864.

Stevens, J., Blixt, O., Tumpey, T.M., Taubenberger, J.K., Paulson, J.C., and Wilson, I.A. (2006c). Structure and receptor specificity of the hemagglutinin from an H5N1 influenza virus. Science *312*, 404–410.

Subbarao, K., and Katz, J. (2000). Avian influenza viruses infecting humans. Cell. Mol. Life Sci. *57*, 1770–1784.

Taubenberger, J.K., and Morens, D.M. (2008). The pathology of influenza virus infections. Annu. Rev. Pathol. *3*, 499–522.

Tharakaraman, K., Jayaraman, A., Raman, R., Viswanathan, K., Stebbins, N.W., Johnson, D., Shriver, Z., Sasisekharan, V., and Sasisekharan, R. (2013a). Glycan receptor binding of the influenza A virus H7N9 hemagglutinin. Cell *153*, 1486–1493.

Tharakaraman, K., Raman, R., Viswanathan, K., Stebbins, N.W., Jayaraman, A., Krishnan, A., Sasisekharan, V., and Sasisekharan, R. (2013b). Structural determinants for naturally evolving H5N1 hemagglutinin to switch its receptor specificity. Cell *153*, 1475–1485.

Tumpey, T.M., Basler, C.F., Aguilar, P.V., Zeng, H., Solorzano, A., Swayne, D.E., Cox, N.J., Katz, J.M., Taubenberger, J.K., Palese, P., *et al.* (2005). Characterization of the reconstructed 1918 Spanish influenza pandemic virus. Science *310*, 77–80.

Tumpey, T.M., Maines, T.R., Van Hoeven, N., Glaser, L., Solorzano, A., Pappas, C., Cox, N.J., Swayne, D.E., Palese, P., Katz, J.M., *et al.* (2007). A two-amino acid change in the hemagglutinin of the 1918 influenza virus abolishes transmission. Science *315*, 655–659.

Van Hoeven, N., Pappas, C., Belser, J.A., Maines, T.R., Zeng, H., Garcia-Sastre, A., Sasisekharan, R., Katz, J.M., and Tumpey, T.M. (2009). Human HA and polymerase subunit PB2 proteins confer transmission of an avian influenza virus through the air. Proc. Natl. Acad. Sci. U.S.A. *106*, 3366–3371.

van Riel, D., Munster, V.J., de Wit, E., Rimmelzwaan, G.F., Fouchier, R.A., Osterhaus, A.D., and Kuiken, T. (2006). H5N1 Virus attachment to lower respiratory tract. Science *312*, 399.

Viswanathan, K., Koh, X., Chandrasekaran, A., Pappas, C., Raman, R., Srinivasan, A., Shriver, Z., Tumpey, T.M., and Sasisekharan, R. (2010). Determinants of glycan receptor specificity of H2N2 influenza A virus hemagglutinin. PLoS ONE *5*, e13768.

Walther, T., Karamanska, R., Chan, R.W., Chan, M.C., Jia, N., Air, G., Hopton, C., Wong, M.P., Dell, A., Malik Peiris, J.S., *et al.* (2013). Glycomic analysis of human respiratory tract tissues and correlation with influenza virus infection. PLoS Pathog. *9*, e1003223.

Wang, C.C., Chen, J.R., Tseng, Y.C., Hsu, C.H., Hung, Y.F., Chen, S.W., Chen, C.M., Khoo, K.H., Cheng, T.J., Cheng, Y.S., *et al.* (2009). Glycans on influenza hemagglutinin affect receptor binding and immune response. Proc. Natl. Acad. Sci. U.S.A. *106*, 18137–18142.

Wang, W., Lu, B., Zhou, H., Suguitan, A.L., Jr., Cheng, X., Subbarao, K., Kemble, G., and Jin, H. (2010). Glycosylation at 158N of the hemagglutinin protein and receptor binding specificity synergistically affect the antigenicity and immunogenicity of a live attenuated H5N1 A/Vietnam/1203/2004 vaccine virus in ferrets. J. Virol. *84*, 6570–6577.

Watanabe, T., Kiso, M., Fukuyama, S., Nakajima, N., Imai, M., Yamada, S., Murakami, S., Yamayoshi, S., Iwatsuki-Horimoto, K., Sakoda, Y., *et al.* (2013). Characterization of H7N9 influenza A viruses isolated from humans. Nature *501*, 551–555.

Xia, B., Kawar, Z.S., Ju, T., Alvarez, R.A., Sachdev, G.P., and Cummings, R.D. (2005). Versatile fluorescent derivatization of glycans for glycomic analysis. Nat. Methods *2*, 845–850.

Xiong, X., Martin, S.R., Haire, L.F., Wharton, S.A., Daniels, R.S., Bennett, M.S., McCauley, J.W., Collins, P.J., Walker, P.A., Skehel, J.J., *et al.* (2013). Receptor binding by an H7N9 influenza virus from humans. Nature *499*, 496–499.

Xu, D., Newhouse, E.I., Amaro, R.E., Pao, H.C., Cheng, L.S., Markwick, P.R., McCammon, J.A., Li, W.W., and Arzberger, P.W. (2009). Distinct glycan topology for avian and human sialopentasaccharide receptor analogues upon binding different hemagglutinins: a molecular dynamics perspective. J. Mol. Biol. *387*, 465–491.

Xu, R., McBride, R., Paulson, J.C., Basler, C.F., and Wilson, I.A. (2010). Structure, receptor binding, and antigenicity of influenza virus hemagglutinins from the 1957 H2N2 pandemic. J. Virol. *84*, 1715–1721.

Yang, H., Carney, P., and Stevens, J. (2010a). Structure and Receptor binding properties of a pandemic H1N1 virus hemagglutinin. PLoS Curr. *2*, RRN1152.

Yang, H., Carney, P.J., Donis, R.O., and Stevens, J. (2012). Structure and receptor complexes of the hemagglutinin from a highly pathogenic H7N7 influenza virus. J. Virol. *86*, 8645–8652.

Yang, H., Chen, L.M., Carney, P.J., Donis, R.O., and Stevens, J. (2010b). Structures of receptor complexes of a North American H7N2 influenza hemagglutinin with a loop deletion in the receptor binding site. PLoS Pathog. *6*, e1001081.

Yen, H.L., Liang, C.H., Wu, C.Y., Forrest, H.L., Ferguson, A., Choy, K.T., Jones, J., Wong, D.D., Cheung, P.P., Hsu, C.H., *et al.* (2011). Hemagglutinin-neuraminidase balance confers respiratory-droplet transmissibility of the pandemic H1N1 influenza virus in ferrets. Proc. Natl. Acad. Sci. U.S.A. *108*, 14264–14269.

Zhang, W., Shi, Y., Qi, J., Gao, F., Li, Q., Fan, Z., Yan, J., and Gao, G.F. (2013). Molecular basis of the receptor binding specificity switch of the hemagglutinins from both the 1918 and 2009 pandemic influenza A viruses by a D225G substitution. J. Virol. *87*, 5949–5958.

Zhu, H., Wang, D., Kelvin, D.J., Li, L., Zheng, Z., Yoon, S.W., Wong, S.S., Farooqui, A., Wang, J., Banner, D., *et al.* (2013). Infectivity, transmission, and pathology of human-isolated H7N9 influenza virus in ferrets and pigs. Science *341*, 183–186.

PB1-F2: A Multifunctional Non-structural Influenza A Virus Protein

7

Eike R. Hrincius and Jonathan A. McCullers

Abstract

A central determinant of pathogenicity for influenza A virus (IAV) infections is the interplay of the invading virus with the host immune system. The host has to recognize and fight the invading pathogen; at the same time the induced immune reaction has to be well balanced and not self-destroying. Influenza viruses have evolved strategies to support their replication and to circumvent host immune responses. The PB1-F2 protein of IAVs, a non-structural protein only found within the infected cell, has had manifold functions attributed to it. The protein's proposed support of virus replication, together with modulation of immune responses, categorize PB1-F2 as a classic multifunctional viral protein. Shortly after its discovery it became obvious that PB1-F2 has the potential to mediate pathogenicity upon primary viral infection and also during bacterial co-infections. This effect appears to be mediated by induction of cell death, promotion of cytokine release and inflammation, and/or modulation of interferon responses in a virus, cell type, and host-specific manner. Because these functions of PB1-F2 are poorly understood and this protein has not been as well studied as other influenza virus proteins, research efforts need to be intensified to clarify the role of PB1-F2 in influenza virus infections.

Introduction and context

The PB1-F2 protein is an accessory protein in influenza A viruses (IAV) and has no known homologue in influenza B viruses (IBV). PB1-F2 was discovered in 2001 during a search for alternative reading frame peptides that are recognized by $CD8^+$ T-cells (Chen *et al.*, 2001). Because of genome restrictions and the need for evolutionary conservation of multiple protein domains, small RNA viruses often express nonstructural multifunctional proteins with high plasticity for fulfilling their replication cycle. The best studied example of such a protein is the nonstructural protein 1 (NS1) of influenza viruses. Research in the last few decades has revealed multiple functions for the NS1 protein, most striking of which is its interferon (IFN) inhibitory capacity (Garcia-Sastre *et al.*, 1998). Accumulating evidence shows that the NS1 protein fulfils its functions almost exclusively by direct binding to proteins of the host cell (Hale *et al.*, 2008). In addition to multistrategic inhibition of the type I IFN system, NS1 mediates the enhancement of viral mRNA translation (de la Luna *et al.*, 1995) and directly regulates multiple signalling pathways within infected cells (Hale *et al.*, 2008). Interestingly, investigations of the PB1-F2 protein since its discovery revealed PB1-F2 as nonstructural protein like NS1 (Shaw *et al.*, 2008) as well as a protein fulfilling manifold functions classifying PB1-F2 as multifunctional protein of IAV. PB1-F2 expression has been implicated in pathogenesis (Alymova *et al.*, 2011; McAuley *et al.*, 2007, 2010a, 2013; Schmolke *et al.*, 2011), but it does not play a major role in replication and viral fitness in mammalian hosts (Schmolke *et al.*, 2011). Interestingly, and even more pronounced than its role in primary viral infection, PB1-F2 can serve as a modifier of severe secondary bacterial infections (Alymova *et al.*, 2011; McAuley *et al.*, 2007, 2010a).

In this chapter, the current knowledge of the complex role of PB1-F2 in IAV infection biology will be summarized and potential concepts for intervention will be discussed. In addition to PB1-F2 protein structure and expression, the evolution and ecology of PB1-F2 will be explicated. Finally, the broad impact of PB1-F2 on pathogenicity will be introduced along with the PB1-F2 functions regulating such impacts.

Structure

The structure of PB1-F2 can vary by IAV strain. PB1-F2 can be up to 90 amino acids in length with a molecular weight of 10.5 kDa. However, multiple truncated versions of PB1-F2 exist in nature, and some IAV do not even express PB1-F2 (Zell *et al.*, 2007) emphasizing a virus strain and even a host-dependent need for PB1-F2 expression. Protein structure analysis has revealed that PB1-F2 proteins consist of two short α-helices at the N-terminus, being connected to a larger helical structure at the C-terminus via a flexible and unstructured linker region (Bruns *et al.*, 2007). A detailed comparison of different PB1-F2 proteins revealed distinct structural signatures for different IAV PB1-F2 proteins, with variability noted especially in the C-terminal region of the protein. Versions of PB1-F2 carrying two C-terminal helical structures connected by a loop occur, and interestingly PB1-F2 proteins of highly pathogenic IAV show this structural modification (Solbak *et al.*, 2013).

PB1-F2 proteins can fold into different structures depending on the environment (Bruns *et al.*, 2007; Chevalier *et al.*, 2010), which emphasizes the plasticity and flexibility of the protein related to function. A structural characterization study revealed that PB1-F2 behaves more as a large random coil peptide in aqueous solutions, but adapts to a α-helical structure in a membrane environment (Bruns *et al.*, 2007). In contrast, another study revealed β-sheet secondary structures of PB1-F2 in membrane environment that were associated with protein oligomerization and amyloid fibre formation of PB1-F2 (Chevalier *et al.*, 2010), but the study reiterated the dependency of PB1-F2 protein structures on the environment. The intrinsic property of PB1-F2 oligomerization is likely responsible for PB1-F2-mediated membrane pore formation (Chanturiya *et al.*, 2004; Zamarin *et al.*, 2005).

In addition to expressing full-length PB1-F2, which occurs with a very high prevalence in highly pathogenic H5N1 IAV (Smith and McCullers, 2013), multiple influenza viruses express N- or C-terminal truncated versions of PB1-F2, especially resulting in partial or total loss of the C-terminal domain (Chakrabarti and Pasricha, 2013; Pasricha *et al.*, 2013; Zell *et al.*, 2007). The molecular consequences of the differential expression of PB1-F2 in different IAV and in different hosts are poorly understood, opening up an opportunity to investigate virus- and host-specific functions of PB1-F2, especially in the context of adaptation and zoonotic potential of IAV from the avian reservoir. In addition to the C-terminal structures of PB1-F2, where most of the biological activity is thought to be located, the N-terminus can be modified by post-translational phosphorylation via the cellular protein kinase C

(PKC), and the phosphorylation sites are linked to cell-specific functions in the IAV life cycle (Mitzner *et al.*, 2009). The possibility that PB1-F2 is a protein with distinct functions in the N- and C-terminal domains emphasizes the need to understand the consequences of the structural flexibility of PB1-F2 in greater detail, even in the context of potential self-regulatory properties of the N- and C-terminal domains of PB1-F2. Taken together, the structure of PB1-F2 can be extremely variable and is characterized by a virus strain and protein environment dependency.

Expression and localization

The PB1-F2 protein is expressed from an overlapping +1 open reading frame (ORF) of the influenza gene segment 2. The gene segment 2 of IAV encodes three different protein products initiating at different start codons on the overlapping ORFs (Fig. 7.1). Several start codons, which differ in the relative strength of their Kozak sequence, have been identified within the PB1 segment for the initiation of protein translation (Wise *et al.*, 2009). The main protein product of segment 2 is the polymerase basic protein 1 (PB1), which is necessary for genome transcription and replication. The initiation of PB1 translation is mediated by the first start codon encoded on gene segment 2. The PB1 ORF has a moderately strong Kozak sequence and the translation of PB1-F2 is regulated by leaky ribosomal scanning. Because

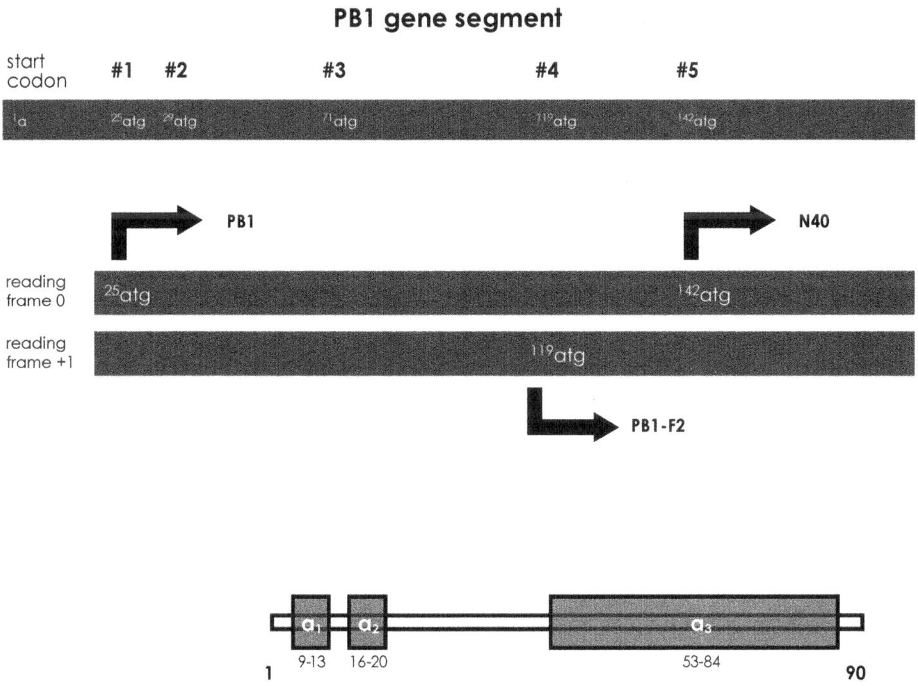

Figure 7.1 Coding schema for the gene segment 2 of influenza A viruses showing initiation of PB1, N40, and PB1-F2 at different start sites, and resulting in production of PB1-F2, pictured as a full-length protein.

of this process, the first three ORFs are bypassed and translation of PB1-F2 is initiated from the fourth start codon in gene segment 2, which has a stronger Kozak sequence than that of ORF1–3 (Chen *et al.*, 2001; Wise *et al.*, 2009). Recently, a third protein product from gene segment 2 was identified and designated as N40. The N40 ORF is in frame with the PB1 ORF and translation is initiated at PB1 codon 40 (start codon five in gene segment 2) by using a very strong Kozak sequence for translation initiating (Wise *et al.*, 2009) (Fig. 7.1). In this way, N40 resembles an N-terminal truncated version of PB1 lacking transcriptase activity but still interacts with PB2 (Wise *et al.*, 2009). Thus, the context and strength of start codons are pivotal for regulation of protein production from gene segment 2 of IAV, which further emphasizes the interdependent regulation of PB1, PB1-F2 and N40 expression. The fine-tuned regulation of protein production from gene segment 2 highlights the complexity of genetic manipulation of gene expression from this gene segment, because blocking the expression of one protein can affect the expression of other proteins (Wise *et al.*, 2009). To study functionalities of the different proteins, sole expression via plasmids can potentially impede such interrelated alterations in protein expression; however this method has its own pitfalls, as it removes the codependency of gene expression from gene segment 2. The regulation of PB1-F2 translation has recently been shown to be even more complex, because two independent regions within the PB1 mRNA, which are located downstream of the PB1-F2 start codon, are involved in this regulation as well. This finding indicates that the analysis for carrying the full-length PB1-F2 ORF may not directly and solely help predict PB1-F2 protein expression (Buehler *et al.*, 2013). These data even more strongly support the complex influenza strain-specific regulation of PB1-F2 expression.

The intracellular localization of proteins after translation is extremely important for their functionality and can help predict their functions. A study tracking the localization of PB1-F2 after infection showed strong differences in PB1-F2 accumulation among different cell types (Chen *et al.*, 2001). The accumulation of PB1-F2 was highest in the mitochondria, but some cytoplasmic and nuclear localization was also detectible after infection; in contrast, overexpressed PB1-F2 was only marginally detected in the nucleus or cytoplasm (Chen *et al.*, 2001). The mitochondrial accumulation, which was associated with morphological changes in the mitochondria and diminished membrane potential linked to cell apoptosis, was mediated by a short mitochondrial targeting sequence (MTS, amino acid 65–87) located in the C-terminus of the protein. The MTS was predicted to form a positively charged amphipathic α-helix needed for targeting the inner mitochondrial membrane and subsequently altering mitochondrial functions (Gibbs *et al.*, 2003). A domain from residue 46–75 within PB1-F2 was found to be necessary and sufficient for the mitochondrial localization of PB1-F2 (Yamada *et al.*, 2004), emphasizing potentially interrelated active domains.

The functions of the nuclear and cytoplasmic fractions of PB1-F2 are poorly understood, and the kinetics of the intracellular distribution of PB1-F2 proteins has not been fully determined. In addition, the change in the localization pattern of PB1-F2 after infection and its overexpression suggest that these features are mediated via its interaction with other viral proteins. Furthermore, the strain-dependent accumulation of PB1-F2 within the infected cells (Chen *et al.*, 2010) makes this scenario even more complex. Finally, it is still debatable whether PB1-F2 exerts extracellular effects after release from dying cells. Studies in which cells were ectopically treated with PB1-F2 peptides suggest that PB1-F2 has the capacity to exert such extracellular effects (McAuley *et al.*, 2007, 2010a).

In sum, the expression of PB1-F2 from an overlapping +1 reading frame of the influenza gene segment 2 is highly regulated and interrelated with PB1 and N40 expression. After translation of the protein, the major proportion of PB1-F2 can be found in the mitochondria, nevertheless, PB1-F2 accumulation demonstrates strain specificity.

Ecology and evolution

IAV have zoonotic potential to cause pandemics in humans, with virulent IAV (e.g. from birds) having the ability to cross the species barrier and infect humans. A pandemic can occur when the general human population does not have preexisting immunity against this virus. Often, avian IAV enter humans after adaptation in intermediate hosts such as domestic poultry or swine. The segmented genome of influenza viruses can lead to the reassortment of gene segments after a host cell is infected with two different IAV, which can produce a new and unique virus variant with devastating potential. Also, genes can evolve in different hosts in parallel, and their mixing together via reassortment events can result in multilineage reassortant influenza viruses, as seen most recently in the 2009 swine flu pandemic (Neumann *et al.*, 2009).

The ecology of PB1-F2 implies virus-, cell- and host-specific functionalities (Table 7.1). In avian IAV, PB1-F2 is typically expressed as a full-length protein (Smith and McCullers, 2013) and its high evolutionary conservation suggests important functions. Viral protein

Table 7.1 PB1-F2 isolates by subtype, host, and length

	Total	101	90	87	80–60	< 60	Varied size
H1N1	2608	1	653	22	40	1891	1
Human	1571	1	52	9	0	1509	0
Swine	737	0	319	1	39	378	0
Avian	293	0	276	12	0	4	1
H2N2	144	1	142	0	0	1	0
Human	75	1	73	0	0	1	0
Swine	0	0	0	0	0	0	0
Avian	68	0	68	0	0	0	0
H3N2	6211	26	5396	74	109	600	6
Human	5339	25	4630	62	64	552	6
Swine	636	0	545	6	41	44	0
Avian	215	1	200	6	4	4	0
H5N1	1319	3	1211	2	4	98	1
Human	163	1	156	0	2	4	0
Swine	14	0	13	0	0	1	0
Avian	1084	2	988	2	2	89	1

functionalities in avian hosts can be different from those in mammalian hosts due to the different tropism of IAV in birds. Primary replication in the avian gut and in mammalian lungs almost certainly require different strategies and viral protein functions. In contrast to the avian host, PB1-F2 seems to be dispensable in mammalian hosts (Table 7.1). Frequent truncations of PB1-F2 with the loss of expression have occurred in swine (Zell *et al.*, 2007) and also during adaptation in humans, especially in the human H1N1 lineage starting in the mid-twentieth century (Chakrabarti and Pasricha, 2013). The onset and persistence of truncated versions of PB1-F2 may reflect a negative selection of full-length PB1-F2 expression during replication in mammalian hosts.

The pandemic strains in 1918, 1957, and 1968 carried gene segment 2 from avian sources, leading to the assumption that pandemic strains are potentially facilitated by carrying new PB1 segments expressing full-length PB1-F2. In line with this possibility, research on the H5N1 PB1-F2 and PB1-F2 proteins from these pandemics has revealed an important role for PB1-F2 in pathogenesis, at least in mice (McAuley *et al.*, 2010a). Interestingly, the 2009 pandemic IAV took its gene segment 2 from triple reassortant swine viruses that underwent PB1-F2 truncation while circulating in swine, resulting in the loss of PB1-F2 expression (Fig. 7.2). Originally, the 2009 PB1-F2 derived from an avian IAV introduced in humans during the 1968 H3N2 pandemic and this H3N2 lineage was introduced in swine in the late 1990 ending in these triple reassortant swine viruses (Fig. 7.2), In general, the H3N2 lineage, in contrast to the H1N1 lineage, does not show evolution towards truncated PB1-F2 proteins;

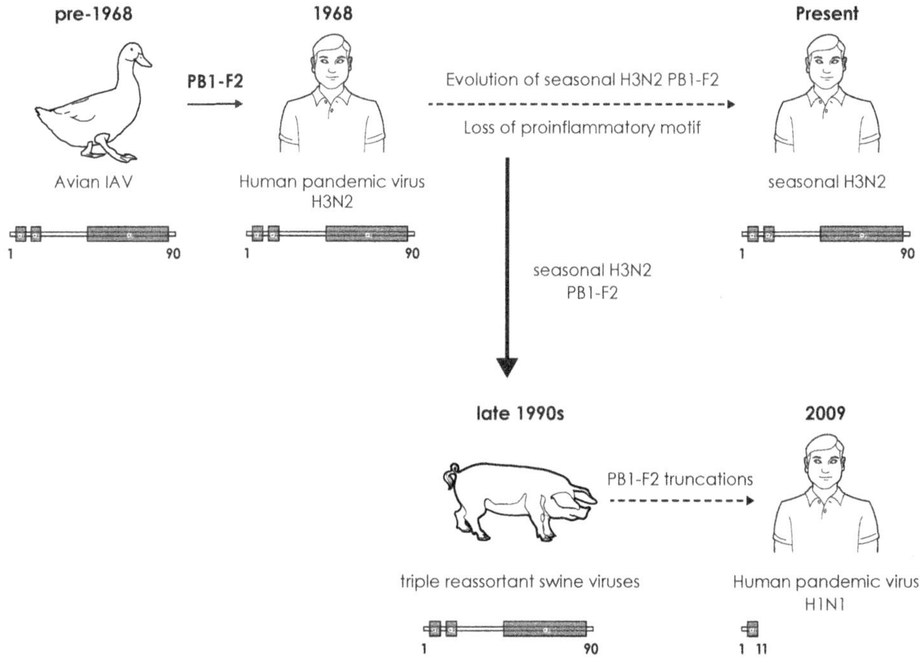

Figure 7.2 The evolutionary history of the PB1-F2 protein of the 2009 H1N1 pandemic strain is show to highlight the complexities of changing length as gene segments move between species and evolve.

however, H3N2 viruses have undergone mutational drift during adaptation, resulting in a considerably changed function and role in pathogenesis (Alymova *et al.*, 2011; McAuley *et al.*, 2010a) (Fig. 7.2).

In addition to the diverse ecology and evolution of PB1-F2 proteins, the effect of PB1-F2 on pathogenesis appears to differ by hosts. In ducks, mutational alteration or depletion of PB1-F2 expression can affect the pathogenicity of avian H5N1 IAV (Marjuki *et al.*, 2010; Schmolke *et al.*, 2011). Also, a study on different H3N2 viruses in swine found a strong virus strain-dependent impact on virulence and pathogenicity (Pena *et al.*, 2012). Most studies on the role of PB1-F2 in pathogenicity have been conducted in mice, illustrating strain dependent contributions to pathogenicity as well (Alymova *et al.*, 2011, 2013; McAuley *et al.*, 2007, 2010a, 2013). Although the mouse model is suitable for understanding the concepts of infection and pathology, the relevance to humans is unclear in the context of prominent virus strains and host-dependent differences of PB1-F2 functionalities.

In summary, while focusing on the ecology and evolution of PB1-F2, influenza virus lineage and host-dependent evolution of PB1-F2 expression need to be considered in the dependency of host-specific functions of PB1-F2.

Multifunctional role in pathogenesis

The PB1-F2 of IAV represents a classic viral multifunctional protein. Evolutionary pressure and the need for rapid adaptation, combined with a small genome size, compel small RNA viruses such as influenza viruses to evolve multifunctional proteins. These proteins have enormous plasticity, carrying spatial and timely well-coordinated functionalities. In the last decade, three major functons for PB1-F2 have been identified (Fig. 7.3): (1) induction of cell death, (2) interactions with the immune system and (3) modulation of replication. These functions may result in PB1-F2-dependent pathogenicity in primary virus infections, although the impact appears to often be much more pronounced in bacterial superinfections.

Induction of cell death

PB1-F2 carries the cell-type-specific ability to cause cell death via a mitochondrial pathway (Fig. 7.3). Interestingly, initially, it was discovered that immune cells such as monocytes are sensitive to PB1-F2 induced apoptosis whereas epithelial cells are protected from it (Chen *et al.*, 2001), leading to the possibility that *in vivo* PB1-F2 specifically depletes IAV-infected immune cells to impair immune responses. PB1-F2-mediated killing of infected cells may be facilitated by the PB1-F2-incorporated MTS, which can drive integration into membranes. This mechanism is likely to participate in apoptosis through one or more canonical pathways that induce cell apoptosis.

During the last few years, several studies have shed light on the mechanism of PB1-F2 induced cell death. Most studies support that PB1-F2 is a pore-forming protein, which can cause permeabilization of the mitochondrial membrane and subsequently apoptosis. In contrast, PB1-F2 can also arrest cells in the S phase, resulting in mitochondrial fragmentation, loss of mitochondrial membrane potential, and subsequently apoptosis (Yamada *et al.*, 2004). Several models have been proposed for PB1-F2-mediated pore formation in the mitochondrial membrane, and all the models have supported cytochrome C release and caspase-mediated apoptosis (Chakrabarti and Pasricha, 2013). A study on synthetic

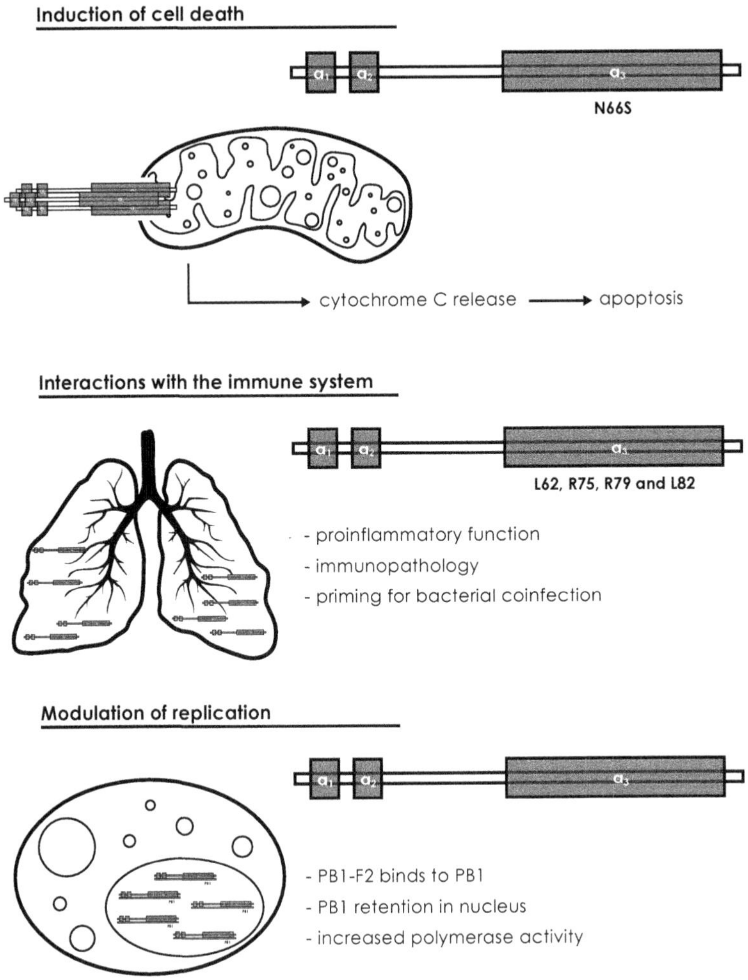

Figure 7.3 Three major proposed mechanisms for the multifunctional influenza A virus protein PB1-F2 are depicted schematically. Highlighted amino acids have been implicated in the described functions.

PB1-F2 revealed that PB1-F2 interacts with negatively charged lipid head group and a transmembrane inner mitochondrial membrane electric field. This results in the incorporation of PB1-F2 into the mitochondrial membrane, causing pore formation, membrane breakdown, and apoptosis (Chanturiya *et al.*, 2004). Another study also revealed that PB1-F2 forms ion channel pores in the mitochondrial membranes via oligomerization of PB1-F2 monomers, which is driven by the α-helical C-terminal domain, leading to disruption of the reticulotubular mitochondrial organization, damage to the inner mitochondrial membrane, and finally apoptosis induction (Henkel *et al.*, 2010).

In addition to protein self-assembly for pore formation, PB1-F2 can also indirectly interact with the mitochondrial membrane via mitochondrial proteins to induce apoptosis (Gibbs *et al.*, 2003; Zamarin *et al.*, 2005). In one study, an interaction of a hydrophobic groove within PB1-F2 with the transporter outer membrane (TOM) receptor was introduced, which facilitates translocation of PB1-F2 α-helical structures through the outer mitochondrial membrane and inner mitochondrial membrane, resulting in disruption of mitochondrial membrane potential and eventually apoptosis (Gibbs *et al.*, 2003). In another study, an indirect interaction of PB1-F2 with the mitochondrial membrane was shown to be mediated by adenine nucleotide translocator 3 (ANT3) and voltage-dependent anion channel 1 (VDAC1), both mitochondrial membrane transport proteins located in the mitochondrial membrane (Zamarin *et al.*, 2005). According to this model, PB1-F2 binds via its C-terminal domain to ANT3 in the inner mitochondrial membrane, whereas the N- and C-terminal domains are crucial for its interaction with VDAC1 in the outer mitochondrial membrane. In conjunction with ANT3 and VDAC1, PB1-F2 forms permeability transition pore complexes (PTPCs) that are involved in mitochondrial permeabilization and cell death induction (Zamarin *et al.*, 2005). A further analysis of the interaction of the C-terminal domain of PB1-F2 with ANT3 and VDAC1 mapped specific sites in both, PB1-F2 and ANT3 and VDAC1 as being responsible for the interaction (Danishuddin *et al.*, 2010).

Another study investigating PB1-F2 from pandemic strains of the twentieth century, a highly pathogenic avian H5N1 strain, human H1N1 virus A/Puerto-Rico/8/34, and seasonal strains showed that the ability of PB1-F2 to manipulate cell fates is strongly dependent on virus strain, with cell death being most strongly induced by the H1N1 PR8 virus (McAuley *et al.*, 2010a). It has been recently shown that the strong aponecrotic potential of PB1-F2 of the H1N1 PR8 virus can be mapped to the residues 68–70 within PB1-F2 (Alymova *et al.*, 2013). This cytotoxic sequence within PB1-F2 is rare and is present in only limited viruses in the animal reservoir. Although this rarity potentially limits the relevance of this for current pandemic planning, the knowledge of the existence of this and other similar motifs in other IAV strains is important. Another study recently showed that an H5N1 PB1-F2 lacking specific residues in the MTS did not localize to mitochondria and subsequently did not induce apoptosis (Chen *et al.*, 2010), again emphasizing the strain specific function of PB1-F2 and that minor amino acid changes within PB1-F2 can significantly affect functionality.

In addition to being virus strain-specific, induction of cell death via PB1-F2 can be host and cell-type-dependent. As mentioned earlier, initial findings suggest that PB1-F2-mediated apoptosis is selectively induced in immune cells but not in epithelial cells (Chen *et al.*, 2001). However, at least the PB1-F2 protein of H1N1 PR8, which carries strong proapoptotic features, induced apoptosis in both immune cells and epithelial cells (McAuley *et al.*, 2010a). Finally, a very recent study proposed an additional model for PB1-F2-induced apoptosis, which involved a non-canonical, caspase 3-independent mechanism (Takahashi *et al.*, 2013).

The current knowledge about PB1-F2 and its ability to induce cell death in host cells clearly supports virus strain specificity and potential host- and cell-type specific functions. Interestingly, asking for the impact of PB1-F2-mediated host cell apoptosis on pathogenicity, several studies have more or less directly linked PB1-F2-induced apoptosis to increased pathogenicity in mice, which mainly occurs by delaying virus clearance. Zamarin *et al.* (2006) speculated that the delayed clearance is due diminished adaptive immune responses due to apoptosis of antigen presenting cells. Furthermore, it has been speculated that PB1-F2 increased the virulence of the 1918 Spanish flu virus by activating cell death pathways of the host (Kash *et al.*, 2006). Transcriptome analyses revealed that PB1-F2 is involved in NK cell dysfunction, epithelial barrier damage, and the expression of genes linked to cell death (Le Goffic *et al.*, 2011; Leymarie *et al.*, 2013), which are potentially the result of cell apoptosis. Interestingly, the recently described novel cytotoxic sequence within PB1-F2 can be a predisposing factor for secondary bacterial infections (Alymova *et al.*, 2013) and an N66S mutation, located in the C-terminal domain and part of the MTS of PB1-F2, interestingly the region linked to apoptosis induction, mediates increased pathogenicity (Conenello *et al.*, 2011), both linking PB1-F2-mediated apoptosis to pathogenicity. The N66S mutation was first detected in the 1918 H1N1 pandemic influenza virus and also in the 1997 H5N1 outbreak in Hong Kong. In the 1918 pandemic virus, the N66S mutation contributes to pathogenicity of primary viral infection and secondary bacterial co-infection (McAuley *et al.*, 2007). Consistent with this finding, the PR8 virus expressing the 1918 PB1-F2 protein showed higher rates of virus production and enhanced cell death, which was confirmed by mathematic modelling, emphasizing an earlier peak in viral load for the 1918 PB1-F2 expressing virus (Smith *et al.*, 2011). Furthermore, Schmolke *et al.* (2011) showed a host-dependent contribution of the N66S polymorphism to pathogenicity using a human H5N1 isolate. In addition, a virus strain-specific contribution was detected in swine (Pena *et al.*, 2012). As will be discussed in detail later, the N66S mutation also reduced the early interferon response (Conenello *et al.*, 2011), indicating a potentially overlapping effect on apoptosis induction and type I IFN induction.

Taken together, the described PB1-F2-mediated apoptosis induction seems to be virus strain and host cell-dependent and several studies connected PB1-F2 induced apoptosis to pathogenicity, however the direct molecular basis for apoptosis-mediated pathogenicity is not solved in detail.

Interactions with the immune system

Proinflammatory domain

In addition to inducing apoptosis, PB1-F2 also has immune modulatory properties. A proinflammatory domain within PB1-F2, which acts independent of the cell death domain, has been discovered and linked to strong proinflammatory action (Fig. 7.3). PB1-F2 of various origins can induce inflammatory responses at the level of proinflammatory cytokines and increased infiltration of immune cells (e.g. macrophages, neutrophils, and dendritic cells), resulting in acute lung injury and mortality in mice (McAuley *et al.*, 2007, 2010a). In addition to primary viral infection, the proinflammatory domain within PB1-F2 facilitates and enhances the severity of secondary bacterial infections (Alymova *et al.*, 2011; McAuley *et al.*, 2007, 2010a). Interestingly, intranasal administration of PB1-F2 peptides covering only the C-terminal region of PB1-F2 is sufficient to induce inflammatory responses (Alymova *et al.*, 2011; McAuley *et al.*, 2007, 2010a). Furthermore, using H3N2 PB1-F2 proteins, the proinflammatory domain has been linked to four defined amino acid positions (L62, R75, R79 and L82) (Alymova *et al.*, 2011). This proinflammatory domain is present in all three twentieth-century pandemic strains and interestingly was lost during adaptation of the H3N2 PB1-F2 lineage in humans resulting in loss of the inflammatory capacity of PB1-F2 (Fig. 7.2). Back introduction of the four amino acids into PB1-F2 of a recently circulating human H3N2 fully recovered the proinflammatory features of the protein (Alymova *et al.*, 2011). Interestingly, the noninflammatory PB1-F2 proteins used in that study showed antimicrobial activity (Alymova *et al.*, 2011) that was potentially mediated by having structural features similar to those of defensins, such as a cationic C-terminal helical domain.

Analysis of the Influenza Research Database for the distribution of the proinflammatory domain among different IAV subtypes revealed that the domain occurred at a high frequency in avian strains, especially in highly pathogenic H5N1 strains (Smith and McCullers, 2013), and had a lower frequency in equine and canine strains. Several types of PB1-F2 sequences exist in swine, but a study on naturally occurring swine IAV revealed that the presence of the proinflammatory domain in PB1-F2 contributed to severity of Gram-positive bacterial coinfections (Weeks-Gorospe *et al.*, 2012). Recent studies on H1N1 IAV found that even partial expression of the proinflammatory motif could be sufficient for proinflammatory effects, thereby emphasizing higher plasticity of this domain.

To identify the mechanism of PB1-F2-induced inflammation, direct recognition of PB1-F2 by pattern recognition receptors of the immune system and its action as chemoattractant have been discussed. A recent study shed light on PB1-F2 triggered inflammation, showing that PB1-F2 protein aggregates are formed and that they finally cause NLRP3 inflammasome activation (McAuley *et al.*, 2013). This activation was dependent on presence of the proinflammatory motif, and NLPR3-deficent mice could not mount inflammatory responses upon peptide administration and viral infection (McAuley *et al.*, 2013). Furthermore, PB1-F2 has been linked to the modulation of NFkB activation, which again depends on the presence and integrity of the proinflammatory domain. These studies show that different residues within the four-amino-acid-spanning domain could have different roles depending on the viral or cellular context. Finally, transcriptome analysis of infected mice lungs revealed that IFN-γ is a central regulator of PB1-F2-regulated genes (Le Goffic *et al.*, 2011) and that PB1-F2 expression is strongly associated with increased transcription of genes encoding chemokines and cytokines (Leymarie *et al.*, 2013), giving rise to PB1-F2 to act as a facilitator of immune cell chemoattractants.

In summary, the proinflammatory action of PB1-F2 has been reported in several independent studies and has been mapped to the C-terminus of PB1-F2. The four amino-acid-spanning proinflammatory domain of PB1-F2-mediated inflammation has been shown as trigger for pathogenicity in primary viral infection, and more markedly, in secondary bacterial challenge.

RIG-I/MAVS pathway

The induction of the type I IFN systems is the most powerful antiviral tool evolved to fight invading pathogens such as viruses. IAV use several strategies to counteract the induction of a general antiviral state mediated by type I IFN. The type I IFN system is activated after the viral RNA is recognized by the RNA helicase retinoic acid–induced gene 1 (RIG-I). RIG-I detects viral ribonucleoprotein complexes (vRNPs) by recognition of RNA secondary base pairing and 5′-triphosphate termini (Rehwinkel *et al.*, 2010). Following detection of vRNPs, RIG-I interacts with the E3 ubiquitin/ISG15 ligase TRIM25 and is recruited to the mitochondria via the mitochondrial antiviral signalling (MAVS) protein. RIG-I recruitment to mitochondria initiates the TANK-binding kinase (TBK) 1/interferon regulatory transcription factor (IRF) 3 signalling pathway finally leading to IFN-β expression (Takaoka and Yanai, 2006). IFN-β is secreted afterwards and induces the expression of multiple IFN-dependent genes after binding and activation of its cell membrane IFN-a/b receptor

(IFNAR) and signalling via the Janus kinase (JAK)/signal transducer and activator of transcription (STAT) signalling pathway.

The main antagonist of the IFN system is the NS1 protein of IAV (Garcia-Sastre *et al.*, 1998; Hale *et al.*, 2008), but PB1-F2 has also been proposed as an IFN antagonist (Conenello *et al.*, 2011; Dudek *et al.*, 2011; Varga *et al.*, 2011). Interestingly, very recently, an even broader influence of the IAV polymerase proteins as IFN antagonists being involved in virulence regulation has been shown (Liedmann *et al.*, 2013). PB1-F2 inhibits type I IFN production at the level of the MAVS protein and PB1-F2 interaction with MAVS has been described as mechanism of type I IFN inhibition (Varga *et al.*, 2011). Thereby, MAVS-dependent signal transduction and subsequently IFN-β expression is hindered by PB1-F2. Interestingly, as introduced before, a known polymorphism in PB1-F2 (N66S) has been mapped to the IFN inhibitory capacity of PB1-F2 (Conenello *et al.*, 2011). This virulence-boosting N66S polymorphism is present in the 1918 pandemic H1N1 IAV and in some highly pathogenic H5N1, but is relative rare in general. The N66S mutation is often associated with the presence of two or three of the four amino acids of the proinflammatory domain, but the occurrence of all the four amino acids in the proinflammatory domain along with N66S, as in the 1918 virus, is rare (Smith and McCullers, 2013).

Taken together, type I IFN antagonistic properties have been attributed to PB1-F2; however, because of the rarity of the N66S polymorphism, a broad contribution of the RIG-I/MAVS pathway inhibition to PB1-F2-mediated pathogenicity remains to be clarified.

Exacerbation of secondary bacterial infections

Because PB1-F2 has an immune modulatory capacity, it can boost the severity of secondary bacterial infections. Compared with the effects on bacterial coinfections, the immune effects of PB1-F2 have been shown to be minor on primary viral pathogenicity in animal models. However, as mentioned previously, conceivable exceptions may be viruses carrying the four residues in the proinflammatory domain together with the N66S polymorphism. These viruses such as the 1918 pandemic H1N1 and some H5N1 strains can show enhanced pathogenicity linked to PB1-F2 during primary viral infection. In animal studies, however, PB1-F2 affects pathogenicity mainly via regulation of secondary bacterial disease. By inducing cell damage and massive inflammation, PB1-F2 can prime the lung for bacterial superinfections. Growing evidence suggests that influenza virus infections alter the lungs so as to promote the adherence and invasion of bacterial pathogens and consequently induction of disease (McCullers, 2006). Depletion or partial loss of epithelial cells due to PB1-F2-mediated apoptosis can result in epithelial barrier breakthrough and potentially decreased production of neutralizers of bacteria such as mucus or defensins.

The induction of cell death specifically in alveolar macrophages can be a priming mechanism for bacterial co-infection as well (Coleman, 2007). Recently, the depletion of alveolar macrophages has been shown to be critical for bacterial coinfection, but there was no clear connection between depletion and PB1-F2 functions (Ghoneim *et al.*, 2013). Many studies indicate that the exacerbation of inflammation during primary viral infection increases the frequency and severity of secondary bacterial infections. PB1-F2 can increase the expression of cytokines and chemokines, resulting in elevated immune cell infiltration; furthermore alveolar epithelial cell hypertrophy and hyperplasia, and fibrin deposition was attributed to PB1-F2 (McAuley *et al.*, 2007). Consistent with these findings, the priming for bacterial coinfections was associated with the number of proinflammatory residues as well as the

N66S polymorphism in PB1-F2 (Weeks-Gorospe *et al.*, 2012). Interestingly, the study also found that the effects on bacterial coinfection were bacterial species and strain-dependent (Weeks-Gorospe *et al.*, 2012), showing that even the pairing of specific IAV and bacterial strains can determine the fate of infection. However, the factors governing bacterial participation in the interplay of influenza infection and bacterial coinfection are extremely poorly understood and require further studies.

Since secondary bacterial infections are a more prominent complication and contributor to death during pandemic outbreaks compared to seasonal influenza, the likelihood of highly inflammatory PB1-F2 proteins to be present in pandemic strains from the avian reservoir may explain this observation. The virus that caused the 2009 pandemic outbreak did not express PB1-F2, which possibly explains the milder disease and less frequent bacterial coinfections during that pandemic.

In summary the effects of PB1-F2 on priming for bacterial coinfections are well documented in mice. Alterations such as airway modulation, inflammatory priming, or desensitization of immune receptors, or the dependency on viral and bacterial pairing have been reported (McCullers, 2006) but need to be studied in more detail future.

Modulation of replication

An additional function for PB1-F2 was introduced by investigating IAV polymerase activity. Initially, the binding of PB1-F2 to PB1 can indirectly regulate polymerase activity (Mazur *et al.*, 2008). The C-terminal domain in PB1-F2 mediates its binding to PB1, and the lack of PB1-F2 expression can result in altered PB1 localization and decreased polymerase activity (Mazur *et al.*, 2008). A recent study confirmed the effects of PB1-F2 on polymerase activity, but attributed it to the N-terminal region of PB1-F2 (Kosik *et al.*, 2011). A PB1-F2-mediated retention of PB1 in the nucleus during later stages of infection caused an increase in polymerase activity. Further studies revealed that PB1-F2 regulates influenza polymerase activity in a virus strain- and cell-type-specific manner (McAuley *et al.*, 2010b). Keeping in mind that the alteration of PB1-F2 expression may impact N40 expression as described earlier (Wise *et al.*, 2009), this idea gives rise to potential unspecific alterations of polymerase activity by unbalancing gene expression from influenza gene segment 2.

Although mathematical modelling of infection kinetics has revealed a potential role for PB1-F2 in early replication and early clearance (Smith *et al.*, 2011), PB1-F2 seems to be dispensable for viral replication and fitness as it is absent in many strains. Experimental data have confirmed that lack of PB1-F2 expression does not affect viral load in mice lungs, suggesting that PB1-F2 has little role in virus replication (McAuley *et al.*, 2010b). Even more, the increase in inflammation driven by PB1-F2 can also affect virus clearance. Thus, increased viral load or delayed clearance of IAV lacking the PB1-F2 protein can be indirectly regulated by less severe inflammation. From an ecological standpoint, it is conceivable that global presence of PB1-F2 full-length expression is more critical for avian IAV, potentially regulating bird-specific functions such as facilitating the systemic spread of IAV in avian hosts or aiding in transmission through increasing secretions from the GI tract.

Taken together, PB1-F2 has been shown to increase IAV polymerase activity and thereby modulates replication. However, these effects are strain specific and almost dispensable for human IAV strains. Thereby, a global impact of the PB1-F2-mediated increase of polymerase activity on regulation of pathogenicity is questionable, however it does not exclude that certain IAV gain advantages from increased polymerase activity.

Implications for treatment and prevention

During an algorithm search for alternative reading frame peptides that are recognized by $CD8^{+}$T-cells (Chen *et al.*, 2001), PB1-F2 was identified to have a $CD8^{+}$ T-cell epitope that seems subdominant to the immune-dominant $CD8^{+}$T-cell epitopes in the nucleoprotein (NP) and acidic polymerase (PA) of IAV (Andreansky *et al.*, 2005; Thomas *et al.*, 2007). Antibodies against PB1-F2 have been found in human serum (Krejnusova *et al.*, 2009). In animal models, antibodies specific for the N-terminal region of PB1-F2 were not protective, whereas those specific for the C-terminus of PB1-F2 partially protected mice from infection (Kosik *et al.*, 2013). Because PB1-F2 is not present in the virion and is dispensable in many IAV, PB1-F2 might not be a promising and globally applicable candidate for drug or vaccine targeting. As inhibition of PB1-F2 does not inhibit virus entry into host cell, targeting PB1-F2 could only have indirect modulatory effects on influenza infections. Nevertheless, PB1-F2 could be a useful secondary target in universal vaccines or vaccines targeting multiple antigens, because the antibody-mediated neutralization of PB1-F2 functions has shown promise in reducing PB1-F2 driven pathogenicity. As PB1-F2 is expressed in many highly pathogenic IAV, it can be a useful target to modulate severe disease caused by highly pathogenic avian IAV or for secondary bacterial infections. In the evolving field of personalized medicine, having a PB1-F2-targeting drug in stock can be a useful strategy to impede the IAV-mediated priming of severe bacterial coinfection, if the invading IAV expresses PB1-F2.

Conclusion and future directions

The PB1-F2 protein of IAV is an example of an accessory viral protein that has high plasticity. Despite being studied for more than a decade, the role of PB1-F2 in pathogenicity remains poorly understood. More studies are required on PB1-F2, especially on translating experimental findings to humans. Although animal models remain the vehicle of choice, well-considered experimental approaches are required to gain further insight on the role of this protein in humans.

Although PB1-F2 is similar to NS1 in that it is a multifunctional protein with several binding partners, it is not as important for viral fitness as NS1, since it is dispensable in mammals. The IFN antagonistic effect of PB1-F2 may be complementary to that of NS1, and can be useful to fine-tune the suppression of IAV-mediated innate immunity. In contrast, the inflammatory function of PB1-F2 may be an undesirable trait in the mammalian lung, as it tends to be lost through negative selection during adaptation in swine and humans. Many highly pathogenic avian IAV strains with pandemic potential, such as H5 and H7 strains, and some swine strains express the full-length PB1-F2 with at least 4 of the residues implicated in pathogenesis.

The ability of IAV to undergo genetic reassortment can result in rapid multilineage reassortant pandemic strains that carry undesirable combinations of protein functions, such as PB1-F2 proteins with high pathogenic potential. The circulation of strains expressing PB1-F2 with strong pathogenic properties needs to be considered during pandemic planning, with efforts focused on increased and more guided surveillance. Because PB1-F2 is almost dispensable for viral fitness in mammalian hosts, its potential contribution to severe IAV pandemics may have been underestimated. However, its contribution in priming for bacterial superinfections is clear in animal models and may be the more important factor. Therefore, resources need to be focused on identifying strains that have the highest potential for causing severe pandemics, such as those that best support secondary bacterial superinfections by using molecular signatures for PB1-F2. Finally, beyond the research needed to further understand the mechanistic basis of PB1-F2 in pathogenesis, PB1-F2 has to be considered as viable target for the modulation of severe infections. Therefore, abrogation of PB1-F2-mediated priming for severe bacterial coinfections might be a promising approach.

References

Alymova, I.V., Green, A.M., van de Velde, N., McAuley, J.L., Boyd, K.L., Ghoneim, H.E., and McCullers, J.A. (2011). Immunopathogenic and antibacterial effects of H3N2 influenza A virus PB1-F2 map to amino acid residues *62, 75, 79*, and 82. J. Virol. *85*, 12324–12333.

Alymova, I.V., Samarasinghe, A., Vogel, P., Green, A.M., Weinlich, R., and McCullers, J.A. (2013). A novel cytotoxic sequence contributes to influenza A protein PB1-F2 pathogenicity and predisposition to secondary bacterial infection. J. Virol. *88*, 503–515.

Andreansky, S.S., Stambas, J., Thomas, P.G., Xie, W., Webby, R.J., and Doherty, P.C. (2005). Consequences of immunodominant epitope deletion for minor influenza virus-specific CD8+-T-cell responses. J. Virol. *79*, 4329–4339.

Bruns, K., Studtrucker, N., Sharma, A., Fossen, T., Mitzner, D., Eissmann, A., Tessmer, U., Roder, R., Henklein, P., Wray, V., *et al.* (2007). Structural characterization and oligomerization of PB1-F2, a proapoptotic influenza A virus protein. J. Biol. Chem. *282*, 353–363.

Buehler, J., Navi, D., Lorusso, A., Vincent, A., Lager, K., and Miller, C.L. (2013). Influenza A virus PB1-F2 protein expression is regulated in a strain-specific manner by sequences located downstream of the PB1-F2 initiation codon. J. Virol. *87*, 10687–10699.

Chakrabarti, A.K., and Pasricha, G. (2013). An insight into the PB1F2 protein and its multi-functional role in enhancing the pathogenicity of the influenza A viruses. Virology *440*, 97–104.

Chanturiya, A.N., Basanez, G., Schubert, U., Henklein, P., Yewdell, J.W., and Zimmerberg, J. (2004). PB1-F2, an influenza A virus-encoded proapoptotic mitochondrial protein, creates variably sized pores in planar lipid membranes. J. Virol. *78*, 6304–6312.

Chen, C.J., Chen, G.W., Wang, C.H., Huang, C.H., Wang, Y.C., and Shih, S.R. (2010). Differential localization and function of PB1-F2 derived from different strains of influenza A virus. J. Virol.. *84*, 10051–10062.

Chen, W., Calvo, P.A., Malide, D., Gibbs, J., Schubert, U., Bacik, I., Basta, S., O'Neill, R., Schickli, J., Palese, P., *et al.* (2001). A novel influenza A virus mitochondrial protein that induces cell death. Nat. Med. *7*, 1306–1312.

Chevalier, C., Al Bazzal, A., Vidic, J., Fevrier, V., Bourdieu, C., Bouguyon, E., Le Goffic, R., Vautherot, J.F., Bernard, J., Moudjou, M., *et al.* (2010). PB1-F2 influenza A virus protein adopts a beta-sheet conformation and forms amyloid fibers in membrane environments. J. Biol. Chem. *285*, 13233–13243.

Coleman, J.R. (2007). The PB1-F2 protein of Influenza A virus: increasing pathogenicity by disrupting alveolar macrophages. Virol. J. *4*, 9.

Conenello, G.M., Tisoncik, J.R., Rosenzweig, E., Varga, Z.T., Palese, P., and Katze, M.G. (2011). A single N66S mutation in the PB1-F2 protein of influenza A virus increases virulence by inhibiting the early interferon response in vivo. J. Virol. *85*, 652–662.

Danishuddin, M., Khan, S.N., and Khan, A.U. (2010). Molecular interactions between mitochondrial membrane proteins and the C-terminal domain of PB1-F2: an in silico approach. J. Mol. Model. *16*, 535–541.

de la Luna, S., Fortes, P., Beloso, A., and Ortin, J. (1995). Influenza virus NS1 protein enhances the rate of translation initiation of viral mRNAs. J. Virol. *69*, 2427–2433.

Dudek, S.E., Wixler, L., Nordhoff, C., Nordmann, A., Anhlan, D., Wixler, V., and Ludwig, S. (2011). The influenza virus PB1-F2 protein has interferon antagonistic activity. Biol. Chem. *392*, 1135–1144.

Garcia-Sastre, A., Egorov, A., Matassov, D., Brandt, S., Levy, D.E., Durbin, J.E., Palese, P., and Muster, T. (1998). Influenza A virus lacking the NS1 gene replicates in interferon-deficient systems. Virology *252*, 324–330.

Ghoneim, H.E., Thomas, P.G., and McCullers, J.A. (2013). Depletion of alveolar macrophages during influenza infection facilitates bacterial superinfections. J. Immunol. *191*, 1250–1259.

Gibbs, J.S., Malide, D., Hornung, F., Bennink, J.R., and Yewdell, J.W. (2003). The influenza A virus PB1-F2 protein targets the inner mitochondrial membrane via a predicted basic amphipathic helix that disrupts mitochondrial function. J. Virol. *77*, 7214–7224.

Hale, B.G., Randall, R.E., Ortin, J., and Jackson, D. (2008). The multi-functional NS1 protein of influenza A viruses. J. Gen. Virol. *89*, 2359–2376.

Henkel, M., Mitzner, D., Henklein, P., Meyer-Almes, F.J., Moroni, A., Difrancesco, M.L., Henkes, L.M., Kreim, M., Kast, S.M., Schubert, U., *et al.* (2010). The proapoptotic influenza A virus protein PB1-F2 forms a nonselective ion channel. PLoS One *5*, e11112.

Kash, J.C., Tumpey, T.M., Proll, S.C., Carter, V., Perwitasari, O., Thomas, M.J., Basler, C.F., Palese, P., Taubenberger, J.K., Garcia-Sastre, A., *et al.* (2006). Genomic analysis of increased host immune and cell death responses induced by 1918 influenza virus. Nature *443*, 578–581.

Kosik, I., Krejnusova, I., Bystricka, M., Polakova, K., and Russ, G. (2011). N-terminal region of the PB1-F2 protein is responsible for increased expression of influenza A viral protein PB1. Acta Virologica *55*, 45–53.

Kosik, I., Krejnusova, I., Praznovska, M., and Russ, G. (2013). The multifaceted effect of PB1-F2 specific antibodies on influenza A virus infection. Virology *447*, 1–8.

Krejnusova, I., Gocnikova, H., Bystricka, M., Blaskovicova, H., Polakova, K., Yewdell, J., Bennink, J., and Russ, G. (2009). Antibodies to PB1-F2 protein are induced in response to influenza A virus infection. Arch. Virol. *154*, 1599–1604.

Le Goffic, R., Leymarie, O., Chevalier, C., Rebours, E., Da Costa, B., Vidic, J., Descamps, D., Sallenave, J.M., Rauch, M., Samson, M., *et al.* (2011). Transcriptomic analysis of host immune and cell death responses associated with the influenza A virus PB1-F2 protein. PLoS Pathog. *7*, e1002202.

Leymarie, O., Jouvion, G., Herve, P.L., Chevalier, C., Lorin, V., Lecardonnel, J., Da Costa, B., Delmas, B., Escriou, N., and Le Goffic, R. (2013). Kinetic characterization of PB1-F2-mediated immunopathology during highly pathogenic avian H5N1 influenza virus infection. PLoS One *8*, e57894.

Liedmann, S., Hrincius, E.R., Anhlan, D., McCullers, J.A., Ludwig, S., and Ehrhardt, C. (2013). New Virulence Determinants Contribute to the Enhanced Immune Response and Reduced Virulence of an Influenza A Virus A/PR8/34 Variant. J. Infect. Dis. *209*, 532-541.

Marjuki, H., Scholtissek, C., Franks, J., Negovetich, N.J., Aldridge, J.R., Salomon, R., Finkelstein, D., and Webster, R.G. (2010). Three amino acid changes in PB1-F2 of highly pathogenic H5N1 avian influenza virus affect pathogenicity in mallard ducks. Arch. Virol. *155*, 925–934.

Mazur, I., Anhlan, D., Mitzner, D., Wixler, L., Schubert, U., and Ludwig, S. (2008). The proapoptotic influenza A virus protein PB1-F2 regulates viral polymerase activity by interaction with the PB1 protein. Cell Microbiol. *10*, 1140–1152.

McAuley, J.L., Chipuk, J.E., Boyd, K.L., Van De Velde, N., Green, D.R., and McCullers, J.A. (2010a). PB1-F2 proteins from H5N1 and 20 century pandemic influenza viruses cause immunopathology. PLoS Pathog. *6*, e1001014.

McAuley, J.L., Hornung, F., Boyd, K.L., Smith, A.M., McKeon, R., Bennink, J., Yewdell, J.W., and McCullers, J.A. (2007). Expression of the 1918 influenza A virus PB1-F2 enhances the pathogenesis of viral and secondary bacterial pneumonia. Cell Host Microbe *2*, 240–249.

McAuley, J.L., Tate, M.D., MacKenzie-Kludas, C.J., Pinar, A., Zeng, W., Stutz, A., Latz, E., Brown, L.E., and Mansell, A. (2013). Activation of the NLRP3 inflammasome by IAV virulence protein PB1-F2 contributes to severe pathophysiology and disease. PLoS Pathog. *9*, e1003392.

McAuley, J.L., Zhang, K., and McCullers, J.A. (2010b). The effects of influenza A virus PB1-F2 protein on polymerase activity are strain specific and do not impact pathogenesis. J. Virol. *84*, 558–564.

McCullers, J.A. (2006). Insights into the interaction between influenza virus and pneumococcus. Clin. Microbiol. Rev. *19*, 571–582.

Mitzner, D., Dudek, S.E., Studtrucker, N., Anhlan, D., Mazur, I., Wissing, J., Jansch, L., Wixler, L., Bruns, K., Sharma, A., *et al.* (2009). Phosphorylation of the influenza A virus protein PB1-F2 by PKC is crucial for apoptosis promoting functions in monocytes. Cell Microbiol. *11*, 1502–1516.

Neumann, G., Noda, T., and Kawaoka, Y. (2009). Emergence and pandemic potential of swine-origin H1N1 influenza virus. Nature *459*, 931–939.

Pasricha, G., Mishra, A.C., and Chakrabarti, A.K. (2013). Comprehensive global amino acid sequence analysis of PB1F2 protein of influenza A H5N1 viruses and the influenza A virus subtypes responsible for the 20th-century pandemics. Influenza Other Resp. Viruses 7, 497–505.

Pena, L., Vincent, A.L., Loving, C.L., Henningson, J.N., Lager, K.M., Li, W., and Perez, D.R. (2012). Strain-dependent effects of PB1-F2 of triple-reassortant H3N2 influenza viruses in swine. J. Gen. Virol. *93*, 2204–2214.

Rehwinkel, J., Tan, C.P., Goubau, D., Schulz, O., Pichlmair, A., Bier, K., Robb, N., Vreede, F., Barclay, W., Fodor, E., *et al.* (2010). RIG-I detects viral genomic RNA during negative-strand RNA virus infection. Cell *140*, 397–408.

Schmolke, M., Manicassamy, B., Pena, L., Sutton, T., Hai, R., Varga, Z.T., Hale, B.G., Steel, J., Perez, D.R., and Garcia-Sastre, A. (2011). Differential contribution of PB1-F2 to the virulence of highly pathogenic H5N1 influenza A virus in mammalian and avian species. PLoS Pathog. 7, e1002186.

Shaw, M.L., Stone, K.L., Colangelo, C.M., Gulcicek, E.E., and Palese, P. (2008). Cellular proteins in influenza virus particles. PLoS Pathog. *4*, e1000085.

Smith, A.M., Adler, F.R., McAuley, J.L., Gutenkunst, R.N., Ribeiro, R.M., McCullers, J.A., and Perelson, A.S. (2011). Effect of 1918 PB1-F2 expression on influenza A virus infection kinetics. PLoS computational biology 7, e1001081.

Smith, A.M., and McCullers, J.A. (2013). Molecular signatures of virulence in the PB1-F2 proteins of H5N1 influenza viruses. Virus Res. *178*, 146–150.

Solbak, S.M., Sharma, A., Bruns, K., Roder, R., Mitzner, D., Hahn, F., Niebert, R., Vedeler, A., Henklein, P., Schubert, U., *et al.* (2013). Influenza A virus protein PB1-F2 from different strains shows distinct structural signatures. Biochim. Biophys. Acta *1834*, 568–582.

Takahashi, T., Takaguchi, M., Kawakami, T., and Suzuki, T. (2013). Sulfatide regulates caspase-3-independent apoptosis of influenza A virus through viral PB1-F2 protein. PLoS One *8*, e61092.

Takaoka, A., and Yanai, H. (2006). Interferon signalling network in innate defence. Cell Microbiol. *8*, 907–922.

Thomas, P.G., Brown, S.A., Keating, R., Yue, W., Morris, M.Y., So, J., Webby, R.J., and Doherty, P.C. (2007). Hidden epitopes emerge in secondary influenza virus-specific CD8+ T cell responses. J. Immunol *178*, 3091–3098.

Varga, Z.T., Ramos, I., Hai, R., Schmolke, M., Garcia-Sastre, A., Fernandez-Sesma, A., and Palese, P. (2011). The influenza virus protein PB1-F2 inhibits the induction of type I interferon at the level of the MAVS adaptor protein. PLoS Pathog. 7, e1002067.

Weeks-Gorospe, J.N., Hurtig, H.R., Iverson, A.R., Schuneman, M.J., Webby, R.J., McCullers, J.A., and Huber, V.C. (2012). Naturally occurring swine influenza A virus PB1-F2 phenotypes that contribute to superinfection with Gram-positive respiratory pathogens. J. Virol. *86*, 9035–9043.

Wise, H.M., Foeglein, A., Sun, J., Dalton, R.M., Patel, S., Howard, W., Anderson, E.C., Barclay, W.S., and Digard, P. (2009). A complicated message: Identification of a novel PB1-related protein translated from influenza A virus segment 2 mRNA. J. Virol. *83*, 8021–8031.

Yamada, H., Chounan, R., Higashi, Y., Kurihara, N., and Kido, H. (2004). Mitochondrial targeting sequence of the influenza A virus PB1-F2 protein and its function in mitochondria. FEBS Lett *578*, 331–336.

Zamarin, D., Garcia-Sastre, A., Xiao, X., Wang, R., and Palese, P. (2005). Influenza virus PB1-F2 protein induces cell death through mitochondrial ANT3 and VDAC1. PLoS Pathog. *1*, e4.

Zamarin, D., Ortigoza, M.B., and Palese, P. (2006). Influenza A virus PB1-F2 protein contributes to viral pathogenesis in mice. J. Virol. *80*, 7976–7983.

Zell, R., Krumbholz, A., Eitner, A., Krieg, R., Halbhuber, K.J., and Wutzler, P. (2007). Prevalence of PB1-F2 of influenza A viruses. J. Gen. Virol. *88*, 536–546.

Avian Influenza H7N9 Virus

Ying Wu, Yi Shi, Jun Liu, Yan Wu and George F. Gao

8

Abstract

In March 2013, the first cases of human infection with a novel reassortant of avian influenza A virus (H7N9) were reported in China. The rapid increase in cases with considerable morbidity and mortality over a subsequent brief time period has posed a great threat to public health globally. In this chapter we present an overview of the current understanding of H7N9 virus from the perspectives of the virus origin, clinical features and treatments of virus infection, host immune responses, virus receptor-binding properties as well as drug resistance. We also provide a snapshot of vaccine development and monoclonal antibody application against H7N9 virus infection and call for precautionary measurements for unpredictable emergence of novel reassortants of influenza viruses, HxNy.

Introduction

Influenza A virus H7 subtype has been reported to cause human infections in combination with different neuraminidase (NA) subtypes, including H7N2, H7N3 and H7N7 (Fouchier *et al.*, 2004; Hirst *et al.*, 2004; Koopmans *et al.*, 2004; Nguyen-Van-Tam *et al.*, 2006; Ostrowsky *et al.*, 2012) before 2013. Those infections are mainly associated with mild diseases, such as conjunctivitis, mild upper respiratory tract illness (uncomplicated influenza-like illness), and a sporadic death in the Netherlands (Fouchier *et al.*, 2004; Hirst *et al.*, 2004; Koopmans *et al.*, 2004; Nguyen-Van-Tam *et al.*, 2006; Ostrowsky *et al.*, 2012). Nevertheless, a new reassortment virus of H7N9 (this is the first time to observe an H7 reassorting with N9 to infect human in China) was diagnosed to cause severe human infections in China in early 2013 (Gao *et al.*, 2013b) and have been in endemic in eastern and southern China in the spring-winter seasons through 2014. Sustained occasional cases were reported during the following two years with more frequent cases in winter and spring seasons each year. As of 23 February 2016, more than 600 laboratory-confirmed cases have been reported, with about 30% case fatality rates (http://who.int/influenza/human_animal_interface/influenza_h7n9/en/).

When you think hard, avian influenza viruses that infect human beings have been increasingly observed since the first human infection event with H5N1 in Hong Kong and H9N2 in mainland China in the mid-1990s (Claas *et al.*, 1998; Peiris *et al.*, 1999). It is believed that the live poultry trade (market) in South-East Asia, especially in China, plays an important role in the virus reassortments and dissemination. Such culture results in poultry coming in close contact with humans, which leads to human infection with avian influenza viruses.

H7N9 is a very good example of such a scenario. After H7N9, we predicted that some new subtypes would arise in China and this indeed has been the case. Human infections with H10N8 and H5N6, albeit sporadic, have since been reported (Bi *et al.*, 2015a; Wang *et al.*, 2014c).

To infect human beings and even cause severe diseases, avian influenza virus must obtain its human receptor binding capability and efficient replication ability in human tissues as both receptors and host replication restriction factors are different in avian and humans (or mammalians in a broader concept). This mechanism has been well studied in H5N1 avian influenza virus (Herfst *et al.*, 2012; Imai *et al.*, 2012; Lu *et al.*, 2013b; Xiong *et al.*, 2013a; Zhang *et al.*, 2013b) and the H7N9 subtype isolated in 2013 provides a unique model of virus adaptation from avian to human *in silico* (Belser *et al.*, 2013; Chen *et al.*, 2013b; Richard *et al.*, 2013; Shi *et al.*, 2013b; Watanabe *et al.*, 2013; Xiong *et al.*, 2013b; Xu *et al.*, 2013b). Luckily we have isolated a few H7N9 viruses from both the patients and fields (including chickens and environment) with different characteristics, in terms of host adaptation (Shi *et al.*, 2014; Yang *et al.*, 2014). First, we have seen the virus strain with a characteristic NA sequence showing five amino acids deletion at the N-terminus, which is the feature for an avian virus to adapt into the terrestrial poultry environment from the migratory/shorebirds waterfowls; second, we have a few virus strains with different amino acid substitutions in haemaglutinin (HA) for differential human versus avian receptor binding affinities; third, we also observed the mammalian-adapted replication restriction mutations in viral polymerase PB2 (notorious E627K mutation); fourth, Tamiflu® (oseltamivir phosphate)-resistant strains with a typical R292K mutation in NA were isolated after the drug was used in the patients.

In this chapter, we summarize our current understanding of H7N9 virus by addressing the virus origin, infection clinical features and host immune response, virus receptor-binding properties and commonly used Tamiflu® drug resistance. We also outline the prospects of vaccine development and monoclonal antibody application for H7N9 virus infection therapy.

Origin, genesis and epidemiology

From the very beginning of the outbreak in the Yangtze River Delta Region in China, virus surveillance and phylogenetic analyses confirm the transmission of the H7N9 infection from poultry to humans (Lam *et al.*, 2013; Lu *et al.*, 2013a; Wu and Gao, 2013). Direct evidence was revealed by an infection case in Jiangsu Province, China, where a female butcher was infected, and a phylogenetically related H7N9 virus was isolated from a chicken cage 1 m away (Wang *et al.*, 2014c). Thus, there was an urgent call to control exposure at poultry farms and live poultry markets. Appropriate measures have been introduced in the most affected areas and the disease has been under control, except for some areas where the live poultry markets are yet kept open.

The novel H7N9 viruses appear to be reassortments with segments from at least three different origins (Lu *et al.*, 2013a): the haemagglutinin (HA) gene from duck H7 viruses, which have been already established in China earlier; the neuraminidase (NA) gene from wild birds in Korea; and internal genes from different lineages of poultry H9N2 viruses. Up to now, a large number of genotypes have been observed, with diverse internal genes from varied H9N2 lineages, but conserved HA and NA genes. Because the H7N9 viruses originated from poultry through genetic reassortment, it is not a surprise that the H7N9 virus could easily reassort with poultry H9N2 viruses under a process called 'dynamic reassortment'. Some distinct virus strains have been isolated with unique characters, e.g. Shanghai-1, Shanghai-5 and Anhui-1 viruses (Wu *et al.*, 2013a). So far none of the H7N9

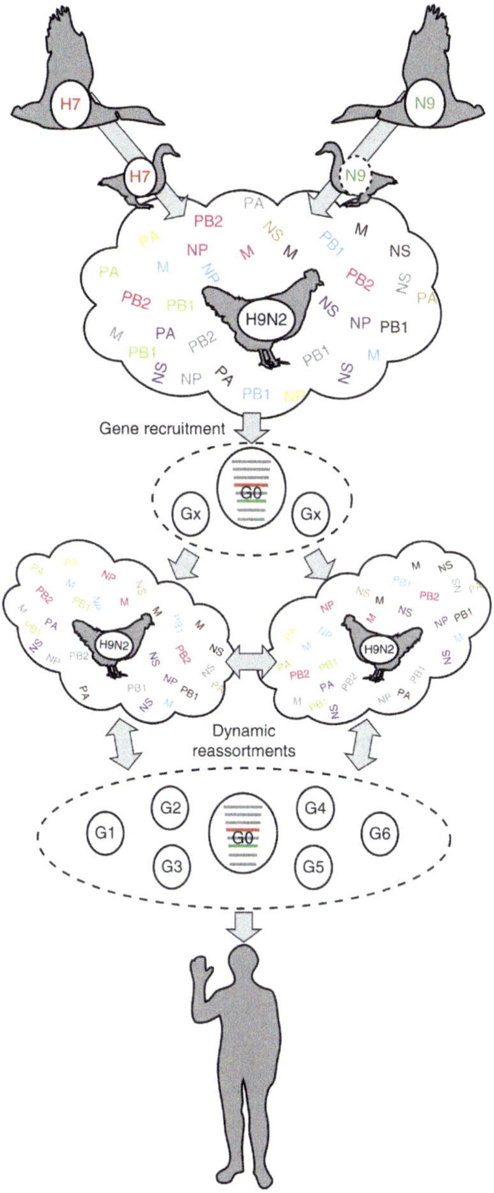

Figure 8.1 Schematics illustrating the formation and dynamic reassortments of the H7N9 influenza viruses. Migratory bird, duck, chicken and human involved in the H7N9 emergence were shown in cartoons. Dashed circle of N9 represents the uncertainty of N9 in ducks due to the lack of surveillance data. Coloured internal gene names in clouds represent diversified H9N2 gene pools.

virus genotypes has gained an overwhelming fitness advantage and that they are still undergoing dynamic reassortment within poultry H9N2 gene pools (Fig. 8.1). Whether a 'super' reassortant fitting the mammalian hosts would appear is unpredictable because genetic reassortment often has major effects on influenza virus replication within cells.

The endemic, so far, is still mainly confined in the Yangtze River Delta Region, though with some areas in central China (Lam *et al.*, 2015). From the current surveillance data, it is believed that the H7N9 has established its niche in the nature and it is difficult to eradicate the virus (Lam *et al.*, 2015). There is a risk of virus dissemination to other areas, especially to South-East Asia.

Clinical features and immunology

Demographic and general medical conditions

Two waves of the H7N9 epidemic have risen since the spring of 2013 in China, and human infected cases are continually reported recently in the 2014 autumn, which may be the prelude of another wave. No significant differences have been discovered between the clinical features of the human cases derived from the first two epidemic waves (Chen *et al.*, 2013a; Wang *et al.*, 2014b). Actually, the generally similar clinical features of H7N9 infections have been described based on hundreds of cases distributed in different provinces of China, e.g. Zhejiang (Chen *et al.*, 2013a; Lv *et al.*, 2013; Sun *et al.*, 2014; Wang *et al.*, 2014a,b; Xia *et al.*, 2014; Xiao *et al.*, 2014), Shanghai (Feng *et al.*, 2014; Huang *et al.*, 2014a; Ren *et al.*, 2014; Wang *et al.*, 2013a, 2014c), Jiangsu (Guo *et al.*, 2014b; Ji *et al.*, 2014; Qi *et al.*, 2014; Qian *et al.*, 2014), Hongkong (Ho *et al.*, 2014; Nicholls *et al.*, 2014), Guangzhou (Kang *et al.*, 2014), Beijing (Song *et al.*, 2014) and Fujian (Yao *et al.*, 2014), although H7N9 viruses isolated in different provinces had distinct reassortments with local H9N2 repertoire (Cui *et al.*, 2014). Generally, the clinical characteristics of the human LPAIV H7N9 virus infections were somewhat comparable to infections of HPAIV H5N1 and severe acute respiratory syndrome coronavirus (SARS-CoV), but also with their distinct characteristics (Chen *et al.*, 2013b; Gao *et al.*, 2013a; To *et al.*, 2014; Wang *et al.*, 2014a). The subjects hospitalized with H7N9 had higher average age (63 years vs. 26 years) and proportion of male (71% vs. 56%) than H5N1 patients. Subjects hospitalized with H7N9 had high prevalence of chronic medical conditions associated with an increased risk of severe influenza disease. Chronic heart disease (CHD) and diabetes were the commonest medical risk factors reported among H7N9 patients, and the prevalence of smoking and hypertension was higher in subjects with H7N9 than in the H5N1 patients (Wang *et al.*, 2014a). Pregnancy has an impact on the pathogenesis and clinical outcome in H7N9 subjects (Qi *et al.*, 2014; Qian *et al.*, 2014), but was less common than in subjects hospitalized with 2009 pH1N1 (Wang *et al.*, 2014a).

Symptoms and laboratory results

Acute H7N9 infection causes severe pneumonia, which typically deteriorates and extends rapidly to involve both lungs. Subjects with H7N9 virus infection were more likely to report a fever (94%), a productive cough (57%), and haemoptysis (24%) than those with H5N1 virus infection (Wang *et al.*, 2014a). Other respiratory and nonspecific symptoms included dyspnoea, sputum production, headache, myalgia, fatigue, vomiting and diarrhoea (Gao *et al.*, 2013a; Sun *et al.*, 2014). Alanine aminotransferase, lactate dehydrogenase, and creatinine kinase were also elevated in H7N9 patients (Gao *et al.*, 2013a; Ji *et al.*, 2014). Disease severity was associated with higher levels of C-reactive protein, serum creatinine and myoglobin (Shen *et al.*, 2014).

Radiologic findings

The typical viral pneumonia-featured imaging findings included ground-glass opacities (GGOs) and consolidations were observed in the chest radiography and thin-section computed tomography (CT) of the patients (Lu *et al.*, 2013a; Wang *et al.*, 2013a). Other characteristics, i.e. air bronchograms, interlobular septal thickening, centrilobular nodules, reticulations, cystic changes, bronchial dilatation and subpleural linear opacities were also observed. The lung lesions involved three or more lobes in most severe cases and were mostly detected in the right lower lobe. The severity of these imaging findings is associated with the mortality in patients with pneumonia (Feng *et al.*, 2014).

Histopathology

Histopathological manifestations of the lung tissues based on H7N9-related autopsy clearly showed the features of direct viral invasion of organs and immunopathology (Nicholls *et al.*, 2014; Wang *et al.*, 2014c; Yu *et al.*, 2013b). Pneumonia was characterized by typical early exudative phase followed by a fibroproliferative phase in H7N9 patients, which was similar to other severe influenza infection. Influenza nucleoprotein positive cells were detected by immunohistochemistry in the lungs through an autopsy study, reflecting a direct infection of the lower respiratory tract by H7N9 (Yu *et al.*, 2013b). In addition to the pulmonary pathological changes, such as diffuse alveolar damage, hyaline membrane formation, widespread intraalveolar haemorrhage, extensive lymphocyte infiltration (Wang *et al.*, 2014c), organizing thrombus and fibrinous serositis, other extrapulmonary features were also observed, including reactive haemophagocytosis, splenic lymphoid atrophy, hepatic spotty necrosis, and renal tubular degeneration (Yu *et al.*, 2013b). These pathological changes were suggestive of the directly infect of multiple organs by H7N9 and the pivotal role of severe immunopathology.

Complications

Acute respiratory distress syndrome (ARDS) is a common complication in H7N9 patients and is associated with a high mortality rate (Gao *et al.*, 2013a; Liu *et al.*, 2013; Zhou *et al.*, 2013). Multivariate analysis revealed that the presence of an underlying medical condition is an independent risk factor for ARDS (Gao *et al.*, 2013a). Many patients had nosocomial bacteraemia and bacterial pneumonia. The increased predisposition to secondary infection in the patients may be related to the deranged immune responses (Wu *et al.*, 2014b). Common nosocomial organisms include *Acinetobacter baumannii*, *Klebsiella pneumoniae* and *Pseudomonas aeruginosa* (Yu *et al.*, 2013b). Pathogens resistant to multiple antibiotics were common implicated in these nosocomial infections, owing to the use of broad-spectrum antibiotics in many patients (Gao *et al.*, 2013a; Zhou *et al.*, 2013). Other severe complications included shock, congestive heart failure, acute kidney injury, liver damage, disseminated intravascular coagulation, rhabdomyolysis, and encephalopathy (Gao *et al.*, 2013a; Huang *et al.*, 2014b; Liu *et al.*, 2013; Wiwanitkit, 2014; Zhou *et al.*, 2013). Some rare complications for influenza infections have also been reported, showing the clinical variability of H7N9 infection. Acute myelitis featured with numbness of the lower limbs, urinary retention and faecal incontinence and magnetic resonance imaging (MRI) of the spinal cord revealed oedema at the thoracic level in one patient (Xia *et al.*, 2014). Immunoneuroendocrine axis dysfunction and vitamin D insufficiency were observed in severe cases (Yao *et al.*, 2014). Brugada syndrome with anteroseptal ST-segment elevation on electrocardiography (ECG) has also been demonstrated associated with H7N9 infection (Wang *et al.*, 2013b).

Mild and asymptomatic infections

Mild or asymptomatic H7N9 infections were described among the population by China's national sentinel surveillance system for influenza-like illness or by the trace of close contacts of H7N9 patients. Based on the recent data, three different populations were prone to present mild or asymptomatic infections:

1. Major H7N9 patients with mild manifestations were children or young persons under 26 years of age (Ip *et al.*, 2013; Kang *et al.*, 2014; Ren *et al.*, 2014; Song *et al.*, 2014), which may associate with the robust immune responses for the quick virus clearance in these subjects.
2. The infections of second cases among the H7N9 family clusters tend to be mild or moderate compared with the index case (Kang *et al.*, 2014; Song *et al.*, 2014).
3. The increasing ratios of the poultry workers with positive haemagglutination inhibition titres based on serological surveillance may imply that many of these seropositive individuals had genuine mild infection of H7N9 (Bai *et al.*, 2013; Lv *et al.*, 2013; Wang *et al.*, 2014a; Yang *et al.*, 2014). The existence of mild, moderate and even asymptomatic H7N9 infections among these populations are concordant with the facts that the underlying medical condition of the aged patients was the only independent risk factor for moderate to severe ARDS (Gao *et al.*, 2013a). The H7N9 virus infections seem to be less serious than initially thought at the beginning of the outbreak (Yu *et al.*, 2013a).

Diagnosis

Thus far, RT-PCR based on the nasopharyngeal specimens has the highest sensitivity for the detection of H7N9 virus and is commonly used in different laboratories of local CDC (Hatchette *et al.*, 2013). However, throat swab has a lower sensitivity than sputum (Chen *et al.*, 2013b). Thus, lower respiratory tract specimens including sputum, bronchoalveolar lavage, and tracheal aspirate specimens should be utilized to test for H7N9 virus, even when the pharyngeal specimens are negative for the virus RNA. Virus RNA can also be positive in serum, urine and stool samples of some patients, though it is not necessary to routinely test these specimens (Song *et al.*, 2014). Immunochromatographic tests and direct immunofluorescence antigen tests are also useful methods for virus detection, but less sensitive compare to RT-PCR (Chan *et al.*, 2013; Kang *et al.*, 2014). Virus culture is significant for charactering the virulence of the viruses and thus manipulated in many different CDCs (Li *et al.*, 2013; Yu *et al.*, 2014). Serological tests play a pivotal complimentary role for the retrospective confirmation of the patients, especially when the RT-PCR results are negative in some asymptomatic infections (Dong *et al.*, 2014). Systematic evaluation using similar clinical specimens demonstrated the limitations of different diagnostic strategies for H7N9 infection. Therefore, clinicians and clinical microbiologists should be alerted to the differences in sensitivity for the various commercially available tests (Chan *et al.*, 2014). In one study, Liao *et al.* (2014) developed a simple decision rule based on clinical data obtainable in 121 H7N9 patients' first clinical presentations. This prediction rule has achieved good model performance in predicting the risk of H7N9 infection and could be useful in guiding important clinical decisions.

Treatment

Neuraminidase inhibitor has confirmative efficacy against H7N9 virus and approved for clinical use widely. Studies indicated that administration of antiviral therapy as early as possible was beneficial for the recovery (Cheng *et al.*, 2012; Yang *et al.*, 2012). Giving of neuraminidase inhibitors more than 3 days after disease onset of H7N9 patients has been proved to be correlated with ARDS (Gao *et al.*, 2013a). The dropping of patient's temperature after treatment (Song *et al.*, 2014) and the shorter median times from the initiation of antiviral therapy to a negative test result on daily real-time RT-PCR assay (Gao *et al.*, 2013a) were observed in the oseltamivir tablet-treated patients. Furthermore, rapid and beneficial clinic and virological responses following intravenous zanamivir therapy in H7N9 patients were also observed (Ho *et al.*, 2014). Antiviral resistant isolates of H7N9 emerged as the predominant quasispecies during the NA inhibitor treatment (Chi *et al.*, 2013), characterized by an Arg294Lys substitution in the virus NA gene, which resulted in loss of inhibitor carboxylate interactions, and consequently the binding of all classical NA inhibitors (Wu *et al.*, 2013b). However, it was found that Arg294Lys substitution led to reduced NA catalytic efficiency along with lower viral fitness, which implies that oseltamivir can still be efficiently used in the treatment of H7N9 infections (Wu *et al.*, 2013b).

Though the efficacy of immunomodulators for severe influenza infection is still conflicting, many H7N9 patients received corticosteroid (Huang *et al.*, 2014a; Wang *et al.*, 2014c; Zhou *et al.*, 2013). The proper use of corticosteroid with moderate dosage may be beneficial during the late or fibroproliferative phase of the disease when the disease is characterized by immunodysregulation. Further, intravenous immune globulin (IVIG) has been used for H7N9 treatment, which was shown the beneficial effects in previous studies on seasonal and avian influenza virus therapies (Zhou *et al.*, 2013). The therapy efficacy of IVIG preparations may be contributed by the broadly cross-reactive antibody-dependent cellular cytotoxicity (ADCC) mediating antibodies induced by seasonal influenza infections (Jegaskanda *et al.*, 2014). Considering the frequent occurrence of nosocomial bacterial infections among H7N9 patients, antibiotic drugs were also widely used (Gao *et al.*, 2013a). In addition, respiratory supports, such as extracorporeal membrane oxygenation (ECMO) has been extensively used and has been shown to be beneficial (Lin *et al.*, 2014; Yu *et al.*, 2013b).

Other exploratory treatments include using of bosentan for refractory hypoxaemia and pulmonary hypertension in a H7N9 patient with ARDS (Guo *et al.*, 2014b). Other drugs are also under development and have been proved to be efficacy in animals. A novel polymerase inhibitor favipirava (T-705) was effective for antivirus in a H7N9 infected mouse model (Cao *et al.*, 2013; Watanabe *et al.*, 2013). Further, DAS181, a recombinant fusion protein with sialidase activity, which removes sialic acid-containing receptor from respiratory epithelial cells, preventing attachment of influenza virus, can effectively inhibits replication of H7N9 and protects mice from lethality (Marjuki *et al.*, 2014). In another study, the H7N9 infected mice treated with oseltamivir plus an immunomodulator fenofibrate had prolonged mean survival time accompanied by significantly lower viral titres and decreased pulmonary inflammation (Xu *et al.*, 2014).

White cell subgroups

As other virus infections, the haemogram results were abnormal in most H7N9 infected patients. On admission, nearly half of the patients (46%) had a low white blood cell counts, while lymphopenia and thrombocytopenia were found in over 88% and 73% of patients, respectively (Gao *et al.*, 2013a). Low proportions of $CD3^+$, $CD4^+$ and $CD8^+$ T-cells were observed in H7N9-infected individuals compared to 2009 pH1N1 patients(Chen *et al.*, 2014a). The T-cell ratios were shown to be negatively correlated with clinical APACHE II scores and H7N9 virus loads in sputum of the patients. A dramatic increase in lymphocyte subgroups was observed in those who survived beyond the early stage of infection, while T-cell levels fluctuated during hospitalization and decreased suddenly on the day of death in those who succumbed to infection (Chen *et al.*, 2014a). However, the percentages of $CD38^+$ or Tim-3^+ T-cells (including both $CD8^+$ and $CD4^+$ T-cells) were significantly increased, which may indicates indicated significant T-cell activation status specifically induced by virus infection (Wu *et al.*, 2014b). The significant reduce of monocytes was also common among H7N9 infections (Diao *et al.*, 2014; Wu *et al.*, 2014b). Particularly, percentages of HLA-DR^+CD14^+ and Tim-3^+CD14^+ monocytes were decreased in patients compared with healthy control subjects. Importantly, the expression of HLA-DR on $CD14^+$ cells were negatively correlated with H7N9 infection severity. Furthermore, the monocytes of patients with severe infection had a lower antigen-presenting capacity than those isolated from patients with mild disease, although the phagocytosis capabilities were similar (Diao *et al.*, 2014). Furthermore, another study elucidated that H7N9 virus induces impaired interferon responses in human monocyte-derived dendritic cells *in vitro* (Arilahti *et al.*, 2014). Likewise, a study indicated that *in vitro* transcriptomic response of human lung epithelial cells to H7N9 virus included the lack of induction of the antigen presentation pathway compared to that with H3N2 (Josset *et al.*, 2014). The dysfunction of host immune cells could lead to efficient virus spread within the infected host, which could have an important impact on the immunogenicity and virulence of H7N9 in humans.

Cytokines and chemokines

Similar to what has been observed for H5N1 infections, immunopathogenetic analysis of H7N9 infection samples revealed high levels of proinflammatory cytokines and chemokines, termed hypercytokinaemia, in the early stage of the infection (Bi *et al.*, 2015b; Chen *et al.*, 2014a; Chi *et al.*, 2013; Shen *et al.*, 2014; Zhou *et al.*, 2013). This was illuminated not only within the protein level in patient plasma, but also within the transcription level tested by transcriptome sequencing of peripheral blood samples from H7N9 patients (Josset *et al.*, 2014; Mei *et al.*, 2014). The concentrations of several cytokines/chemokines, including MIP-1β, IL-6 and IL-8, were even higher than those of previously reported H5N1 infection cases (Zhou *et al.*, 2013). Furthermore, the hypercytokinemia is correlated with disease severity for H7N9 infection. Higher levels of IL-6, IL-8, IL-10, IP-10, IL-18, TNF-α and MIP-1β were detected in fatal cases compared to survivors from H7N9 infections (Chen *et al.*, 2014a; Diao *et al.*, 2014; Huang *et al.*, 2014b; Wang *et al.*, 2014c; Guo *et al.*, 2015c). The degree of liver damage in these patients significantly correlated with their serum levels of Th2 cytokines IL-4 and IL-9 (Huang *et al.*, 2014b). Our recent study discovered that

34 of the 48 cytokines and chemokines examined were significantly elevated in the plasma samples from H7N9-infected patients. The levels of MIF, SCF, MCP-1, HGF, SCGF-beta were highly positively linked to disease severity and the profile of these mediators was an independent outcome predictor. Nevertheless, two independent studies indicated that IFN-γ levels were significantly lower in the patients with severe disease than in those with mild disease, which implies a protective role of IFN-γ in H7N9 infection (Chi *et al.*, 2013; Diao *et al.*, 2014). Our data also indicate that plasma levels of angiotensin II were correlated with disease severity and could predict fatal outcomes in H7N9-infected patients (Huang *et al.*, 2014a). Simultaneous measurement of serum sCD40L during the acute phase of H7N9 infection showed a significant suppression in H7N9 patients compared to healthy human controls (Huang *et al.*, 2014b).

Despite this progress, two important issues remain: (1) to profile the sequential connections of these cytokines/chemokines and clarify the key factors in the infection process, particularly in the local mucosal tissues of the lungs of H7N9 patients; and (2) to determine the immunopathogenic or immunoprotection roles (or both) of different mediators, especially when considering that many cytokines/chemokines are directly associated with the viral load in the patients (Chen *et al.*, 2014a; Huang *et al.*, 2014b; Shen *et al.*, 2014).

Antibody responses

Most H7N9 patients displayed a robust serological response after the onset of the disease, as revealed by antibody reactivity kinetics (Yang *et al.*, 2014; Zhang *et al.*, 2013a). Detectable H7N9-specific antibodies appeared in the sera of survivors earlier than in fatal cases. In addition, the highest antibody titres in fatal cases were also lower than in survivors (Yu *et al.*, 2013b). Among the survivors of H7N9 infections, the group with higher antibody titres time from the onset of the disease to recovery was shorter (Yang *et al.*, 2014; Zhang *et al.*, 2013a). These data indicate that an earlier and robust H7N9-specific humoral response provides a protective effect and improves clinical outcomes in patients. Interestingly, an IgG against H3 titrated by ELISA with recombinant H3 HA antigens was boosted in H7N9 patients after infection, and IgG level against H3 in acute-phase samples correlated with that against H7 in convalescent-phase samples. This could be contributed by a heterosubtypic HA antibody response, especially considering the conserved HA stalk region of H3 and H7 subtypes, which both belong to subgroup 2 of HAs (Guo *et al.*, 2014a).

Specific T-cell responses

Direct data on H7N9-specific T-cell responses in patients are still lacking. However, immunoinformatics analysis of H7N9 proteins indicates that conservation of T-cell epitopes with other recently circulating strains of influenza is very limited (De Groot *et al.*, 2013, 2014; He *et al.*, 2014). Though the extent of conservation between endemic human seasonal influenza and avian influenza H7N9 was comparable to that with the avian influenza H5N1 and H9N2 (Mao *et al.*, 2014), the role of the non-conserved peptides in the immunogenicity variety of these viruses has not been determined. Approximately 60% of the previously well-defined major histocompatibility complex class I (MHC I)-restricted T-cell epitopes have substitutions in the corresponding sequences in H7N9 as revealed by the comparison of H7N9 with 2009 pH1N1. Furthermore, a study of human leucocyte antigen (HLA)-typed healthy subjects demonstrates that seasonal influenza virus-specific T-cells poorly cross-react to individual H7N9 variant epitopes, apart from the recognition of the whole virus (van de

Sandt *et al.*, 2014). It is also indicated that cross-$CD8^+$ T-cell immunity to the H7N9 varies across different ethnic groups based on the MHC I gene background (Quinones-Parra *et al.*, 2014). This is concordant with the population coverage analysis across different ethnicities using commonly conserved $CD4^+$ T-cell epitopes and corresponding MHC II alleles, which also indicates a susceptibility of North American and Australian indigenous peoples vulnerable to H7N9 infection (Duvvuri *et al.*, 2014). Further investigations into the features of the H7N9-specific T-cell responses in patients and a comparison of $CD8^+$ and $CD4^+$ T-cell-related immunogenic variance of H7N9 to other currently circulating influenza viruses, e.g. 2009 pH1N1, should be performed.

Other host factors

It is elucidated that the human single nucleotide polymorphism (SNP) rs12252-C, which is associated with dysfunctional interferon induced transmembrane protein-3 (IFITM3), plays a crucial genetic role in early hypercytokinaemia development in H7N9-infected patients (Wang *et al.*, 2014c). Meanwhile, H7N9 virus-induced IFITM3 levels remained extremely low compared with the levels seen in human H3N2 virus-infected monocyte-derived dendritic cells (Arilahti *et al.*, 2014). Recent studies in mouse model demonstrated that host protease TMPRSS2 plays a major role in the replication of H7N9 and seasonal influenza viruses, which mainly use this specific protease for HA cleavage *in vivo* (Sakai *et al.*, 2014; Tarnow *et al.*, 2014). The replication and pathogenicity of H5N1 virus *in vivo* are not dependent the TMPRSS2, which may indicate the dependence on other proteases ofH5N1 HA.

The investigation of serum microRNA (miRNA) profile among the H7N9 patients showed that miR-17, miR-20a, miR-106a and miR-376c were significantly elevated in patients compared with healthy individuals (Zhu *et al.*, 2014). These significant alterations in serum miRNA expression following virus infection could act a potential marker for the diagnosis of viral diseases. However, the physiological functions of these miRNA within the H7N9 infection need to be determined.

Molecular basis of the 'host jump'

The molecular basis which enables the avian-origin influenza virus to 'jump' to infect humans is an important scientific question that remains to be fully understood (Shi *et al.*, 2014). The receptor binding preference shift is one of the key factors responsible for the influenza virus 'host jump' and the virus obtains such ability by a few amino acid substitutions in the receptor-binding site of the haemagglutinin (HA). The H7N9 strains isolated during the epidemic provided a unique chance for us to explore the adaptation process of this subtype of virus to gradually bind human-like receptor for human infection. A process of 'genetic tuning' is under way for the molecular adaptation.

During the adaption of the avian influenza viruses to humans, the receptor binding properties of the influenza viruses can be classified into three types: human receptor binding, avian receptor binding and dual receptor binding. For example, seasonal influenza virus has adapted to humans, and preferentially binds to the human receptor, α2,6-linked sialic acid (SA). By contrast, highly pathogenic avian H5N1 influenza virus infects humans by occasion, and preferentially binds to the avian receptor, α2,3-linked SA (Shi *et al.*, 2014; Wu *et al.*, 2014c). As for the newly occurring avian H7N9 influenza virus in China, it can infect humans, but has not been adapted to humans for efficient transmission and can only cause limited probable human to human transmission (not yet definitively confirmed), if any (Chen *et al.*, 2013b; Richard *et al.*, 2013; Shi *et al.*, 2013b; Watanabe *et al.*, 2013; Xu *et al.*, 2013b). The dominant endemic virus strain, AH1-H7N9 (A/Anhui/1/2013)-like virus, shows dual receptor binding properties, though with higher binding affinity to avian-like receptor (Shi *et al.*, 2013b). Whereas the early strain, SH1-H7N9 virus (A/Shanghai/1/2013), preferentially binds avian-like receptor (Shi *et al.*, 2013b). We suspect that there might be an evolutionary link between SH1-H7N9 and AH1-H7N9, and SH5-H7N9 (A/Shanghai/5/2013) might be intermediate virus strain in the evolutionary process (Fig. 8.2). It is plausible that AH1-H7N9 could acquire the ability to bind human receptor and thus spread well in the human population. There are eight amino acid substitutions between the SH1-H7N9 and AH1-H7N9 HAs, of which four residues (S138A, G186V, T221P and Q226L) are in the receptor binding site. By mutagenesis assay, the amino acid substitution Q226L has been found not to be solely responsible for the HA of AH1-H7N9 acquiring the ability to bind human receptors. This is different from H5N1 influenza virus mentioned above consequently, other amino acids around the receptor binding site are also very important. We considered that the human receptor-binding properties probably arise from the introduction of two bulky hydrophobic residues by the substitutions Q226L and G186V (Shi *et al.*, 2013b; Xiong *et al.*, 2013b). The structures of SH1-H7N9, AH1-H7N9 and its L226Q mutant, in their free forms and in complex with the avian or human receptor

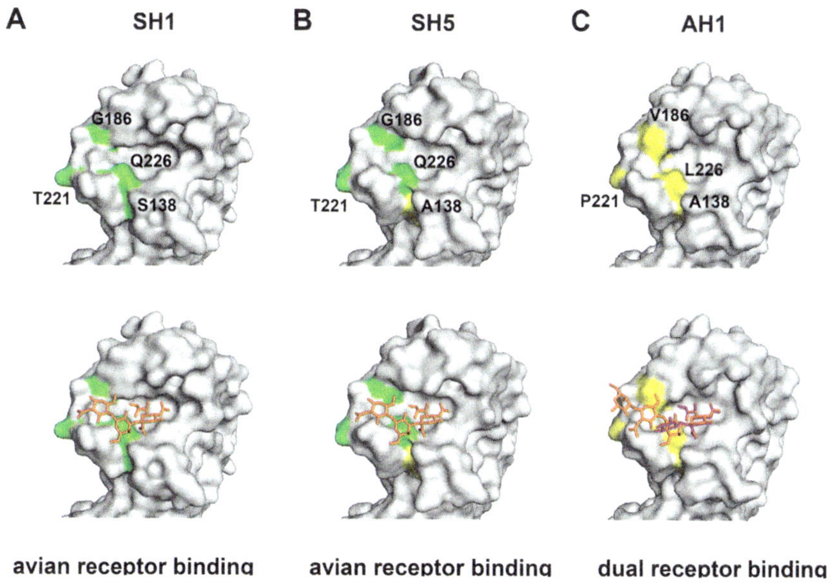

Figure 8.2 Evolutionary analysis of receptor binding properties of H7N9 influenza viruses. Three representative H7N9 virus strains are chosen to show the evolutional process, including A/Shanghai/1/2013 (SH1), A/Shanghai/5/2013 (SH5) and A/Anhui/1/2013 (AH1). The residues at position 138, 186, 221 and 226 are important for the receptor binding change. SH1 and SH5 display preferential avian receptor binding capacity, while AH1 shows dual receptor binding capacity (avian and human receptor binding). The HA structure of SH5 is obtained through homology-modelling under SWISS-MODEL server using HA structure of SH1 as a template.

analogues, were solved to illuminate the structural basis of receptor binding shift(Shi *et al.*, 2013b). The four substitutions are able to create a hydrophobic region on the receptor binding site of AH1-H7N9, which is favourable for the human receptor binding. For the first time, two conformations (*cis* or *trans*) of avian receptor analogue were seen in SH1-HA/avian receptor and AH1-HA mutant/avian receptor complex structures, despite of the same hydrophilic amino acid Q226. It is reported (Breg *et al.*, 1989; Merritt *et al.*, 1994; Poppe *et al.*, 1992; Sabesan *et al.*, 1991; Stehle and Harrison, 1996; Wright and Jaeger, 1993) that the avian receptor analogue can exist with two conformations in water solution while the human receptor analogue mainly exists in the *cis* conformation. In the future, we should bear this in mind that the avian receptor is not simply in a *trans* conformation, when studying receptor binding properties of HA.

Virulence and drug resistance

The contribution of the H7 protein to the pathogenicity for human infection in the newly emergent H7N9 has been discussed in the section 'host jump'. In this section, we discuss about the contribution of the N9 protein and six internal genes to the virulence of H7N9.

It is known that the internal genes of influenza A viruses play important roles in virus replication, interspecies transmission and virulence to mammals. The NP and M genes are critical for virus replication and transmission (Lakdawala *et al.*, 2011; Tada *et al.*, 2011), the PA, PB2, and NP genes impact viral pathogenicity (Mok *et al.*, 2011; Naffakh *et al.*, 2008; Song *et al.*, 2009; Tada *et al.*, 2011; Wang *et al.*, 2012; Zhu *et al.*, 2012), and the PB1 gene induces apoptosis and regulates the cellular interferon response of host cells (Zamarin *et al.*, 2005). NS1 inhibits both interferon production and the activity of several interferon-induced genes (Jiao *et al.*, 2008). NS2, also called NEP, functions as a mediator to export the vRNPs from the host cell nucleus and is able to confer a significant replicative advantage during mammalian adaptation of an highly pathogenic avian influenza virus (Manz *et al.*, 2012). It has been revealed that the PB2, M, and NP genes of the novel H7N9 virus play important roles in its high replication ability and virulence *in vitro* and *in vivo* (Bi *et al.*, 2015b). Further, the RNP complexes containing H7N9 PB2 presented remarkably high polymerase activities in both 293T and DF-1 cells, and the reassortant containing H7N9 PB2 displayed the highest replication ability in MDCK cells and pathogenicity in mice, suggesting that the H7N9-PB2 gene is the key factor for the adaptation of the H7N9 virus to avian and human cells and is critical for the high pathogenicity of H7N9 in mammals.

It is clear that N9 proteins from early clinical isolates are divergent and an oseltamivir-resistant K294-containing N9 was identified from the first few isolates. N9 from Shanghai-1 is the prototype and the patient from whom the virus was isolated was initially treated with Tamiflu®. In some further clinical cases of H7N9 infection treated with oseltamivir, viruses carrying an R294K substitution have also been isolated (Hu *et al.*, 2013). R294 is one of the three key conserved active site arginines that surround the carboxylate group of sialic acid. This tri-arginyl cluster is thought to be a major factor for distorting the sialic acid pyranose ring from a chair to a boat conformation, a critical step for influenza NA to catalyse the hydrolytic cleavage of terminal sialic acid from α2,3- or α2,6 -linked glycoconjugates (Varghese *et al.*, 1992; Vavricka *et al.*, 2013). Therefore, it is not surprising that N9 from Shanghai-1 H7N9 has much lower NA activity and R294K has never before been found in a wild-type N9 variant, though laboratory artificial drug-present passages yielded a R294K N9.

Vaccine development

Traditional split-virus vaccine

To meet the urgent challenge of vaccine development against H7N9 infection, different approaches, including the traditional split-virus vaccine, are under investigation in animal models or have already been approved to proceed to clinical trials. Although the efficacy of several vaccines has been investigated in different phase 1 or 2 clinical trials, no vaccine has yet been approved for use. Traditional strategies for influenza virus vaccine development based on the inactivated virus have been manipulated among mice and ferrets. A reassortant virus that contained the HA and NA genes from wild-type H7N9 and six genes encoding internal proteins from the A/Puerto Rico/8/34 (PR8) virus can completely protected mice from lethal wild-type H7N9 virus challenge only under two doses of at least 15 μg (Duan *et al.*, 2014). A vaccine utilizing whole inactivated H7N9 virus confers protection from severe disease but not infection in ferrets (Wong *et al.*, 2014).

Other strategies

In considering of the low immunogenicity and ineffective protection in animals, diverse unconventional approaches for influenza vaccine development have been explored, including live recombinant viral vector-based vaccines, live attenuated influenza vaccines, universal DNA vaccines and virus-like particles (VLPs). One vaccine containing recombinant Newcastle disease virus expressing North American lineage H7 subtype haemagglutinin could induce cross-reactive antibodies to H7N9 virus (Goff *et al.*, 2013). Immunization with modified vaccinia virus Ankara (MVA)-based vaccine afforded protection in the H7N9-infected ferret models (Kreijtz *et al.*, 2015). It is also illuminated that co-expression of IL-15 as an adjuvant in multivalent vaccinia-based vaccine can improve the heterosubtypic protection for H7N9 challenge in mice (Valkenburg *et al.*, 2014).

To avoid the pathogenicity of H7N9, the development of live attenuated vaccines was majorly focused on different H7 subtypes, e.g. H7N1, H7N3 and H7N7, which have been elucidated to provide a heterosubtypic reactivity and protection to the current H7N9 virus (Carter *et al.*, 2015; Jiang *et al.*, 2014; Krammer *et al.*, 2014a; Rudenko *et al.*, 2013; Rudenko *et al.*, 2014; Xu *et al.*, 2013a). By means of reassortment with cold-adapted influenza virus A/Ann Arbor/6/60 (AA ca) and multiple substitutions in the HA head, a high-yield live attenuated H7N9 vaccine was generated, which could provide protection against H7 wild-type viruses in ferrets (Chen *et al.*, 2014b). A phase I clinical trial using H7N3 live attenuated influenza vaccine demonstrated a good safety profile in human and the vaccine induced H7N9-specific antibodies responses, $CD4^+$ and $CD8^+$ memory T cells among the majority (86.2%) of vaccinated recipients (Rudenko *et al.*, 2014).

Synthetic consensus DNA vaccine represents a new tool for targeting emerging infection for the rapid deployment of vaccines. One study in mice model indicated that a synthetic DNA vaccine expressing HA from H7N9 could elicit high-titre HAI and potent polyfunctional effector $CD4^+$ and $CD8^+$ T cell memory responses against the H7N9 viruses (Yan *et al.*, 2014). Also, universal DNA vaccines based on antibodies targeting the HA stalk region were examined as a possible candidate to prevent H7N9 infection. The H3 stalk-based vaccine was able to elicit antibodies reactive with H7 proteins and also protects mice from H7N9 challenge (Krammer *et al.*, 2014b).

In addition, insect cell-derived VLPs containing HA and NA from H7N9 display promising protection in mice against H7N9 (Klausberger *et al.*, 2014; Smith *et al.*, 2013). Indeed, shortly after these animal experiments, enrolment of 284 adults was initiated for a phase 1 clinical trial of a monovalent VLP (H7N9) vaccine candidate with and without adjuvant (Fries *et al.*, 2013). The clinical trial suggests that VLPs in the presence of adjuvant induce an immune response at a low dosage.

Adjuvants

To identify an effective adjuvant is also a pivotal way to settle the problem of the low immunogenicity of H7N9 in vaccine development. A squalene-based adjuvant (AddaVAX) formulated H7N9 split-virus based vaccines could elicit significantly higher humoral immune response in mice against H7N9 virus compared to formulations with aluminium hydroxide $Al(OH)_3$(Wu *et al.*, 2014a). During stage I of a phase 1/2 clinical trial, intranasal seasonal influenza vaccine adjuvanted with a TLR-3 agonist, rintatolimod, induced cross-reactive IgA antibody against H7N9. MF59 (Novartis Vaccines) is a well-established oil-in-water emulsion adjuvant shown to significantly augment the immune response to both pandemic and seasonal influenza vaccines licensed in the European Union and other countries (Clark *et al.*, 2009). In a phase 1 trial, MF59-adjuvanted H7N9 vaccine is immunogenic in adults (Bart *et al.*, 2014). However, within a phase 2 clinical trial, administration of two doses of H7N9 vaccine with MF59 adjuvant produced seroconversion in only 59% of participants (Mulligan *et al.*, 2014).

Although no vaccine for H7N9 has been approved for using, all of these efforts to develop effective H7N9 influenza vaccines with traditional or new techniques are attempting to increase the vaccine immunogenicity and meet the manufacturing requirements for rapid deployment.

Conclusion and perspectives

The emergence of the novel reassortant H7N9 has pointed to the role of live poultry market (trading) in arising of new subtypes of influenza viruses (Gao, 2014). In addition to the traditional notion that swine are regarded as mixing vessel for newly emerging influenza viruses, poultry (chicken) in the live poultry markets are recognized as a new mixing vessel for the emergence of novel influenza virus (Liu *et al.*, 2014). This is especially worrisome, as live poultry markets/trading are still very popular in China and South-East Asia. Amid the endemic of H7N9 in mainland China, a human infection case of H6N1 was reported in Taiwan with mild symptoms (Shi *et al.*, 2013a). As more than a decade has passed since the introduction of vaccination of chickens against both H9N2 and H5N1 in China and other countries (Vietnam, Egypt, etc.), rather than culling, H9N2 and H5N1 have become established in the poultry population in the vaccinated areas. H9N2 virus can easily, though lowly pathogenic, isolated in the poultry, especially from the chickens in the live poultry markets. The virus is regarded now as gene pool source for reassortant subtypes/strains of novel influenza viruses (Liu *et al.*, 2014). Truly, novel human-infecting H10N8 and H5N6 have been isolated in China (Bi *et al.*, 2015a; Wang *et al.*, 2014c) since the outbreak of H7N9 in China and we are expecting more novel reassortants of influenza virus arising, HxNy. Therefore close and extensive surveillance of influenza viruses, especially the viruses carried by migratory birds and poultry, is required.

It is the H7N9 virus that provides a unique chance for us, for the first time, to see the host-adaptation process of mutations of the receptor binding site of HA to suit for the human receptor binding. From Shanghai-5, to Shanghai-1 and then Anhui-1, the virus gradually increases its human receptor binding affinity by amino acids substitutions to fit the different configurations of avian versus human receptors. It is clear that different amino acids are used for different subtypes of HA to fit differential receptor bindings. Further work should be focused on the molecular basis of receptor binding preference from different HA subtypes.

It is also noted that genomes of two influenza-like viruses, H17N10 and H18N11, were identified from bats in southern America (Wu *et al.*, 2014c). Their public health significance should be closely watched in the future.

References

Arilahti, V., Makela, S.M., Tynell, J., Julkunen, I., and Osterlund, P. (2014). Novel avian influenza A (H7N9) virus induces impaired interferon responses in human dendritic cells. PLoS One *9*, e96350.

Bai, T., Zhou, J., and Shu, Y. (2013). Serologic study for influenza A (H7N9) among high-risk groups in China. N. Engl. J. Med. *368*, 2339–2340.

Bart, S.A., Hohenboken, M., Della Cioppa, G., Narasimhan, V., Dormitzer, P.R., and Kanesa-Thasan, N. (2014). A cell culture-derived MF59-adjuvanted pandemic A/H7N9 vaccine is immunogenic in adults. Sci. Transl. Med. *6*, 234–255.

Belser, J.A., Gustin, K.M., Pearce, M.B., Maines, T.R., Zeng, H., Pappas, C., Sun, X., Carney, P.J., Villanueva, J.M., Stevens, J., *et al.* (2013). Pathogenesis and transmission of avian influenza A (H7N9) virus in ferrets and mice. Nature *501*, 556–559.

Bi, Y., Mei, K., Shi, W., Liu, D., Yu, X., Gao, Z., Zhao, L., Gao, G.F., Chen, J., and Chen, Q. (2015a). Two novel reassortants of avian influenza A (H5N6) virus in China. J. Gen. Virol. *96*, 975–981.

Bi, Y., Xie, Q., Zhang, S., Li, Y., Xiao, H., Jin, T., Zheng, W., Li, J., Jia, X., Sun, L., *et al.* (2015b). Assessment of the internal genes of influenza A (H7N9) virus contributing to high pathogenicity in mice. J. Virol. *89*, 2–13.

Breg, J., Kroon-Batenburg, L.M., Strecker, G., Montreuil, J., and Vliegenthart, J.F. (1989). Conformational analysis of the sialyl alpha(2----3/6)N-acetyllactosamine structural element occurring in glycoproteins, by two-dimensional NOE 1H-NMR spectroscopy in combination with energy calculations by hard-sphere exo-anomeric and molecular mechanics force-field with hydrogen-bonding potential. Eur. J. Biochem. *178*, 727–739.

Cao, R.Y., Xiao, J.H., Cao, B., Li, S., Kumaki, Y., and Zhong, W. (2013). Inhibition of novel reassortant avian influenza H7N9 virus infection in vitro with three antiviral drugs, oseltamivir, peramivir and favipiravir. Antivir. Chem. Chemother. *23*, 237–240.

Carter, D.M., Bloom, C.E., Kirchenbaum, G.A., Tsvetnitsky, V., Isakova-Sivak, I., Rudenko, L., and Ross, T.M. (2015). Cross-protection against H7N9 influenza strains using a live-attenuated H7N3 virus vaccine. Vaccine 33, 108–116.

Chan, K.H., To, K.K., Chan, J.F., Li, C.P., Chan, K.M., Chen, H., Ho, P.L., and Yuen, K.Y. (2014). Assessment of antigen and molecular tests with serial specimens from a patient with influenza A(H7N9) infection. J. Clin. Microbiol. *52*, 2272–2274.

Chan, K.H., To, K.K., Chan, J.F., Li, C.P., Chen, H., and Yuen, K.Y. (2013). Analytical sensitivity of seven point-of-care influenza virus detection tests and two molecular tests for detection of avian origin H7N9 and swine origin H3N2 variant influenza A viruses. J. Clin. Microbiol. *51*, 3160–3161.

Chen, E., Chen, Y., Fu, L., Chen, Z., Gong, Z., Mao, H., Wang, D., Ni, M.Y., Wu, P., Yu, Z., *et al.* (2013a). Human infection with avian influenza A(H7N9) virus re-emerges in China in winter 2013. Euro. Surveill. *18*, 1–10.

Chen, Y., Li, X., Tian, L., Zheng, S., Yang, S., Dong, Y., Wang, Y., Cui, D., Liu, X., Liang, W., *et al.* (2014a). Dynamic behavior of lymphocyte subgroups correlates with clinical outcomes in human H7N9 infection. J. Infect. *69*, 358–365.

Chen, Y., Liang, W., Yang, S., Wu, N., Gao, H., Sheng, J., Yao, H., Wo, J., Fang, Q., Cui, D., *et al.* (2013b). Human infections with the emerging avian influenza A H7N9 virus from wet market poultry: clinical analysis and characterisation of viral genome. Lancet *381*, 1916–1925.

Chen, Z., Baz, M., Lu, J., Paskel, M., Santos, C., Subbarao, K., Jin, H., and Matsuoka, Y. (2014b). Development of a high-yield live attenuated H7N9 influenza virus vaccine that provides protection against homologous and heterologous H7 wild-type viruses in ferrets. J. Virol. *88*, 7016–7023.

Cheng, V.C., To, K.K., Tse, H., Hung, I.F., and Yuen, K.Y. (2012). Two years after pandemic influenza A/2009/H1N1: what have we learned? Clin. Microbiol. Rev. *25*, 223–263.

Chi, Y., Zhu, Y., Wen, T., Cui, L., Ge, Y., Jiao, Y., Wu, T., Ge, A., Ji, H., Xu, K., *et al.* (2013). Cytokine and chemokine levels in patients infected with the novel avian influenza A (H7N9) virus in China. J. Infect. Dis. *208*, 1962–1967.

Claas, E.C., Osterhaus, A.D., van Beek, R., De Jong, J.C., Rimmelzwaan, G.F., Senne, D.A., Krauss, S., Shortridge, K.F., and Webster, R.G. (1998). Human influenza A H5N1 virus related to a highly pathogenic avian influenza virus. Lancet *351*, 472–477.

Clark, T.W., Pareek, M., Hoschler, K., Dillon, H., Nicholson, K.G., Groth, N., and Stephenson, I. (2009). Trial of 2009 influenza A (H1N1) monovalent MF59-adjuvanted vaccine. N. Engl. J. Med. *361*, 2424–2435.

Cui, L., Liu, D., Shi, W., Pan, J., Qi, X., Li, X., Guo, X., Zhou, M., Li, W., Li, J., *et al.* (2014). Dynamic reassortments and genetic heterogeneity of the human-infecting influenza A (H7N9) virus. Nat. Commun. *5*, 3142.

De Groot, A.S., Ardito, M., Terry, F., Levitz, L., Ross, T., Moise, L., and Martin, W. (2013). Low immunogenicity predicted for emerging avian-origin H7N9: implication for influenza vaccine design. Hum. Vaccin. Immunother. *9*, 950–956.

De Groot, A.S., Moise, L., Liu, R., Gutierrez, A.H., Terry, F., Koita, O.A., Ross, T.M., and Martin, W. (2014). Cross-conservation of T-cell epitopes: now even more relevant to (H7N9) influenza vaccine design. Hum. Vaccin. Immunother. *10*, 256–262.

Diao, H., Cui, G., Wei, Y., Chen, J., Zuo, J., Cao, H., Chen, Y., Yao, H., Tian, Z., and Li, L. (2014). Severe H7N9 infection is associated with decreased antigen-presenting capacity of CD14+ cells. PLoS One *9*, e92823.

Dong, L., Bo, H., Bai, T., Gao, R., Dong, J., Zhang, Y., Guo, J., Zou, S., Zhou, J., Zhu, Y., *et al.* (2014). A combination of serological assays to detect human antibodies to the avian influenza A H7N9 virus. PLoS One *9*, e95612.

Duan, Y., Gu, H., Chen, R., Zhao, Z., Zhang, L., Xing, L., Lai, C., Zhang, P., Li, Z., Zhang, K., *et al.* (2014). Response of mice and ferrets to a monovalent influenza A (H7N9) split vaccine. PLoS One *9*, e99322.

Duvvuri, V.R., Duvvuri, B., Alice, C., Wu, G.E., Gubbay, J.B., and Wu, J. (2014). Preexisting CD4+ T-cell immunity in human population to avian influenza H7N9 virus: whole proteome-wide immunoinformatics analyses. PLoS One *9*, e91273.

Feng, F., Jiang, Y., Yuan, M., Shen, J., Yin, H., Geng, D., Xu, J., Hua, Y., Shi, J., Shi, Y., *et al.* (2014). Association of radiologic findings with mortality in patients with avian influenza H7N9 pneumonia. PLoS One *9*, e93885.

Fouchier, R.A., Schneeberger, P.M., Rozendaal, F.W., Broekman, J.M., Kemink, S.A., Munster, V., Kuiken, T., Rimmelzwaan, G.F., Schutten, M., Van Doornum, G.J., *et al.* (2004). Avian influenza A virus (H7N7) associated with human conjunctivitis and a fatal case of acute respiratory distress syndrome. Proc. Natl. Acad. Sci. U.S.A. *101*, 1356–1361.

Fries, L.F., Smith, G.E., and Glenn, G.M. (2013). A recombinant viruslike particle influenza A (H7N9) vaccine. N. Engl. J. Med. *369*, 2564–2566.

Gao, G.F. (2014). Influenza and the live poultry trade. Science *344*, 235.

Gao, H.N., Lu, H.Z., Cao, B., Du, B., Shang, H., Gan, J.H., Lu, S.H., Yang, Y.D., Fang, Q., Shen, Y.Z., *et al.* (2013a). Clinical findings in 111 cases of influenza A (H7N9) virus infection. N. Engl. J. Med. *368*, 2277–2285.

Gao, R., Cao, B., Hu, Y., Feng, Z., Wang, D., Hu, W., Chen, J., Jie, Z., Qiu, H., Xu, K., *et al.* (2013b). Human infection with a novel avian-origin influenza A (H7N9) virus. N. Engl. J. Med. *368*, 1888–1897.

Goff, P.H., Krammer, F., Hai, R., Seibert, C.W., Margine, I., Garcia-Sastre, A., and Palese, P. (2013). Induction of cross-reactive antibodies to novel H7N9 influenza virus by recombinant Newcastle disease virus expressing a North American lineage H7 subtype hemagglutinin. J. Virol. *87*, 8235–8240.

Guo, L., Zhang, X., Ren, L., Yu, X., Chen, L., Zhou, H., Gao, X., Teng, Z., Li, J., Hu, J., *et al.* (2014a). Human antibody responses to avian influenza A(H7N9) virus, 2013. Emerg. Infect. Dis. *20*, 192–200.

Guo, Q., Huang, J.A., and Fraidenburg, D.R. (2014b). Bosentan as rescue treatment in refractory hypoxemia and pulmonary hypertension in a patient with ARDS and H7N9 influenza virus infection. Lung *192*, 635–636.

Guo, J., Huang, F., Liu, J., Chen, Y., Wang, W., Cao, B., Zou, Z., Liu, S., Pan, J., Bao, C., et al. (2015c). The serum profile of hypercytokinemia factors identified in H7N9-infected patients can predict fatal outcomes. Sci. Rep. *5*, 10942.

Hatchette, T.F., Drews, S.J., Bastien, N., Li, Y., German, G., Antonishyn, N., Charest, H., Mazzulli, T., Fonseca, K., Krajden, M., *et al.* (2013). Detection of influenza H7N9 virus: all molecular tests are not equal. J. Clin. Microbiol. *51*, 3835–3838.

He, L., De Groot, A.S., Gutierrez, A.H., Martin, W.D., Moise, L., and Bailey-Kellogg, C. (2014). Integrated assessment of predicted MHC binding and cross-conservation with self reveals patterns of viral camouflage. BMC Bioinformatics *15(Suppl 4)*, S1.

Herfst, S., Schrauwen, E.J., Linster, M., Chutinimitkul, S., de Wit, E., Munster, V.J., Sorrell, E.M., Bestebroer, T.M., Burke, D.F., Smith, D.J., *et al.* (2012). Airborne transmission of influenza A/H5N1 virus between ferrets. Science *336*, 1534–1541.

Hirst, M., Astell, C.R., Griffith, M., Coughlin, S.M., Moksa, M., Zeng, T., Smailus, D.E., Holt, R.A., Jones, S., Marra, M.A., *et al.* (2004). Novel avian influenza H7N3 strain outbreak, British Columbia. Emerg. Infect. Dis. *10*, 2192–2195.

Ho, P.L., Sin, W.C., Chan, J.F., Cheng, V.C., and Chan, K.H. (2014). Severe influenza A H7N9 pneumonia with rapid virological response to intravenous zanamivir. Eur. Respir. J. *44*, 535–537.

Hu, Y., Lu, S., Song, Z., Wang, W., Hao, P., Li, J., Zhang, X., Yen, H.L., Shi, B., Li, T., *et al.* (2013). Association between adverse clinical outcome in human disease caused by novel influenza A H7N9 virus and sustained viral shedding and emergence of antiviral resistance. Lancet *381*, 2273–2279.

Huang, F., Guo, J., Zou, Z., Liu, J., Cao, B., Zhang, S., Li, H., Wang, W., Sheng, M., Liu, S., *et al.* (2014a). Angiotensin II plasma levels are linked to disease severity and predict fatal outcomesin H7N9-infected patients. Nat. Commun. *5*, 3595.

Huang, R., Zhang, L., Gu, Q., Zhou, Y.H., Hao, Y., Zhang, K., Liu, Y., Dong, D., Wang, S., Huang, Z., *et al.* (2014b). Profiles of acute cytokine and antibody responses in patients infected with avian influenza A H7N9. PLoS One *9*, e101788.

Imai, M., Watanabe, T., Hatta, M., Das, S.C., Ozawa, M., Shinya, K., Zhong, G., Hanson, A., Katsura, H., Watanabe, S., *et al.* (2012). Experimental adaptation of an influenza H5 HA confers respiratory droplet transmission to a reassortant H5 HA/H1N1 virus in ferrets. Nature *486*, 420–428.

Ip, D.K., Liao, Q., Wu, P., Gao, Z., Cao, B., Feng, L., Xu, X., Jiang, H., Li, M., Bao, J., *et al.* (2013). Detection of mild to moderate influenza A/H7N9 infection by China's national sentinel surveillance system for influenza-like illness: case series. BMJ *346*, f3693.

Jegaskanda, S., Vandenberg, K., Laurie, K.L., Loh, L., Kramski, M., Winnall, W.R., Kedzierska, K., Rockman, S., and Kent, S.J. (2014). Cross-reactive influenza-specific antibody-dependent cellular cytotoxicity in intravenous immunoglobulin as a potential therapeutic against emerging influenza viruses. J. Infect. Dis. *210*, 1811–1822.

Ji, H., Gu, Q., Chen, L.L., Xu, K., Ling, X., Bao, C.J., Tang, F.Y., Qi, X., Wu, Y.Q., Ai, J., *et al.* (2014). Epidemiological and clinical characteristics and risk factors for death of patients with avian influenza A H7N9 virus infection from Jiangsu Province, Eastern China. PLoS One *9*, e89581.

Jiang, W.M., Wang, S.C., Liu, H.L., Yu, J.M., Du, X., Hou, G.Y., Li, J.P., Liu, S., Wang, K.C., Zhuang, Q.Y., *et al.* (2014). Evaluation of avian influenza virus isolated from ducks as a potential live vaccine candidate against novel H7N9 viruses. Vaccine *32*, 6433–6439.

Jiao, P., Tian, G., Li, Y., Deng, G., Jiang, Y., Liu, C., Liu, W., Bu, Z., Kawaoka, Y., and Chen, H. (2008). A single-amino-acid substitution in the NS1 protein changes the pathogenicity of H5N1 avian influenza viruses in mice. J. Virol. *82*, 1146–1154.

Josset, L., Zeng, H., Kelly, S.M., Tumpey, T.M., and Katze, M.G. (2014). Transcriptomic characterization of the novel avian-origin influenza A (H7N9) virus: specific host response and responses intermediate between avian (H5N1 and H7N7) and human (H3N2) viruses and implications for treatment options. mBio *5*, e01102–01113.

Kang, K., Chen, L., Zhao, X., Qin, C., Zhan, Z., Wang, J., Li, W., Dzakah, E.E., Huang, W., Shu, Y., *et al.* (2014). Development of rapid immunochromatographic test for hemagglutinin antigen of H7 subtype in patients infected with novel avian influenza A (H7N9) virus. PLoS One *9*, e92306.

Klausberger, M., Wilde, M., Palmberger, D., Hai, R., Albrecht, R.A., Margine, I., Hirsh, A., Garcia-Sastre, A., Grabherr, R., and Krammer, F. (2014). One-shot vaccination with an insect cell-derived low-dose influenza A H7 virus-like particle preparation protects mice against H7N9 challenge. Vaccine *32*, 355–362.

Koopmans, M., Wilbrink, B., Conyn, M., Natrop, G., van der Nat, H., Vennema, H., Meijer, A., van Steenbergen, J., Fouchier, R., Osterhaus, A., *et al.* (2004). Transmission of H7N7 avian influenza A virus to human beings during a large outbreak in commercial poultry farms in the Netherlands. Lancet *363*, 587–593.

Krammer, F., Albrecht, R.A., Tan, G.S., Margine, I., Hai, R., Schmolke, M., Runstadler, J., Andrews, S.F., Wilson, P.C., Cox, R.J., *et al.* (2014a). Divergent H7 immunogens offer protection from H7N9 virus challenge. J. Virol. *88*, 3976–3985.

Krammer, F., Margine, I., Hai, R., Flood, A., Hirsh, A., Tsvetnitsky, V., Chen, D., and Palese, P. (2014b). H3 stalk-based chimeric hemagglutinin influenza virus constructs protect mice from H7N9 challenge. J. Virol. *88*, 2340–2343.

Kreijtz, J.H., Wiersma, L.C., De Gruyter, H.L., Vogelzang-van Trierum, S.E., van Amerongen, G., Stittelaar, K.J., Fouchier, R.A., Osterhaus, A.D., Sutter, G., and Rimmelzwaan, G.F. (2015). A single immunization with modified vaccinia virus ankara-based influenza virus H7 vaccine affords protection in the influenza A(H7N9) pneumonia ferret model. J. Infect. Dis. *211*, 791–800.

Lakdawala, S.S., Lamirande, E.W., Suguitan, A.L., Jr., Wang, W., Santos, C.P., Vogel, L., Matsuoka, Y., Lindsley, W.G., Jin, H., and Subbarao, K. (2011). Eurasian-origin gene segments contribute to the transmissibility, aerosol release, and morphology of the 2009 pandemic H1N1 influenza virus. PLoS Pathog. *7*, e1002443.

Lam, T.T., Wang, J., Shen, Y., Zhou, B., Duan, L., Cheung, C.L., Ma, C., Lycett, S.J., Leung, C.Y., Chen, X., *et al.* (2013). The genesis and source of the H7N9 influenza viruses causing human infections in China. Nature *502*, 241–244.

Lam, T.T., Zhou, B., Wang, J., Chai, Y., Shen, Y., Chen, X., Ma, C., Hong, W., Chen, Y., Zhang, Y., *et al.* (2015). Dissemination, divergence and establishment of H7N9 influenza viruses in China. Nature *522*, 102–105.

Li, J., Yu, X., Pu, X., Xie, L., Sun, Y., Xiao, H., Wang, F., Din, H., Wu, Y., Liu, D., *et al.* (2013). Environmental connections of novel avian-origin H7N9 influenza virus infection and virus adaptation to the human. Sci. China Life Sci. *56*, 485–492.

Liao, Q., Ip, D.K., Tsang, T.K., Cao, B., Jiang, H., Liu, F., Zheng, J., Peng, Z., Wu, P., Huai, Y., *et al.* (2014). A clinical prediction rule for diagnosing human infections with avian influenza A(H7N9) in a hospital emergency department setting. BMC Med. *12*, 127.

Lin, P.H., Chao, T.L., Kuo, S.W., Wang, J.T., Hung, C.C., Lin, H.C., Yang, Z.Y., Ho, S.Y., Chang, C.K., Huang, M.S., *et al.* (2014). Virological, serological, and antiviral studies in an imported human case of avian influenza A(H7N9) virus in Taiwan. Clin. Infect. Dis. *58*, 242–246.

Liu, D., Shi, W., and Gao, G.F. (2014). Poultry carrying H9N2 act as incubators for novel human avian influenza viruses. Lancet *383*, 869.

Liu, S., Sun, J., Cai, J., Miao, Z., Lu, M., Qin, S., Wang, X., Lv, H., Yu, Z., Amer, S., *et al.* (2013). Epidemiological, clinical and viral characteristics of fatal cases of human avian influenza A (H7N9) virus in Zhejiang Province, China. J. Infect. *67*, 595–605.

Lu, S., Zheng, Y., Li, T., Hu, Y., Liu, X., Xi, X., Chen, Q., Wang, Q., Cao, Y., Wang, Y., *et al.* (2013a). Clinical findings for early human cases of influenza A(H7N9) virus infection, Shanghai, China. Emerg. Infect. Dis. *19*, 1142–1146.

Lu, X., Shi, Y., Zhang, W., Zhang, Y., Qi, J., and Gao, G.F. (2013b). Structure and receptor-binding properties of an airborne transmissible avian influenza A virus hemagglutinin H5 (VN1203mut). Protein Cell *4*, 502–511.

Lv, H., Han, J., Zhang, P., Lu, Y., Wen, D., Cai, J., Liu, S., Sun, J., Yu, Z., Zhang, H., *et al.* (2013). Mild illness in avian influenza A(H7N9) virus-infected poultry worker, Huzhou, China, April 2013. Emerg. Infect. Dis. *19*, 1885–1888.

Manz, B., Brunotte, L., Reuther, P., and Schwemmle, M. (2012). Adaptive mutations in NEP compensate for defective H5N1 RNA replication in cultured human cells. Nat. Commun. *3*, 802.

Mao, H., Yen, H.L., Liu, Y., Lau, Y.L., Malik Peiris, J.S., and Tu, W. (2014). Conservation of T cell epitopes between seasonal influenza viruses and the novel influenza A H7N9 virus. Virol. Sin. *29*, 170–175.

Marjuki, H., Mishin, V.P., Chesnokov, A.P., De La Cruz, J.A., Fry, A.M., Villanueva, J., and Gubareva, L.V. (2014). An investigational antiviral drug, DAS181, effectively inhibits replication of zoonotic influenza A virus subtype H7N9 and protects mice from lethality. J. Infect. Dis. *210*, 435–440.

Mei, B., Ding, X., Xu, H.Z., and Wang, M.T. (2014). Global gene expression changes in human peripheral blood after H7N9 infection. Gene *551*, 255–260.

Merritt, E.A., Sarfaty, S., van den Akker, F., L'Hoir, C., Martial, J.A., and Hol, W.G. (1994). Crystal structure of cholera toxin B-pentamer bound to receptor GM1 pentasaccharide. Protein Sci. *3*, 166–175.

Mok, C.K., Yen, H.L., Yu, M.Y., Yuen, K.M., Sia, S.F., Chan, M.C., Qin, G., Tu, W.W., and Peiris, J.S. (2011). Amino acid residues 253 and 591 of the PB2 protein of avian influenza virus A H9N2 contribute to mammalian pathogenesis. J. Virol. *85*, 9641–9645.

Mulligan, M.J., Bernstein, D.I., Winokur, P., Rupp, R., Anderson, E., Rouphael, N., Dickey, M., Stapleton, J.T., Edupuganti, S., Spearman, P., *et al.* (2014). Serological responses to an avian influenza A/H7N9 vaccine mixed at the point-of-use with MF59 adjuvant: a randomized clinical trial. JAMA *312*, 1409–1419.

Naffakh, N., Tomoiu, A., Rameix-Welti, M.A., and van der Werf, S. (2008). Host Restriction of Avian Influenza Viruses at the Level of the Ribonucleoproteins. Annu. Rev. Microbiol. *62*, 403–424.

Nguyen-Van-Tam, J.S., Nair, P., Acheson, P., Baker, A., Barker, M., Bracebridge, S., Croft, J., Ellis, J., Gelletlie, R., Gent, N., *et al.* (2006). Outbreak of low pathogenicity H7N3 avian influenza in UK, including associated case of human conjunctivitis. Euro Surveill. *11*, E060504.

Nicholls, J.M., Tsai, P.N., Chan, R.W., Hui, K.P., Chan, M.C., Malik Peiris, J.S., Chan, K.H., Yuen, K.Y., and To, K.K. (2014). Fatal H7N9 pneumonia complicated by viral infection of a prosthetic cardiac valve – An autopsy study. J. Clin. Virol. *61*, 466–469.

Ostrowsky, B., Huang, A., Terry, W., Anton, D., Brunagel, B., Traynor, L., Abid, S., Johnson, G., Kacica, M., Katz, J., *et al.* (2012). Low pathogenic avian influenza A (H7N2) virus infection in immunocompromised adult, New York, U.S.A., 2003. Emerg. Infect. Dis. *18*, 1128–1131.

Peiris, M., Yuen, K.Y., Leung, C.W., Chan, K.H., Ip, P.L., Lai, R.W., Orr, W.K., and Shortridge, K.F. (1999). Human infection with influenza H9N2. Lancet *354*, 916–917.

Poppe, L., Stuike-Prill, R., Meyer, B., and van Halbeek, H. (1992). The solution conformation of sialyl-alpha (2----6)-lactose studied by modern NMR techniques and Monte Carlo simulations. J. Biomol. NMR *2*, 109–136.

Qi, X., Cui, L., Xu, K., Wu, B., Tang, F., Bao, C., Zhu, Y., Zhou, M.H., and Wang, H. (2014). Avian influenza A(H7N9) virus infection in pregnant woman, China, 2013. Emerg. Infect. Dis. *20*, 333–334.

Qian, W., Jiang, P.C., Qian, J., Jin, Z.C., Yang, J., Lin, J., Wen, X.M., Han, F.A., Mao, L.X., Yang, J., *et al.* (2014). Kinetic analysis of the immunity in a pregnant patient infected with avian influenza H7N9. Int. J. Clin. Exp. Med. *7*, 1768–1774.

Quinones-Parra, S., Grant, E., Loh, L., Nguyen, T.H., Campbell, K.A., Tong, S.Y., Miller, A., Doherty, P.C., Vijaykrishna, D., Rossjohn, J., *et al.* (2014). Preexisting CD8+ T-cell immunity to the H7N9 influenza A virus varies across ethnicities. Proc. Natl. Acad. Sci. U.S.A. *111*, 1049–1054.

Ren, L., Yu, X., Zhao, B., Wu, F., Jin, Q., Zhang, X., and Wang, J. (2014). Infection with possible precursor of avian influenza A(H7N9) virus in a child, China, 2013. Emerg. Infect. Dis. *20*, 1362–1365.

Richard, M., Schrauwen, E.J., de Graaf, M., Bestebroer, T.M., Spronken, M.I., van Boheemen, S., de Meulder, D., Lexmond, P., Linster, M., Herfst, S., *et al.* (2013). Limited airborne transmission of H7N9 influenza A virus between ferrets. Nature *501*, 560–563.

Rudenko, L., Isakova-Sivak, I., and Donina, S. (2013). H7N3 live attenuated influenza vaccine has a potential to protect against new H7N9 avian influenza virus. Vaccine *31*, 4702–4705.

Rudenko, L., Kiseleva, I., Naykhin, A.N., Erofeeva, M., Stukova, M., Donina, S., Petukhova, G., Pisareva, M., Krivitskaya, V., Grudinin, M., *et al.* (2014). Assessment of human immune responses to H7 avian influenza virus of pandemic potential: results from a placebo-controlled, randomized double-blind phase I study of live attenuated H7N3 influenza vaccine. PLoS One *9*, e87962.

Sabesan, S., Bock, K., and Paulson, J.C. (1991). Conformational analysis of sialyloligosaccharides. Carbohydr. Res. *218*, 27–54.

Sakai, K., Ami, Y., Tahara, M., Kubota, T., Anraku, M., Abe, M., Nakajima, N., Sekizuka, T., Shirato, K., Suzaki, Y., *et al.* (2014). The host protease TMPRSS2 plays a major role in in vivo replication of emerging H7N9 and seasonal influenza viruses. J. Virol. *88*, 5608–5616.

Shen, Z., Chen, Z., Li, X., Xu, L., Guan, W., Cao, Y., Hu, Y., and Zhang, J. (2014). Host immunological response and factors associated with clinical outcome in patients with the novel influenza A H7N9 infection. Clin. Microbiol. Infect. *20*, O493–500.

Shi, W., Shi, Y., Wu, Y., Liu, D., and Gao, G.F. (2013a). Origin and molecular characterization of the human-infecting H6N1 influenza virus in Taiwan. Protein Cell *4*, 846–853.

Shi, Y., Wu, Y., Zhang, W., Qi, J., and Gao, G.F. (2014). Enabling the 'host jump': structural determinants of receptor-binding specificity in influenza A viruses. Nat. Rev. Microbiol. *12*, 822–831.

Shi, Y., Zhang, W., Wang, F., Qi, J., Wu, Y., Song, H., Gao, F., Bi, Y., Zhang, Y., Fan, Z., *et al.* (2013b). Structures and receptor binding of hemagglutinins from human-infecting H7N9 influenza viruses. Science *342*, 243–247.

Smith, G.E., Flyer, D.C., Raghunandan, R., Liu, Y., Wei, Z., Wu, Y., Kpamegan, E., Courbron, D., Fries, L.F., 3rd, and Glenn, G.M. (2013). Development of influenza H7N9 virus like particle (VLP) vaccine: homologous A/Anhui/1/2013 (H7N9) protection and heterologous A/chicken/Jalisco/CPA1/2012 (H7N3) cross-protection in vaccinated mice challenged with H7N9 virus. Vaccine *31*, 4305–4313.

Song, M.S., Pascua, P.N., Lee, J.H., Baek, Y.H., Lee, O.J., Kim, C.J., Kim, H., Webby, R.J., Webster, R.G., and Choi, Y.K. (2009). The polymerase acidic protein gene of influenza a virus contributes to pathogenicity in a mouse model. J. Virol. *83*, 12325–12335.

Song, R., Pang, X., Yang, P., Shu, Y., Zhang, Y., Wang, Q., Chen, Z., Liu, J., Cheng, J., Jiao, Y., *et al.* (2014). Surveillance of the first case of human avian influenza A (H7N9) virus in Beijing, China. Infection *42*, 127–133.

Stehle, T., and Harrison, S.C. (1996). Crystal structures of murine polyomavirus in complex with straight-chain and branched-chain sialyloligosaccharide receptor fragments. Structure *4*, 183–194.

Sun, J., Gong, Z., Lv, H., Chen, Z., Chai, C., Liu, S., Ling, F., Lu, Y., Cai, J., Yu, Z., *et al.* (2014). Comparison of characteristics between patients with H7N9 living in rural and urban areas of Zhejiang Province, China: a preliminary report. PLoS One *9*, e93775.

Tada, T., Suzuki, K., Sakurai, Y., Kubo, M., Okada, H., Itoh, T., and Tsukamoto, K. (2011). Emergence of avian influenza viruses with enhanced transcription activity by a single amino acid substitution in the nucleoprotein during replication in chicken brains. J. Virol. *85*, 10354–10363.

Tarnow, C., Engels, G., Arendt, A., Schwalm, F., Sediri, H., Preuss, A., Nelson, P.S., Garten, W., Klenk, H.D., Gabriel, G., *et al.* (2014). TMPRSS2 is a host factor that is essential for pneumotropism and pathogenicity of H7N9 influenza A virus in mice. J. Virol. *88*, 4744–4751.

To, K.K., Chan, J.F., and Yuen, K.Y. (2014). Viral lung infections: epidemiology, virology, clinical features, and management of avian influenza A(H7N9). Curr. Opin. Pulm. Med. *20*, 225–232.

Valkenburg, S.A., Li, O.T., Mak, P.W., Mok, C.K., Nicholls, J.M., Guan, Y., Waldmann, T.A., Peiris, J.S., Perera, L.P., and Poon, L.L. (2014). IL-15 adjuvanted multivalent vaccinia-based universal influenza vaccine requires CD4+ T cells for heterosubtypic protection. Proc. Natl. Acad. Sci. U.S.A. *111*, 5676–5681.

van de Sandt, C.E., Kreijtz, J.H., de Mutsert, G., Geelhoed-Mieras, M.M., Hillaire, M.L., Vogelzang-van Trierum, S.E., Osterhaus, A.D., Fouchier, R.A., and Rimmelzwaan, G.F. (2014). Human cytotoxic T lymphocytes directed to seasonal influenza A viruses cross-react with the newly emerging H7N9 virus. J. Virol. *88*, 1684–1693.

Varghese, J.N., McKimm-Breschkin, J.L., Caldwell, J.B., Kortt, A.A., and Colman, P.M. (1992). The structure of the complex between influenza virus neuraminidase and sialic acid, the viral receptor. Proteins *14*, 327–332.

Vavricka, C.J., Liu, Y., Kiyota, H., Sriwilaijaroen, N., Qi, J., Tanaka, K., Wu, Y., Li, Q., Li, Y., Yan, J., *et al.* (2013). Influenza neuraminidase operates via a nucleophilic mechanism and can be targeted by covalent inhibitors. Nat. Commun. *4*, 1491.

Wang, J., Sun, Y., Xu, Q., Tan, Y., Pu, J., Yang, H., Brown, E.G., and Liu, J. (2012). Mouse-adapted H9N2 influenza A virus PB2 protein M147L and E627K mutations are critical for high virulence. PLoS One *7*, e40752.

Wang, Q., Zhang, Z., Shi, Y., and Jiang, Y. (2013a). Emerging H7N9 influenza A (novel reassortant avian-origin) pneumonia: radiologic findings. Radiology *268*, 882–889.

Wang, S.Y., Ren, S.H., Huang, M.X., Yu, D.J., Shen, Q., Zhao, H.F., Lu, Q.H., and Qian, S.X. (2013b). Clinical variability in onset of influenza A (H7N9) infection. Chin. Med. J. *126*, 4194–4196.

Wang, X., Fang, S., Lu, X., Xu, C., Cowling, B.J., Tang, X., Peng, B., Wu, W., He, J., Tang, Y., *et al.* (2014a). Seroprevalence to avian influenza A(H7N9) virus among poultry workers and the general population in southern China: a longitudinal study. Clin. Infect. Dis. *59*, e76–83.

Wang, X.Y., Chai, C.L., Li, F.D., He, F., Yu, Z., Wang, X.X., Shang, X.P., Liu, S.L., and Lin, J.F. (2014b). Epidemiology of human infections with avian influenza A(H7N9) virus in the two waves before and after October 2013 in Zhejiang province, China. Epidemiol. Infect. *143*, 1839–1845.

Wang, Z., Zhang, A., Wan, Y., Liu, X., Qiu, C., Xi, X., Ren, Y., Wang, J., Dong, Y., Bao, M., *et al.* (2014c). Early hypercytokinemia is associated with interferon-induced transmembrane protein-3 dysfunction and predictive of fatal H7N9 infection. Proc. Natl. Acad. Sci. U.S.A. *111*, 769–774.

Watanabe, T., Kiso, M., Fukuyama, S., Nakajima, N., Imai, M., Yamada, S., Murakami, S., Yamayoshi, S., Iwatsuki-Horimoto, K., Sakoda, Y., *et al.* (2013). Characterization of H7N9 influenza A viruses isolated from humans. Nature *501*, 551–555.

Wiwanitkit, V. (2014). Thrombohemostatic disorders in the new emerging H7N9 influenza. Rev. Bras. Hematol. Hemoter. *36*, 235–236.

Wong, S.S., Jeevan, T., Kercher, L., Yoon, S.W., Petkova, A.M., Crumpton, J.C., Franks, J., Debeauchamp, J., Rubrum, A., Seiler, P., *et al.* (2014). A single dose of whole inactivated H7N9 influenza vaccine confers protection from severe disease but not infection in ferrets. Vaccine *32*, 4571–4577.

Wright, C.S., and Jaeger, J. (1993). Crystallographic refinement and structure analysis of the complex of wheat germ agglutinin with a bivalent sialoglycopeptide from glycophorin A. J. Mol. Biol. *232*, 620–638.

Wu, A., Su, C., Wang, D., Peng, Y., Liu, M., Hua, S., Li, T., Gao, G.F., Tang, H., Chen, J., *et al.* (2013a). Sequential reassortments underlie diverse influenza H7N9 genotypes in China. Cell Host Microbe *14*, 446–452.

Wu, C.Y., Chang, C.Y., Ma, H.H., Wang, C.W., Chen, Y.T., Hsiao, P.W., Chang, C.C., Chan, C.H., Liu, C.C., and Chen, J.R. (2014a). Squalene-adjuvanted H7N9 virus vaccine induces robust humoral immune response against H7N9 and H7N7 viruses. Vaccine *32*, 4485–4494.

Wu, W., Shi, Y., Gao, H., Liang, W., Sheng, J., and Li, L. (2014b). Immune derangement occurs in patients with H7N9 avian influenza. Crit. Care *18*, R43.

Wu, Y., Bi, Y., Vavricka, C.J., Sun, X., Zhang, Y., Gao, F., Zhao, M., Xiao, H., Qin, C., He, J., *et al.* (2013b). Characterization of two distinct neuraminidases from avian-origin human-infecting H7N9 influenza viruses. Cell Res. *23*, 1347–1355.

Wu, Y., and Gao, G.F. (2013). Lessons learnt from the human infections of avian-origin influenza A H7N9 virus: live free markets and human health. Sci. China Life Sci. *56*, 493–494.

Wu, Y., Tefsen, B., Shi, Y., and Gao, G.F. (2014c). Bat-derived influenza-like viruses H17N10 and H18N11. Trends Microbiol. *22*, 183–191.

Xia, J.B., Zhu, J., Hu, J., Wang, L.M., and Zhang, H. (2014). H7N9 influenza A-induced pneumonia associated with acute myelitis in an adult. Intern. Med. *53*, 1093–1095.

Xiao, Y.Y., Cai, J., Wang, X.Y., Li, F.D., Shang, X.P., Wang, X.X., Lin, J.F., and He, F. (2014). Prognosis and survival of 128 patients with severe avian influenza A(H7N9) infection in Zhejiang province, China. Epidemiol. Infect. *143*, 1833–1838.

Xiong, X., Coombs, P.J., Martin, S.R., Liu, J., Xiao, H., McCauley, J.W., Locher, K., Walker, P.A., Collins, P.J., Kawaoka, Y., *et al.* (2013a). Receptor binding by a ferret-transmissible H5 avian influenza virus. Nature *497*, 392–396.

Xiong, X., Martin, S.R., Haire, L.F., Wharton, S.A., Daniels, R.S., Bennett, M.S., McCauley, J.W., Collins, P.J., Walker, P.A., Skehel, J.J., *et al.* (2013b). Receptor binding by an H7N9 influenza virus from humans. Nature *499*, 496–499.

Xu, L., Bao, L., Li, F., Gu, S., Lv, Q., Yuan, J., Xu, Y., Zhu, H., Deng, W., Li, Y., *et al.* (2014). Combinations of Oseltamivir and Fibrates Prolong the Mean Survival Time of Mice Infected with the Lethal H7N9 Influenza Virus. J. Gen. Virol. *96*, 46–51.

Xu, Q., Chen, Z., Cheng, X., Xu, L., and Jin, H. (2013a). Evaluation of live attenuated H7N3 and H7N7 vaccine viruses for their receptor binding preferences, immunogenicity in ferrets and cross reactivity to the novel H7N9 virus. PLoS One *8*, e76884.

Xu, R., de Vries, R.P., Zhu, X., Nycholat, C.M., McBride, R., Yu, W., Paulson, J.C., and Wilson, I.A. (2013b). Preferential recognition of avian-like receptors in human influenza A H7N9 viruses. Science *342*, 1230–1235.

Yan, J., Villarreal, D.O., Racine, T., Chu, J.S., Walters, J.N., Morrow, M.P., Khan, A.S., Sardesai, N.Y., Kim, J.J., Kobinger, G.P., *et al.* (2014). Protective immunity to H7N9 influenza viruses elicited by synthetic DNA vaccine. Vaccine 32, 2833–2842.

Yang, S., Chen, Y., Cui, D., Yao, H., Lou, J., Huo, Z., Xie, G., Yu, F., Zheng, S., Yang, Y., *et al.* (2014). Avian-origin influenza A(H7N9) infection in influenza A(H7N9)-affected areas of China: a serological study. J. Infect. Dis. *209*, 265–269.

Yang, S.G., Cao, B., Liang, L.R., Li, X.L., Xiao, Y.H., Cao, Z.X., Jia, H.Y., Yu, H.J., Xu, Z., Gu, L., *et al.* (2012). Antiviral therapy and outcomes of patients with pneumonia caused by influenza A pandemic (H1N1) virus. PLoS One *7*, e29652.

Yao, J., Liu, L., Chen, G., and Lin, L. (2014). Two severe cases of H7N9 pneumonia patients with immunoneuroendocrine axis dysfunction and vitamin D insufficiency. BMC Infect. Dis. *14*, 44.

Yu, H., Cowling, B.J., Feng, L., Lau, E.H., Liao, Q., Tsang, T.K., Peng, Z., Wu, P., Liu, F., Fang, V.J., *et al.* (2013a). Human infection with avian influenza A H7N9 virus: an assessment of clinical severity. Lancet *382*, 138–145.

Yu, L., Wang, Z.M., Chen, Y., Ding, W., Jia, H.Y., Chan, J.F.W., To, K.K.W., Chen, H.L., Yang, Y.D., Liang, W.F., *et al.* (2013b). Clinical, Virological, and Histopathological Manifestations of Fatal Human Infections by Avian Influenza A (H7N9) Virus. Clin. Infect. Dis. *57*, 1449–1457.

Yu, X., Jin, T., Cui, Y., Pu, X., Li, J., Xu, J., Liu, G., Jia, H., Liu, D., Song, S., *et al.* (2014). Influenza H7N9 and H9N2 viruses: coexistence in poultry linked to human H7N9 infection and genome characteristics. J. Virol. *88*, 3423–3431.

Zamarin, D., Garcia-Sastre, A., Xiao, X.Y., Wang, R., and Palese, P. (2005). Influenza virus PB1-F2 protein induces cell death through mitochondrial ANT3 and VDAC1. PLoS Pathog. *1*, 40–54.

Zhang, A., Huang, Y., Tian, D., Lau, E.H., Wan, Y., Liu, X., Dong, Y., Song, Z., Zhang, X., Zhang, J., *et al.* (2013a). Kinetics of serological responses in influenza A(H7N9)-infected patients correlate with clinical outcome in China, 2013. Euro Surveill. *18*, 20657.

Zhang, W., Shi, Y., Lu, X., Shu, Y., Qi, J., and Gao, G.F. (2013b). An airborne transmissible avian influenza H5 hemagglutinin seen at the atomic level. Science *340*, 1463–1467.

Zhou, J., Wang, D., Gao, R., Zhao, B., Song, J., Qi, X., Zhang, Y., Shi, Y., Yang, L., Zhu, W., *et al.* (2013). Biological features of novel avian influenza A (H7N9) virus. Nature *499*, 500–503.

Zhu, W.F., Zhu, Y., Qin, K., Yu, Z.J., Gao, R.B., Yu, H.Y., Zhou, J.F., and Shu, Y.L. (2012). Mutations in polymerase genes enhanced the virulence of 2009 pandemic H1N1 influenza virus in mice. PLoS One *7*, e33383.

Zhu, Z., Qi, Y., Ge, A., Zhu, Y., Xu, K., Ji, H., Shi, Z., Cui, L., and Zhou, M. (2014). Comprehensive characterization of serum microRNA profile in response to the emerging avian influenza A (H7N9) virus infection in humans. Viruses *6*, 1525–1539.

Index

V